Clinical Manual of Pediatric Consultation-Liaison Psychiatry

Second Edition

T0176395

Clinical Manual of Pediatric Consultation-Liaison Psychiatry

Second Edition

Richard J. Shaw, M.B., B.S.
Professor of Psychiatry and Pediatrics
Stanford University School of Medicine
Medical Director, Pediatric Psychiatry Consult Service at
Lucile Packard Children's Hospital
Stanford, California

David R. DeMaso, M.D.
Psychiatrist-in-Chief and Leon Eisenberg Chair in
Psychiatry, Boston Children's Hospital;
George P. Gardner–Olga E. Monks Professor of
Child Psychiatry & Professor of Pediatrics
Harvard Medical School, Boston, Massachusetts

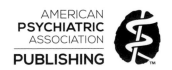

AMERICAN
PSYCHIATRIC
ASSOCIATION
PUBLISHING

Note: The authors have worked to ensure that all information in this book is accurate at the time of publication and consistent with general psychiatric and medical standards, and that information concerning drug dosages, schedules, and routes of administration is accurate at the time of publication and consistent with standards set by the U.S. Food and Drug Administration and the general medical community. As medical research and practice continue to advance, however, therapeutic standards may change. Moreover, specific situations may require a specific therapeutic response not included in this book. For these reasons and because human and mechanical errors sometimes occur, we recommend that readers follow the advice of physicians directly involved in their care or the care of a member of their family.

Books published by American Psychiatric Association Publishing represent the findings, conclusions, and views of the individual authors and do not necessarily represent the policies and opinions of American Psychiatric Association Publishing or the American Psychiatric Association.

If you wish to buy 50 or more copies of the same title, please go to www.appi.org/specialdiscounts for more information.

Copyright © 2020 American Psychiatric Association Publishing
ALL RIGHTS RESERVED
Second Edition
Manufactured in the United States of America on acid-free paper
23   22   21   20   19   5   4   3   2   1
American Psychiatric Association Publishing
800 Maine Avenue SW
Suite 900
Washington, DC 20024-2812
www.appi.org

Library of Congress Cataloging-in-Publication Data
Names: Shaw, Richard J., author. | DeMaso, David R. (David Ray), author. | American Psychiatric Association, issuing body.
Title: Clinical manual of pediatric consultation-liaison psychiatry / Richard J. Shaw, David R. DeMaso.
Other titles: Clinical manual of pediatric psychosomatic medicine
Description: Second edition. | Washington, D.C. : American Psychiatric Association Publishing, [2020] | Preceded by: Clinical manual of pediatric psychosomatic medicine / Richard J. Shaw, David R. DeMaso. 1st ed. c2006. | Includes bibliographical references and index.
Identifiers: LCCN 2019031846 (print) | ISBN 9781615372317 (paperback) | ISBN 9781615372799 (ebook)
Subjects: MESH: Mental Disorders—diagnosis | Mental Disorders—therapy | Child | Adolescent | Child, Hospitalized—psychology | Pediatrics | Referral and Consultation
Classification: LCC RC454 (print) | LCC RC454 (ebook) | NLM WS 350.6 | DDC 616.89—dc23
LC record available at https://lccn.loc.gov/2019031846
LC ebook record available at https://lccn.loc.gov/2019031847
British Library Cataloguing in Publication Data
A CIP record is available from the British Library.

Contents

PART I
Overview

PART II

Specific Psychiatric Symptoms
and Disorders

PART III
Treatment and Intervention

Preface

Pediatric consultation-liaison psychiatry (CLP) refers to a specialized area of psychiatry whose practitioners have particular expertise in the diagnosis and management of psychiatric disorders in children and adolescents with complex physical illnesses (Gitlin et al. 2004). Patients commonly fall primarily into one of three descriptive categories: 1) those with comorbid emotional and physical illnesses that complicate each other's management; 2) those with distressing somatic symptoms plus abnormal thoughts, feelings, and behavior in response to these symptoms; and 3) those with psychiatric symptoms that are a direct consequence of a physical illness and/or its treatment.

Over time, CLP has been designated by several names, including *medical-surgical psychiatry, pediatric psychiatry, psychological medicine, behavioral psychology, pediatric psychology,* and *pediatric psychosomatic medicine.* The term *psychosomatic* was first introduced by Johann Heinroth in 1818, and the term *psychosomatic medicine* was first used by Felix Deutsch in 1922 (Lipsitt 2001). In 1930, in a practice led by Leo Kanner, pediatric psychiatry fellowships were established for pediatricians who went on to develop child psychiatry units within pediatrics. An influential 1932 report on the relationship between pediatrics and psychiatry advocated for greater integration of mental health disciplines into the pediatric hospital setting. As a result of this report, CLP programs were developed across the United States to help increase awareness of the psychological issues affecting physically ill children and adolescents (Fritz 1993; Work 1989). In 1935, the Rockefeller Foundation funded the development of several psychosomatic medicine inpatient units in teaching hospitals throughout the country. Further growth occurred in the 1970s and 1980s as the National Institute of Mental Health funded new training and research grants in the specialty of CLP. In 2003, psychosomatic medicine was established as a subspecialty by the American Board of Psychiatry and Neurology (ABPN). Currently, training in pediatric CLP is a mandatory requirement of training for all ABPN-accredited child and adolescent psychiatry residencies.

Parallel to psychiatry, the fields of psychology and pediatrics also have focused on psychological issues in physically ill children. In 1967, pediatric psychology emerged as a field defined by the concerns of psychologists and allied professionals who work in interdisciplinary settings such as children's hospitals, developmental clinics, and pediatric or medical group practices, as well as traditional clinical child or academic arenas (Wright 1967). The Society of Pediatric Psychology (also known as Division 54 of the American Psychological Association) was founded in 1968 to focus on the rapidly expanding role of behavioral medicine and health psychology in the care of children and adolescents. Currently, Division 54 has an annual forum for research and practice presentations in child health psychology. In 1982, the Society for Developmental and Behavioral Pediatrics was founded with a focus on the developmental and psychosocial aspects of pediatric health care. In 2002, pediatricians with special pediatric fellowship training in emotional and behavioral problems became eligible to receive American Board of Pediatrics certification in the specialty of developmental-behavioral pediatrics.

A number of national and international organizations are dedicated to the specialty of CLP, including the Academy of Consultation-Liaison Psychiatry, the American Psychosomatic Society, the European Association of Psychosomatic Medicine, and the International Organization for Consultation-Liaison Psychiatry. The American Academy of Child and Adolescent Psychiatry (AACAP) has two standing committees that focus on the CLP interface with children, families, and their health care providers—the Physically Ill Child Committee and the Collaborative and Integrated Care Committee.

There are a number of journals that specialize in topics related to the field, including *Psychosomatic Medicine, Psychosomatics, Journal of Psychosomatic Research,* and *Journal of Pediatric Psychology,* as well as more specialized journals that focus on specific disorders (e.g., oncology and transplant psychiatry). A number of outstanding textbooks on CLP are available, including *The American Psychiatric Association Publishing Textbook of Psychosomatic Medicine and Consultation-Liaison Psychiatry*, Third Edition (Levenson 2019), the *Clinical Manual of Psychopharmacology in the Medically Ill,* Second Edition (Levenson and Ferrando 2017), and the *Handbook of Pediatric Psychology,* Fifth Edition (Roberts and Steel 2018). The *Textbook of Pediatric Psychosomatic Medicine* (Shaw and DeMaso 2010) has helped contribute to the pediatric CLP knowledge base, as have a number of excellent disease-specific textbooks, including *Pediatric Psycho-Oncology: A Quick Reference on the Psychosocial Dimensions of Cancer Symptom Management,* Second Edition (Wiener et al. 2015).

Since the publication of the first edition of the *Clinical Manual of Pediatric Psychosomatic Medicine* (Shaw and DeMaso 2006), much has changed in the field of pediatric CLP. In 2018, following a national poll of CLP psychiatrists, the ABPN announced the decision to change the name of their psychosomatic medicine subspecialty to consultation-liaison psychiatry, stating that the latter name "better describes the discipline's key focus of treating behavioral conditions in patients with medical and surgical problems" (Faulkner 2017). The 2013 publication of DSM-5, the fifth edition of the *Diagnostic and Statistical Manual of Mental Disorders* (American Psychiatric Association 2013), has also necessitated significant changes in the classification system of common psychiatric disorders seen in the medical setting.

Another exciting development has been the growth of enthusiasm and interest among practitioners of pediatric CLP. This is most evident in the core missions of the AACAP's Physically Ill Child Committee: 1) to enhance the visibility, commitment, and productivity of child and adolescent psychiatrists involved in research with children in the pediatric setting; 2) to foster collaborative research between child and adolescent psychiatrists at different children's hospitals through the exchange of ideas; 3) to facilitate collaboration between child and adolescent psychiatrists and other groups and organizations involved in relevant research; and 4) to ensure a pediatric CLP programmatic focus at the AACAP Annual Meeting. This committee has an active listserv made up of more than 200 national and international child and adolescent psychiatrists, many of whom direct programs in pediatric CLP. Committee work has generated a number of useful psychoeducational materials, including Facts for Families, which are available on the AACAP website (https://www.aacap.org).

This second edition, retitled the *Clinical Manual of Pediatric Consultation-Liaison Psychiatry,* aims to provide practitioners with concise and pragmatic ways of organizing the key issues that arise in psychiatric consultation with physically ill children and their families as well as to provide a set of templates to help guide clinical assessment and management. This manual is organized into three parts. Chapters 1–4 provide an overview of pediatric CLP, including legal and forensic issues and a discussion of assessment principles. Chapters 5–14 are devoted to specific psychiatric symptoms and disorders in physically ill children and adolescents. Chapters 15–18 address issues related to treatment and intervention.

Richard J. Shaw, M.B., B.S.
David R. DeMaso, M.D.

References

American Psychiatric Association: Diagnostic and Statistical Manual of Mental Disorders, 5th Edition. Arlington, VA, American Psychiatric Association, 2013

Faulkner LR: Memorandum. American Board of Psychiatry and Neurology, November 28, 2017. Available at: https://www.abpn.com/wp-content/uploads/2017/11/PSM-Name-Change-Memo.pdf. Accessed March 13, 2019.

Fritz GK: The hospital: an approach to consultation, in Child and Adolescent Mental Health Consultation in Hospitals, Schools, and Courts. Edited by Fritz GK, Mattison RE, Nurcombe B, et al. Washington, DC, American Psychiatric Press, 1993, pp 7–24

Gitlin DF, Levenson JL, Lyketsos CG: Psychosomatic medicine: a new psychiatric subspecialty. Acad Psychiatry 28(1):4–11, 2004 15140802

Levenson JL (ed): The American Psychiatric Association Publishing Textbook of Psychosomatic Medicine and Consultation-Liaison Psychiatry, 3rd Edition. Washington, DC, American Psychiatric Publishing, 2019

Levenson JL, Ferrando SJ: Clinical Manual of Psychopharmacology in the Medically Ill, 2nd Edition. Washington, DC, American Psychiatric Press, 2017

Lipsitt DR: Consultation-liaison psychiatry and psychosomatic medicine: the company they keep. Psychosom Med 63(6):896–909, 2001 11719628

Roberts MC, Steel RC (eds): Handbook of Pediatric Psychology, 5th Edition. New York, Guilford, 2018

Shaw RJ, DeMaso DR: Clinical Manual of Pediatric Psychosomatic Medicine: Consultation With Physically Ill Children and Adolescents. Washington, DC, American Psychiatric Publishing, 2006

Shaw RJ, DeMaso DR (eds): Textbook of Pediatric Psychosomatic Medicine. Washington, DC, American Psychiatric Publishing, 2010

Wiener LS, Pao MMD, Anne E, et al (eds): Pediatric Psycho-Oncology A: Quick Reference on the Psychosocial Dimensions of Cancer Symptom Management, 2nd Edition. New York, Oxford University Press, 2015

Work HH: The "menace of psychiatry" revisited: the evolving relationship between pediatrics and child psychiatry. Psychosomatics 30(1):86–93, 1989 2643810

Wright L: The pediatric psychologist: a role model. Am Psychol 22(4):323–325, 1967 6041092

Acknowledgments

There are innumerable people whom we wish to thank for their encouragement, advice, and support in preparing this book. We cannot mention them all, but we hope they know of our gratitude. In particular, we acknowledge Dr. Laura Roberts, editor-in-chief of American Psychiatric Association (APA) Publishing; Dr. Hans Steiner in the Department of Psychiatry at Stanford University School of Medicine; and Dr. Heather Walter in the Department of Psychiatry at Boston Children's Hospital and Harvard Medical School.

We have had many critical teachers and mentors who have supported our work on the interface of psychiatry and pediatrics. In psychiatry, there have been Drs. William Beardslee, Myron Belfer, Keith Brodie, Leon Eisenberg, Carl Feinstein, Gregory Fritz, Frederick Melges, and Margaret Stuber. In pediatrics, there have been Drs. Frederick Lovejoy, Alexander Nadas, and Jane Newburger. All of our colleagues and collaborators have been truly invaluable, although Drs. Lourival Baptista-Neto, Michelle Brown, John Campo, Eugene D'Angelo, Stuart Goldman, Joseph Gonzalez-Heydrich, Sally Horwitz, Patricia Ibeziako, Richard Martini, Maryland Pao, Chase Samsel, and Beth Steinberg stand out.

We are especially grateful to John McDuffie, Publisher of APA Publishing, for his support throughout the development and creation of this manual, and to Erika Parker, Acquisitions Coordinator. We thank our families, who have helped in many practical as well as inspirational ways.

Finally, this book could not have been written without the many children and families with whom we have had the privilege of working. It is through the sharing of their lives with us in our work in pediatric consultation-liaison psychiatry that we learned about the adversity and resilience found in children and adolescents facing physical illnesses. It is our understanding of and responses to the stories of these families that form the bedrock of this manual.

PART I

Overview

1

Pediatric Consultation-Liaison Psychiatry

Pediatric consultation-liaison psychiatry (CLP), also known as *pediatric psychosomatic medicine*, is the subspecialty of child and adolescent psychiatry that focuses on providing mental health services to physically ill children and adolescents. Consultants specializing in this field must have in-depth knowledge regarding the way medical, neurological, and other conditions; medications; and metabolic problems interact to cause psychiatric symptoms. Also important is the ability to understand the interaction between psychiatric and medical issues and to recommend the most appropriate treatments (American Academy of Consultation-Liaison Psychiatry 2019).

The field of CLP or psychosomatic medicine has existed for many decades (Ali et al. 2006; Shaw et al. 2010). It has also been designated by other names, including medical psychiatry, medical-surgical psychiatry, psychological medicine, behavioral psychology, and pediatric psychology (Shaw et al. 2010). The field has overlaps with the pediatric specialty of developmental and behavioral pediatrics.

In 2003, the American Board of Psychiatry and Neurology (ABPN) granted psychiatry subspecialty recognition for *psychosomatic medicine*. In 2017 (effective January 1, 2018), the ABPN changed the official subspecialty name from *psychosomatic medicine* to *consultation-liaison psychiatry*. This name change occurred in the context of concern that use of the term *psychosomatics* was thought to suggest that the field's sole focus was on somatic symptom disorders as opposed to the field's much broader approach that integrates biological, psychological, social, and developmental factors into a whole-person multifactorial approach to patients facing physical illnesses (Boland et al. 2018). It is this developmental biopsychosocial framework that lies at the foundation of this clinical manual and our interchangeable use of the terms *pediatric consultation-liaison psychiatry* and *pediatric psychosomatic medicine*.

Building a Collaborative Care Bridge to Pediatrics

The term *consultation* generally refers to activities that involve patient-focused evaluations and recommendations that occur at bedside. By contrast, *liaison* describes activities that focus on the pediatric team and its relationship with the patient. In its broadest interpretation, *liaison* may also include ongoing programmatic developments, policy and protocol issues, and collaborative research.

In bringing together these two activities, consultants serve as bridges for the provision of collaborative mental health care services in the pediatric setting. Ranging along a spectrum from minimal to full collaboration, the following collaborative care models are generally used: 1) *coordinated care*, in which the consultant and pediatric team are in separate facilities with separate systems, communicating intermittently as initiated by the pediatric team; 2) *co-located care*, in which the consultant and pediatric team are in the same facility with some shared systems and communicate frequently about shared patients, although care may still not be coordinated; and 3) *integrated care*, in which the consultant and pediatric team are in the same space within the same facility with shared systems and communicate regularly in person, with resultant practice change (Heath et al. 2013).

Across these bridging models, the framework for collaborative mental health care ideally matches the level of complexity of a patient's needs (de Voursney and Huang 2016). Most commonly, this framework is characterized by a stepped care approach whereby the "right person" in the "right place" delivers the "right care" at the "right time" (Collins et al. 2010; Garrity 2016; Walter et al. 2018). Within this framework, the intensity of treatment ascends based on the severity of the patient's presentation. For example, patients with mild-to-moderate psychiatric disorders are treated within the pediatric setting, whereas those with nonresponsive mild-to-moderate disorders or severe psychiatric disorders are referred for specialty psychiatric assessment and treatment (Collins et al. 2010; Garrity 2016; Walter et al. 2018).

Consultants are thought to be most effective when they work in co-located or integrated care models, whether in outpatient specialty programs or in inpatient hospital settings. Within these bridging models, consultants must appreciate the roles of the professional disciplines involved in the care of physically ill children or adolescents (Table 1–1).

Roles of the Consultant

The consultant has a complex position within the pediatric setting that requires flexibility and adaptability to perform several interrelated roles: assessment and management, patient and family advocacy, liaison activities with pediatric team, and clinical innovation and research.

Assessment and Management

The consultant's primary role is to provide psychiatric assessment and management of physically ill children and adolescents. The American Academy of Child and Adolescent Psychiatry's clinician-oriented practice parameter has outlined core principles (see Chapter 3, "Assessment in Pediatric Consultation-Liaison Psychiatry") to guide consultants in approaching pediatric patients and their families who are facing physical illnesses (DeMaso et al. 2009).

In the assessment, consultants aim to identify comorbid psychiatric illness as well as to recognize the direct effects of physical illnesses that mimic emotional symptoms and physical symptoms that are associated with emotional distress (DeMaso et al. 2009). Consultants can recognize maladaptive coping styles and behaviors that interfere with a patient's health care as well as strengths that promote resilience (DeMaso et al. 2009). Assessment and management are facilitated when consultants assume an engaging and spontaneous

Table 1–1.   Professional disciplines in the pediatric hospital setting

Professional discipline[a]	Roles	Comments
Primary team members		
Attending physician	Leader of pediatric team	May have long-established relationships with patient and family
	Develops diagnostic formulation and treatment interventions	Oriented toward immediate concerns of patient
	Has final medical responsibility for patient	Potential for ambivalent feelings toward the consultant
Resident	Frontline clinician involved in assessment and management	Short-term clinical rotations with lack of continuity
	Has trainee status as participant in residency training program	Frequently dealing with time constraints and excessive burden of clinical work
		Lack of familiarity with role of the consultant
Nurse	Implements bedside treatment interventions	Most frequent, direct contact
	Provides education of patient and family	Closest exposure to physical and emotional distress of the patient
	Provides psychosocial support for patient and family	Lack of continuity due to shift changes and staffing issues
	Serves as liaison between family and pediatric team	

Table 1–1. Professional disciplines in the pediatric hospital setting (*continued*)

Professional discipline[a]	Roles	Comments
Ancillary team members		
Physician (including psychiatrist) consultants	Consult to primary team to provide specialty input into patient's care	May be part of primary team in integrated/colocated care models
Social worker	Assists with basic social services for family	May be part of primary team in integrated/colocated care models
	Serves as liaison with outside agencies, including child protective agencies in cases of abuse and neglect	May have long-established relationship with patient and family
	Provides psychosocial support for patient and family	Has established relationship with pediatric team
	Provides individual and family therapy	Potential for "turf" issues with consultant due to overlap in clinical role
	Oversees referral to and coordination of outpatient services	
Case manager	Coordinates resources and services inside facilities, outside facilities, and between care environments	Generally, case manager is a nurse, although behavioral health support may fall to a social worker and/or a resource specialist
	Works with patients, families, and other professionals to ensure proper resources and service utilization	
	Serves as liaison with insurance companies for authorization of medical/behavioral health services	

Table 1–1.   Professional disciplines in the pediatric hospital setting *(continued)*

Professional discipline[a] Roles	Comments
Ancillary team members *(continued)*	
Occupational and physical therapists	Provides support with activities of daily living
	Oversees rehabilitation of patients after surgery and medical illness
	Provides treatment of feeding difficulties
Nutritionist	Provides nutritional counseling and assists with calculation of caloric needs	Has an important role in treatment of patients with eating disorders and pediatric feeding disorders
Child life specialist	Helps with coping with challenges of hospitalization, surgery, and disability
	Coordinates hospital-based play and recreation services
Chaplain	Provides spiritual assessment of patients and families
	Provides psychosocial and religious support for patient and family

[a]Primary care team is the core team responsible for the care of the patient; ancillary care team comprises those specialists who may or may not be brought into the care of an individual patient.
Source.   Adapted from Fritz 1993.

therapeutic stance that deviates from the more traditional anonymity, abstinence, and neutrality of therapy (DeMaso and Meyer 1996).

Referral Questions

Three types of consultation requests are made of consultants by pediatric practitioners and/or teams: 1) diagnostic (e.g., differential diagnosis of somatic symptoms, depression, delirium, or anxiety—*What does this patient have?*); 2) management (e.g., procedural distress, disruptive behavior, pain management, nonadherence, parental adjustment to illness, or medication—*Please take care of this patient's behavior*); and 3) disposition (e.g., suicide assessment and psychiatric hospitalization—*Please move this patient into a mental health setting*) (DeMaso et al. 2009). These requests are often interrelated, with the relative importance of each request to the individual pediatric practitioner or team varying on a case-to-case basis.

Classification Framework

Figure 1–1 shows a useful framework for consultants to use in organizing the psychiatric issues in physically ill youth by considering the issue of comorbidity. The term *coincidental comorbidity* is used when patients have unrelated psychiatric and physical illnesses, whereas the term *causal comorbidity* is used when the psychiatric disorder is a direct result of physical illness and/or has a significant impact on the course or severity of the physical illness. *Causal comorbidity* also captures psychological symptoms that develop as a direct result of the stress of the illness or its treatment.

Coincidental comorbidity refers to cases in which an emotional disorder that developed before or after the onset of the physical illness is related to factors other than the illness itself. Functionally impairing psychiatric disorders have been estimated to occur in one of every five youth in the United States (Merikangas et al. 2010). When these disorders in youth are untreated, they persist over time, becoming less responsive to treatment while causing progressively greater academic, social, and economic consequences (Copeland et al. 2015). In addition to these findings, evidence indicates that youth with chronic pediatric conditions and co-occurring psychiatric disorders have more than twice the annual medical payments of those with pediatric conditions alone; in this context, psychiatric consultation as a means for early identification and intervention has become an increasingly important consideration for youth facing chronic physical illnesses (Perrin et al. 2019).

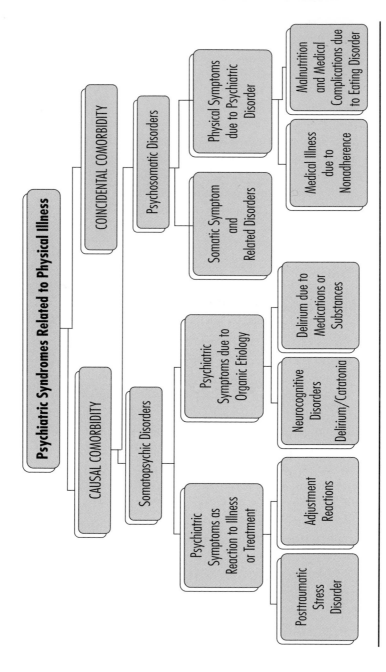

Figure 1–1.   Comorbidity of psychiatric syndromes related to physical illness.

Causal comorbidity refers to instances in which psychiatric symptoms either contribute to or result from the onset of physical illness. Disorders may be classified as psychosomatic or somatopsychic. Patients are diagnosed with *psychosomatic disorders* when physical symptoms are caused by psychiatric illness. Examples include patients with eating disorders who develop medical complications as a result of malnutrition or patients who develop medical complications as a result of failure to adhere to their medical treatment. Similarly, patients with somatic symptom and related disorders have physical symptoms that are primarily a manifestation of underlying psychiatric issues with no demonstrable medical etiology.

Somatopsychic illnesses involve the production of psychiatric symptoms as a direct consequence of a physical illness and/or its treatment. Consultants should be particularly alert to this possibility when psychiatric symptoms develop suddenly, worsen or persist over time, are unresponsive to treatment, and/or have atypical clinical features. One category of patients with somatopsychic illness includes those who develop psychiatric symptoms for which the underlying etiology is medical or medication related. This category includes patients with delirium or a mood disorder due to a medical condition. A second category of patients with somatopsychic illness includes those who develop symptoms of an adjustment disorder or medically related posttraumatic stress disorder as a result of the stress of the physical illness.

Consultant Interventions

Hospital-based treatment interventions are often limited by the lack of time and staff available for their implementation, in addition to the challenge of coordinating the child's care with the large number of hospital staff involved in the patient's overall care. In many cases the consultation is limited to triage and referral to outside agencies. The three most common treatment interventions have been reported to be the use of psychoactive medications, supportive psychotherapy, and assistance with discharge planning by referral or transfer to another facility. Also, consultations have often been reported to involve family therapy, preparation for procedures, and behavioral modification (Ramchandani et al. 1997).

Psychiatric consultants must have a strong grounding in the use of psychotropic medications, including knowledge of potential drug interactions and the need to adjust dosages in patients with physical illnesses (Brown et al. 2000). Common medication requests include the management of delirium, acute symptoms of anxiety or agitation, and insomnia, as well as the use of adjunctive pain medications (see Chapter 5, "Delirium"; Chapter 6, "Neurocognitive Disturbances"; Chapter 7, "Depressive Symptoms and Disorders"; Chapter 8, "Anxiety Symptoms and Trauma/Stress Reactions"; Chapter 10, "Pediatric Pain"; and Chapter 17, "Psychopharmacological Approaches and Considerations").

Psychotherapy by consultants is affected by the current realities of a patient's physical illness and its treatment (O'Dowd and Gomez 2001). Other constraints are the frequent interruptions and the lack of privacy in the hospital setting. As a result, psychotherapy in the inpatient setting is generally supportive in nature. Adjunctive family therapy may also be useful for parents and siblings and to help resolve conflicts that arise between family members (see Chapter 15, "Psychotherapy in the Pediatric Setting," and Chapter 16, "Family Interventions").

Hospital-based behavior modification can be a simple yet effective treatment intervention. Examples include programs to facilitate cooperation with medical procedures, feeding issues, and activities of daily living. Patients with chronic pain or physical disabilities may respond to programs that are presented as part of inpatient rehabilitation treatment. General principles of behavior modification include positive reinforcement of desired behaviors, ignoring negative behaviors, and consistency in the implementation of the program.

Guided imagery, relaxation, and mindfulness interventions are potentially useful in the treatment of pain, anxiety, and insomnia. Patients who are admitted for stressful procedures may benefit from early referral for these services. Hypnosis may be useful for patients with refractory issues of procedural anxiety or pain management (see Chapter 18, "Preparation for Procedures").

Consultants will commonly educate the family regarding what to expect regarding a child's emotional reaction to his or her physical illness. Hospitalization is generally a stressful time in which the family experiences feelings of loss and a lack of control. Education may include information about regression as well as about how a child's level of development affects his or her understanding of the illness.

Patient and Family Advocacy

Advocacy for the child or adolescent serves an important function in supporting and enhancing the provision of patient- and/or family-centered care. Using their biopsychosocial lens, consultants are in the unique position of being able to provide to the family and pediatric team insight into a patient's view of his or her illness, which is influenced by the patient's developmental stage. Adolescents with terminal illness, for example, may wish to be told about their prognosis or have strong opinions about whether to continue their treatment but may find it difficult to convey these thoughts to the pediatric team. Consultants can be a useful conduit for this information and can help promote consideration of and attunement to each patient's perspective. Similarly, consultants are also uniquely positioned to advocate on behalf of the family in their relationship with the pediatric team.

An increasingly important critical advocacy area for consultants involves supporting the patient's health care transition from adolescence to adulthood. The transition from pediatric, parent-supervised health care to more independent, patient-centered adult care represents risk and vulnerability to many patients (White et al. 2018). Those with complex pediatric conditions pose special challenges that might require refinements in the transition process, including flexibility in age of transfer to adult medical care, delayed scheduling of specialist transfers, condition-specific protocols, and/or pediatric consultation arrangements (White et al. 2018). Consultants can be helpful in developing an effective transition program through their attunement to and understanding of the developmental psychosocial needs of individual patients combined with their knowledge of both pediatric and adult health care settings.

Liaison Activities With Pediatric Team

Consultants can help support pediatric practitioners and/or teams during the difficult clinical situations that frequently arise with physically ill youth. This support might involve helping the individual pediatric practitioner or team stay engaged with patients who are acting out or rejecting treatment. Liaison activities may involve work with terminally ill children where feelings of guilt and hopelessness may result in avoidance on the part of practitioners. Referrals for consultation may carry an implied request that the consultant assist in sharing the emotional burden that may be involved in the management of a physically ill child.

Consultants are well positioned to educate the pediatric team in approaching and managing patients' mental health issues. Consultants can help pediatric practitioners to better understand the behavior of patients and to provide guidance on how to work more effectively with them and their families. Education serves to raise practitioners' awareness of the biopsychosocial issues faced by physically ill patients and to encourage early and appropriate referrals. At times, consultants can help individual practitioners to better manage their countertransference reactions and thereby reduce the risk of responding adversely to patients whom they find difficult to approach and manage.

Given that half of U.S. physicians may have symptoms of burnout (work-related emotional exhaustion, depersonalization, and sense of diminished accomplishment), consultants should be alert for this phenomenon, particularly given its adverse impact on patient care (Rotenstein et al. 2018; Rothenberger 2017; Shenoi et al. 2018). It is not unusual for consultants to be sought out by their pediatric and nursing colleagues for personal advice and support. Thoughtful listening and problem solving, with referrals as indicated, are often well received by individual practitioners.

Clinical Innovation and Research

Consultants may have the opportunity to collaborate with pediatric colleagues in quality improvement and/or research initiatives. For example, the significant improvements in pediatric care over the last few decades that have resulted in most children surviving into adulthood have been accompanied by ongoing efforts to better understand and optimize health-related quality of life in children and their families. By bringing their psychiatric expertise into innovative clinical performance improvement initiatives and/or research studies, consultants have the opportunity to significantly impact ongoing patient care while simultaneously enhancing the integration of their own positions into the pediatric setting and advancing their own academic interests.

Practice Patterns in Pediatric Consultation-Liaison Psychiatry

An understanding of national practice patterns in pediatric CLP can be gained from the results of a 2016 survey of 89 academic pediatric CLP programs in the United States and Canada (Shaw et al. 2016). With a 52.5% response rate, this survey revisited a previous 2006 survey to describe the service composition, clinical consultation services, service demand, and service funding and challenges encountered by these CLP programs (Shaw et al. 2006, 2016).

Service Composition

Of pediatric CLP programs responding to the survey, 96% had an attending psychiatrist (Shaw et al. 2016). The average number of psychiatrists was 2.19± 1.79 in small hospitals (<100 beds) and 2.23±1.72 in large hospitals (>100 beds). In terms of full-time faculty equivalents (FTE), 78.2% of small hospitals indicated that the total number for psychiatrists was 0.5–1.0 FTE, with the remainder having >1.0 FTE. Of the large hospital programs, 64.3% indicated that the total for psychiatrists was 0.5–1.0 FTE, with the remainder having >1.0 FTE. There was no significant difference in the number of psychiatrists stratified by hospital size.

Nearly half (46.2%) of surveyed programs had a staff clinical psychologist, with a mean of 2.23 psychologists in small hospitals and 2.48 in large hospitals. Only 25.9% of the programs reported employing social workers, with means of 2.60 and 2.36 social workers (when present) in small and large hospitals, respectively. Advanced practice nurses were employed by 7.8% of the surveyed programs. Most programs utilized trainees—child and adolescent psychiatry fellows (82.7%), general psychiatry residents (25.3%), psychology interns (38.7%), and postdoctoral psychology fellows (15.1%)—with means ranging from 1.13 to 1.52 for each type of trainee when present.

Although most programs reported increased staffing in the past 5 years, it is evident that pediatric CLP services are on average covered by part-time clinicians who also work in other clinical settings.

Clinical Consultation Services

The most frequent reasons for referral to the surveyed pediatric CLP programs were suicide assessment (78.5%), differential diagnosis of medically unexplained symptoms (72.3%), adjustment to illness with depressed mood (58.5%) or anxiety (55.4%), psychotropic medication evaluation (49.2%), delirium (29.2%), and treatment nonadherence (24.6%). The management of psychiatric patients admitted to medical beds because of lack of intensive psychiatric services ("psychiatric boarding") was reported by 23.1% of the programs. Among small hospitals, most programs (70.4%) reported 1–5 new consults per

week on average, whereas large hospitals experienced a wider distribution—
32.5% reported 1–5 consults per week, 30.0% reported 6–10 per week, 17.5%
reported 11–14 per week, and 20.0% reported having greater than 15 consults
per week.

The most frequent services offered were assessment (100.0%), parent psychoeducation (100.0%), psychiatric medications (98.4%), patient psychoeducation (96.9%), liaison activities (89.1%), supportive psychotherapy
(87.5%), coordination with outside provider (85.9%), facilitating outpatient
and inpatient psychiatric referrals (78.1% and 71.9%, respectively), behavioral modification interventions (67.2%), and cognitive-behavioral therapy
(64.1%). There was a high average frequency of collateral contacts with other
providers, including outpatient providers and primary care physicians; daily
(38.8%) or more than daily (41.8%) collateral contacts were common. All
programs reportedly respond to consults within 24 hours, with the majority
(59.7%) responding on the same day.

Only 39.1% of surveyed programs rely on screening tools as part of routine assessment. The most frequently used screening tools included the Screen
for Child Anxiety Related Disorders (52.0%), Vanderbilt Assessment Scales
(32.0%), Children's Depression Inventory (28.0%), Cornell Assessment of
Pediatric Delirium (16.0%), and Pediatric Health Questionnaire (16.0%).
Only 8.1% of programs reportedly use outcome measures, the most frequent
being the Children's Global Assessment Scale. Nearly half of the programs surveyed (45.3%) were actively involved in independent or collaborative research, with the most common areas of investigation being chronic physical
illness, health service delivery, somatic symptom disorders, and/or delirium.

Service Demand

The majority (89.2%) of surveyed pediatric CLP programs reported an increase
in the number of new consults compared with 5 years earlier, with the most
cited reasons for the increase being increased demand for mental health services (87.9%), increased psychiatric boarding on pediatric units (43.1%), and
expansion of hospital/institutional clinical services to all patients (27.6%). Of
programs reporting the increased demand, 54.5% noted that the demand
resulted in less direct patient time; decreased time for liaison, teaching, and
research activities; and increased consultant burnout.

The significant increase in psychiatric boarding comes in the context of children and adolescents seeking acute psychiatric care in larger numbers along with a dramatic reduction in the number of available psychiatric beds (Gallagher et al. 2017). The assessment and management of these boarding patients, who are generally either suicidal or behaviorally out of control, are not reviewed in this manual given this volume's predominant focus on physically ill youth as well as the readily available alternative sources of information regarding the assessment of suicidal and at-risk youth (Walter and DeMaso 2018). Nevertheless, the time demands and emotional impact on consultants who must manage the care of these acutely ill patients represent a growing dimension to and time demand on their work in the pediatric setting.

Service Funding and Challenges

Although hospital support for CLP programs increased significantly from 8% in 2006 to 60.0% in 2016 (Shaw et al. 2006, 2016), departments of psychiatry and pediatrics continued to provide the majority of the financial support. Changes in reimbursement rates were fairly evenly split between those programs reporting either an increase or a decrease.

The CLP program funding issues reported in 2016—including poor rates of reimbursement (41.7%), inadequate or decreased funding (31.1% and 24.6%, respectively), and reliance on professional fees (14.8%)—remain a common challenge, as they were in the 2006 survey (Shaw et al. 2006, 2016). Access to outpatient psychiatry services (50%), lack of space (24.6%), inadequate service staffing (36.1%), and lack of administrative support (24.6%) are additional program challenges. Many (28.3%) of the programs reported a negative effect related to the management of medical boarders.

Conclusion

The field of pediatric CLP is in an increasingly stronger position in that the demand for psychiatric consultation for children and adolescents facing physical illnesses has increased over the past decade (Shaw et al. 2016). Pediatric care providers, whether they be primary care or specialty care physicians or large health care enterprises, have become increasingly aware of the importance of responsive pediatric CLP consultants to help with the diagnosis, management, and disposition of patients with complex pediatric conditions, along with the need to include mental health services in programs designated as a center of pediatric health care excellence.

The time-honored maxim for psychiatric consultants to follow has long been to *"be available, be understandable, be practical,"* while taking care to avoid psychiatric jargon (DeMaso and Meyer 1996; DeMaso et al. 2009). The subsequent chapters in this manual honor this maxim by supporting psychiatric consultants as they work to build bridges into pediatric care in order to reach children and adolescents facing troubling physical and psychiatric issues.

References

Ali S, Ernst C, Pacheco M, et al: Consultation-liaison psychiatry: how far have we come? Curr Psychiatry Rep 8(3):215–222, 2006 19817072

American Academy of Consultation-Liaison Psychiatry: What is consultation-liaison psychiatry? 2019. Available at: https://www.clpsychiatry.org/about-aclp/whatis-clp/. Accessed March 13, 2019.

Boland RJ, Rundell J, Epstein S, et al: Consultation-liaison psychiatry vs psychosomatic medicine: what's in a name change? Psychosomatics 59(3):207–210, 2018 29254807

Brown TM, Stoudemire A, Fogel BS, et al: Psychopharmacology in the medical patient, in Psychiatric Care of the Medical Patient, 2nd Edition. Edited by Stoudemire A, Fogel BS, Greenberg DB. New York, Oxford University Press, 2000, pp 373–394

Collins C, Hewson D, Munger R, et al: Evolving models of behavioral health integration. The Milbank Quarterly, May 25, 2010. Available at: https://www.milbank.org/publications/evolving-models-of-behavioral-health-integration-in-primary-care/. Accessed March 13, 2019.

Copeland WE, Wolke D, Shanahan L, et al: Adult functional outcomes of common childhood psychiatric problems: a prospective, longitudinal study. JAMA Psychiatry 72(9):892–899, 2015 26176785

DeMaso DR, Meyer EC: A psychiatric consultant's survival guide to the pediatric intensive care unit. J Am Acad Child Adolesc Psychiatry 35(10):1411–1413, 1996 8885596

DeMaso DR, Martini DR, Cahen LA, et al; Work Group on Quality Issues: Practice parameter for the psychiatric assessment and management of physically ill children and adolescents. J Am Acad Child Adolesc Psychiatry 48(2):213–233, 2009 20040826 de Voursney D, Huang LN: Meeting the mental health needs of children and youth through integrated care: a systems and policy perspective. Psychol Serv 13(1):77–91, 2016 26845491

Fritz GK: The hospital: an approach to consultation, in Child and Adolescent Mental Health Consultation in Hospitals, Schools, and Courts. Edited by Fritz GK, Mattison RE, Nurcombe B, et al. Washington, DC, American Psychiatric Press, 1993, pp 7–24

Gallagher KAS, Bujoreanu IS, Cheung P, et al: Psychiatric boarding in the pediatric inpatient medical setting: a retrospective analysis. Hosp Pediatr 7(8):444–450, 2017 28716803

Garrity M: Evolving models of behavioral health integration: evidence update 2010–2015. The Milbank Quarterly, May 12, 2016. Available at: https://www.milbank.org/publications/evolving-models-of-behavioral-health-integration-evidence-update-2010–2015/. Accessed March 13, 2019.

Heath B, Wise R, Reynolds K: A review and proposed standard framework for levels of integrated healthcare for SAMHSA-HRSA center for integrated health solutions. March 2013. Available at: https://www.integration.samhsa.gov/integrated-care-models/A_Standard_Framework_for_Levels_of_Integrated_Healthcare.pdf. Accessed March 13, 2019.

Merikangas KR, He JP, Brody D, et al: Prevalence and treatment of mental disorders among U.S. children in the 2001–2004 NHANES. Pediatrics 125(1):75–81, 2010 20008426

O'Dowd MA, Gomez MF: Psychotherapy in consultation-liaison psychiatry. Am J Psychother 55(1):122–132, 2001 11291188

Perrin JM, Asarnow JR, Stancin T, et al: Mental health conditions and healthcare payments for children with chronic medical conditions. Acad Pediatr 19(1):44–50, 2019 30315948

Ramchandani D, Lamdan RM, O'Dowd MA, et al: What, why, and how of consultation-liaison psychiatry: an analysis of the consultation process in the 1990s at five urban teaching hospitals. Psychosomatics 38(4):349–355, 1997 9217405

Rotenstein LS, Torre M, Ramos MA, et al: Prevalence of burnout among physicians: a systematic review. JAMA 320(11):1131–1150, 2018 30326495

Rothenberger DA: Physician burnout and well-being: a systematic review and framework for action. Dis Colon Rectum 60(6):567–576, 2017 28481850

Shaw RJ, Wamboldt M, Bursch B, et al: Practice patterns in pediatric consultation-liaison psychiatry: a national survey. Psychosomatics 47(1):43–49, 2006 16384806

Shaw RJ, Bassols AMS, Berelowitz M, et al: Pediatric psychosomatic medicine, in Textbook of Pediatric Psychosomatic Medicine. Edited by Shaw RJ, DeMaso, MD. Washington, DC, American Psychiatric Publishing, 2010, pp 3–20

Shaw RJ, Pao M, Holland JE, et al: Practice patterns revisited in pediatric psychosomatic medicine. Psychosomatics 57(6):576–585, 2016 27393387

Shenoi AN, Kalyanaraman M, Pillai A, et al: Burnout and psychological distress among pediatric critical care physicians in the United States. Crit Care Med 46(1):116–122, 2018 29016364

Walter HJ, DeMaso DR: Psychiatric emergencies: agitation, suicidality, and other psychiatric emergencies, in Mental Health Care in of Children and Adolescents. Edited by Foy JM. Itasca, IL, American Academy of Pediatrics, 2018, pp 399–432

Walter HJ, Kackloudis G, Trudell EK, et al: Enhancing pediatricians' behavioral health competencies through child psychiatry consultation and education. Clin Pediatr (Phila) 57(8):958–969, 2018 29082768

White PH, Cooley WC; Transitions Clinical Report Authoring Group, et al: Supporting the health care transition from adolescence to adulthood in the medical home. Pediatrics 142(5):e20182587, 2018 30348754

2

Coping and Adaptation in Physically Ill Children

Pediatric and public health innovations have led to substantial reductions in infectious diseases and greatly improved survival rates for children with cancer, congenital heart disease, cystic fibrosis, and other chronic health conditions (Perrin et al. 2014). Most children (>90%) with significant physical illnesses now survive into adulthood, resulting in a heightened focus on understanding the factors affecting their adaptation and coping (Snell and DeMaso 2010).

Although most health conditions are relatively mild and interfere little with normal activities, more than 8% of youth have health conditions that consistently affect their daily activities (Perrin et al. 2014). This represents a nearly fourfold rise over the past 50 years, a change that is primarily due to increases in asthma, obesity, mental health conditions, and neurodevelopmental disorders. The care of youth with other complex physical conditions (e.g., diabetes, cystic fibrosis, cancer, epilepsy) is concentrated in regional subspecialty care centers, with youth having less complex conditions being increasingly cared for in primary or specialty outpatient care settings (Perrin et al. 2014).

Chronic physical illnesses have been defined as conditions that last for a substantial period of time and have persistent and debilitating sequelae. More specifically, chronic illnesses interfere with daily functioning for more than 3 months in a year or cause more frequent hospitalizations, home health care, and/or extensive medical care (Compas et al. 2012). Effective management of chronic conditions can optimize health outcomes and reduce unnecessary health care utilization and costs (Miller et al. 2016). The importance of psychiatric consultant involvement in this care is underscored by the fact that individuals with chronic medical conditions and coexisting behavioral health disorders have much higher health care costs than those with chronic medical conditions alone (Perrin et al. 2019).

Childhood chronic illnesses affect daily functioning via the *direct effects* of a physical illness and/or its medical treatment—these include pain, discomfort, or medication effects (Snell and DeMaso 2010). In addition, youth may develop *indirect effects* to an illness—that is, emotional and behavioral responses, including maladaptive coping strategies, that may last for hours, days, months, or years. Most chronic illnesses require intermittent pediatric services, such as for diagnosis, frequent follow-up appointments, and/or intermittent medical crises. Parents or other primary caregivers play central roles in the day-to-day management of these illnesses and are not spared the stress of responding and living with the children's health conditions. Siblings, relatives, friends, and/or teachers to varying degrees experience the impact of childhood physical illnesses.

To enable consultants to understand a child's adaptation to physical illnesses and thereby enhance their ability to intervene effectively, we address in this chapter the correlates that shape children's emotional and behavioral responses to physical illnesses that must be faced each and every day.

Conceptualization of Physical Illness: Categorical Versus Noncategorical

There has been much discussion in the literature regarding the utilization of categorical versus noncategorical approaches to conceptualizing the childhood illness experience (Snell and DeMaso 2010; van der Lee et al. 2007). In a *categorical* approach, illnesses are grouped in terms of specific physical illnesses, such as congenital heart disease, diabetes mellitus, or cystic fibrosis. This approach considers the different rates and presentations of psychological problems in childhood within each category of illness. This method has the advantage of being able to identify important differences between conditions and to identify specific targets for intervention. Nevertheless, an alternative focus has been placed on the characteristics that specific illnesses have in common, and efforts have been made to categorize these conditions along a variety of dimensions.

In a *noncategorical* approach, physical illnesses are classified on the basis of general dimensions that are considered common to the illness experience regardless of the specific condition a child has, such as whether the condition is visible versus invisible or fatal versus nonfatal. This approach takes into account premorbid emotional functioning and developmental stage, as well as the degree of psychosocial stress. A noncategorical approach views the stressors that physically ill children and families experience as being due to a variety of factors that are not related to a specific condition. This chapter takes a noncategorical approach to understanding coping and adaptation in the face of chronic physical illnesses.

Correlates of Adjustment to Physical Illness

Consultants are well served to consider the following interrelated correlates of adjustment in approaching the assessment and management of children and adolescents with chronic physical illnesses (Figure 2–1).

Coping Style

Coping can be viewed as a collection of purposeful, volitional efforts that are directed at the regulation of aspects of the self and the environment under stress (Compas et al. 2012). A child's coping style is defined as the set of his or her cognitive, emotional, and behavioral responses to stressors (Van Horn et al. 2001a). Coping involves a child's consistent use of particular strategies for managing stressors across contexts. The style a child adopts depends on the interaction between a child's automatic temperamentally based ways of reacting to stress (stress response) and a child's purposeful coping responses that aim to manage and adapt to stress and that emerge later in development (coping re-

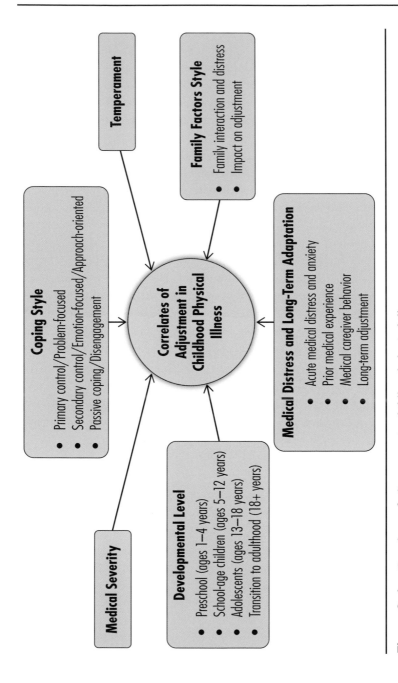

Figure 2–1.   Correlates of adjustments in childhood physical illness.

sponse) (Compas et al. 2012; Rudolph et al. 1995). The intent of the coping response is stress reduction (coping goal) (Folkman and Lazarus 1988; Snell and DeMaso 2010).

A model of perceived control outlines three types of coping responses that are central to understanding successful adaptation in childhood chronic illness (Compas et al. 2012; Rudolph et al. 1995): 1) *primary control* refers to coping efforts that are intended to influence objective events or conditions, 2) *secondary control* or *accommodative coping* involves coping aimed at maximizing one's fit to current conditions, and 3) *passive coping* or *disengagement* refers to the absence of any coping attempt.

Children's coping styles have also been categorized in a number of related subtypes, again based on the central role of controllability. *Approach-oriented coping* (primary and secondary control) refers to behaviors and thoughts directed at addressing or managing the stressor or the feelings it elicits. This style includes asking questions, displaying interest in medical play and equipment, and seeking emotional and social support prior to procedures. *Avoidance-oriented coping* (passive coping) refers to thoughts and behaviors designed to avoid experiencing the stressor at the physical, cognitive, or emotional level. Examples of this coping style include going to sleep, daydreaming, and refusing to ask or answer questions (Rudolph et al. 1995). Another method of categorizing coping responses identifies children's strategies as *problem-focused coping* (primary control) versus *emotion-focused coping* (secondary control) (Folkman and Lazarus 1988; Snell and DeMaso 2010). Problem-focused coping strategies are directed at altering the stressor or associated external circumstances, whereas emotion-focused coping strategies are aimed at regulating emotional responses to the stressor.

Many studies have examined associations between particular coping responses and outcomes based on hypotheses that specific coping approaches would be reliably associated with better adaptation (Compas et al. 2012; Rudolph et al. 1995). Although research results have been inconsistent, perhaps in part because of variations in the conceptualizations of coping styles and the times at which they are assessed, considerable evidence shows that secondary control coping is related to better adjustment through the use of acceptance, cognitive reappraisal, and distraction, which are cognitive strategies that maximize one's fit with the demands of an illness (Compas et al. 2012). The use of avoidance, denial, and wishful thinking in passive coping is related to poorer adjustment, as emotional distress regulation is undermined and may disrupt engagement coping strategies aimed at reducing stress (Compas et al. 2012).

The evidence for primary control has been less consistent, because this approach may not be a good fit for different sources of stress (Compas et al. 2012). It may not prove adaptive in the context of acute medical stressors in which a stressor is largely uncontrollable. Primary control has, however, been found to be useful for long-term adaptation, as has been demonstrated through enhanced treatment regimen adherence, such as in diabetes management (Snell and DeMaso 2010).

Developmental Level

Developmental level has an impact on adaptation, affecting not only the coping responses available to youth but also their ability to process and benefit from health-related information and to adhere to medical regimens (Snell and DeMaso 2010). Although this impact is most apparent in the midst of an acute physical illness, studies have not consistently demonstrated age effects on long-term psychosocial adjustment in physically ill youth.

Preschool Children (Ages 1–4 Years)

Preschool children may fail to understand why their parents do not protect them from the perceived threat of medical procedures and may feel threatened by forced separations during procedures because of normative anxieties about physical safety, separation from parents, and encounters with unfamiliar people. Magical thinking and associative logic characterize their cognition, and therefore preschool children often attribute events in their lives to their own thoughts, feelings, and behaviors and infer causal links between events that occur in close physical or temporal proximity. Pediatric procedures can easily be misinterpreted as "punishment" for bad behavior. Children at this age have difficulty comprehending abstract concepts such as duration (e.g., "It will only last a minute") and quantity (e.g., "This will only hurt a little bit"). Because of their limited verbal and attention abilities, they are less likely to be able to recall and comprehend information intended to prepare them for procedures. Because preschool children are unable to use self-generated primary or secondary coping strategies, they are more likely to engage in passive coping strategies when faced with procedural stressors.

School-Age Children (Ages 5–12 Years)

Because mastery is a primary developmental task of school-age children, the loss of control experienced during a physical illness and its treatment challenges basic emotional needs and can elicit feelings of anxiety and helplessness. Similarly, advances in cognitive skills at this age can sensitize children to new aspects of pediatric encounters. School-age children may become focused on the effects of interventions on their bodies and begin to display fears of bodily harm and death. They are prone to misinterpretations and worries about painful procedures. Fortunately, children's coping repertoires tend to expand during this developmental period, which may be the reason that overall levels of pediatric fear decrease with age. The adaptive use of secondary coping responses increases with age and has been associated with declines in negative emotional and behavioral responses to procedures.

Adolescents (Ages 13–18 Years)

Adolescents face the task of developing a sense of autonomy from family, often through the formation of close peer relationships that foster a sense of identity and belonging. Rapid physical changes associated with puberty engender heightened self-awareness and preoccupation with appearance. Procedures can impinge on adolescents' emerging sense of autonomy and bodily integrity, particularly when the procedures involve a potential loss of functioning or alteration in physical appearance. The acceptance of authority and relinquishing of control required to undergo procedures can be difficult and may foster feelings of helplessness and dependence. Adolescents may become more resistant and less adherent to needed pediatric treatment if their need for control and independence is challenged. The cognitive advances of adolescence are both an asset and a liability in terms of pediatric interventions. Because adolescents are capable of abstract thinking, they may experience greater fears about potential outcomes and implications of their physical conditions; however, their cognitive skills allow them to draw upon an even wider range of coping responses to address these fears.

Transition to Adulthood (18+ Years)

The transition from adolescence to young adulthood involves tasks that include moving away from family, becoming independent, developing one's identity, and learning to handle more complex relationships (White et al. 2018). Individuals of this age can face the challenges of starting college and/or moving into the working world. There is the required transition from pediatric, parent-supervised health care to more independent, patient-centered adult health care, which is more difficult in the context of a physical illness (White et al. 2018). The following are potential barriers that transitioning patients might experience: fear of a new health care system and/or hospital, not wanting to leave the previous pediatric practitioner/team and institution, anxiety about relinquishing control around managing their condition, less interest in health compared with broader life questions, and/or inadequate preparation by or support from clinicians in the patients' transition process to an adult model of health care (White et al. 2018).

Medical Severity

The immediate impact of pain or other direct effects of acutely presenting medical illness in a novel setting, such as an emergency room, are readily observed. However, the long-term impact of a physical illness on a child's adjustment may prove problematic, despite being less apparent. For example, both critical congenital heart conditions and inflammatory bowel disease have direct effects on the brain with an associated increased risk for emotional disorders and neurodevelopment impairments (DeMaso et al. 2014, 2017; Holland et al. 2017; Szigethy et al. 2014). These impairments may be associated with problems in the ability of children to use the types of complex cognitive coping strategies (Compas et al. 2012) that are needed to effectively cope with stress, as well as problems in academic and peer functioning. Finally, illnesses with complex treatment regimens, unpredictable treatment courses, and/or longer disease duration may also increase the risk for an adverse adaptation to an illness.

Consultants must also be alert to coincidental comorbidity, in which the patient has unrelated psychiatric and physical illnesses occurring together (see Chapter 1, "Pediatric Consultation-Liaison Psychiatry"). This occurrence is captured in the old medical school adage designed to ensure that all diagnoses are considered: "A patient can have as many diseases as he [or she] damn well pleases." This consideration is pertinent in the hospital setting, because higher rates of co-occurring physical and psychiatric illnesses are associated with longer hospital stays and higher hospital costs (Doupnik et al. 2016; Gerteis et al. 2014; Mitchell et al. 2017).

Temperament

Temperamental difficulties have been found to predict poor behavioral and emotional adjustment in children with chronic pediatric illnesses (Snell and DeMaso 2010; Wallander et al. 2003). More anxious children may choose techniques such as distraction to avoid experiencing the stressor, whereas less anxious children may be more likely to seek information about the stressor. These factors are important to consider because evidence suggests that the fit between child temperament and environmental influences may be important in determining adjustment.

Medical Distress and Long-Term Adaptation

Acute Distress and Anxiety

The experience of acute distress and anxiety is a common problem that has been associated with behavior management and adherence problems. Prevalence estimates are as high as 7%, and estimates of resultant behavior management problems range from 9% to 11% (Van Horn et al. 2001a). Overt emotional and behavioral distress (e.g., verbal/physical protests or refusal to cooperate) often reflects the child's efforts to avoid frightening and unpleasant situations, serving as a protective response to an external threat. Only 60% of children who reported significant fear displayed uncooperative behaviors during treatment (Rudolph et al. 1995). This means that many children may become withdrawn and uncommunicative when faced with anxiety-provoking situations and are seemingly cooperative, yet they may actually be overwhelmed with disabling anxiety.

Consultants are well served to keep in mind that assessing the adequacy of a child's coping response is complicated in that different people involved in a health care encounter may have different perspectives on the most desired outcome. Parents may focus on minimizing observed distress in a child, whereas health care providers may focus on maximizing adherence (Rudolph et al. 1995). As a result, having multiple sources of information on whether a coping response is adaptive is recommended.

Child's Prior Medical Experience

Consultants should be attuned to a pediatric patient's history of difficult, painful, and/or unsuccessful medical experiences and the child's reactions to them because such a history may fuel the patient's expectations of later similar experiences and result in accompanying anxiety. Studies suggest that children who have had prior experiences of hospitalization may display more anxiety during subsequent procedures (Dahlquist et al. 1986; Lerwick 2016). Having knowledge of a child's prior pediatric health care experiences may help the consultant determine which interventions might help a child to cope with anxiety. For example, preparation programs that emphasize information giving, modeling, and demonstration may not have the same protective benefits for children who have previous experience with the procedure as they do for those without previous experience.

Pediatric Caregiver Behavior

Pediatric practitioners should consider the critical importance of their own behavior in supporting and working with patients and their families. The pediatric caregiver who provides excessive explanation and reassurance during medical procedures tends not to be effective and may inadvertently validate and magnify the aversive experience. On the other hand, the pediatric caregiver who denies or minimizes expressed fears and worries also tends to be ineffective. The caregiver who works somewhere between these extremes is more likely to create an effective working partnership with patients and families.

Long-Term Adjustment

Over the long term, pediatric patients and their families appear remarkably resilient in adapting to challenges presented by physical illnesses (Snell and DeMaso 2010). Yet there remains a significant number who are at risk for subclinical or subthreshold psychiatric problems as well as diagnosable psychiatry disorders (DeMaso et al. 2014, 2017; Holland et al. 2017; Szigethy et al. 2014). The rate of emotional disorders in children younger than 18 years with medical illnesses is estimated to be approximately 25%, whereas the rate in physically healthy children is 20% (Wallander et al. 2003). Children with chronic physical illness present primarily with internalizing syndromes, such as anxiety and depression, that can persist over time (DeMaso et al. 2014, 2017; Holland et al. 2017; Szigethy et al. 2014; Thompson et al. 1990).

Family Factors

Simply put, parenting a child with a chronic physical illness is stressful. Family concerns include those related to medical prognosis (immediate prognosis and treatment), psychosocial functioning (emotional and social adjustment), effect on the family (impact on family life and functioning), quality of life (functional limitations due to medical involvement), and financial issues (short- and long-term costs) (Snell et al. 2010; Van Horn et al. 2001b). Depending on the immediate circumstances of an illness, it is common for parents to be fearful to varying degrees and to manifest this fear in the forms of anxiety, guilt, depression, and/or even anger.

Family Interaction and Acute Distress

Parents are commonly managing three essential questions, which generally go unexpressed: 1) Will my child get better? 2) How long will it take? and 3) How much will it cost? Consultants are well served to be alert to these questions because when they go unanswered (or are unanswerable), levels of parental uncertainty and stress rise appreciably. Many parents have described this phenomenon as analogous to being on an emotional roller coaster and not knowing when they will get off.

Parental trait anxiety has been associated with parental distress during procedures (Melamed 1993). Parental distress can interfere with parents' ability to respond to the emotional needs of their children and their ability to help their children generate effective coping strategies and can affect both immediate and long-term outcomes, as well as negatively affecting their working relationships with their medical caregivers (DeMaso and Bujoreanu 2013). Children who have highly anxious mothers often exhibit lower levels of distress when their mothers are absent during a procedure. Distress-promoting behaviors tend to involve criticism of the child's emotional reactions or behaviors, threats, and punitiveness (Dolgin and Katz 1988). Excessive parental attention to a child's distress through reassurance, empathy, apologies, and/or relinquishing control to the child is associated with increased behavioral distress (Blount et al. 1989), just as excessive attention from pediatric team members, as discussed in the earlier subsection "Pediatric Caregiver Behavior," can result in less successful outcomes.

Impact on Adjustment

Maternal depression and anxiety play important roles in child adjustment to chronic illnesses, just as they do in a child's behavior during procedures (DeMaso et al. 1991; Wallander et al. 2003). Family adjustment and perceptions play important roles in mother-reported behavior problems and in child-reported psychiatric symptoms. Of note, parental/family functioning appears to be a greater predictor of a child's emotional adjustment than the medical severity of the child's illness (DeMaso et al. 1991, 2000, 2004a, 2004b, 2014).

Conclusion

Children and adolescents face a wide variety of chronic physical illnesses that may impinge on their development and their emotional, cognitive, behavioral, and social functioning. In assessing the adaptation and coping of a child facing a chronic physical illness, consultants should integrate the correlates of adjustment—coping style, developmental level, medical severity, temperament, medical distress and long-term adaptation, and family factors—into a biopsychosocial formulation that helps build an effective intervention strategy that minimizes the impact of physical illness and promotes the health and wellness of the patient and the family.

References

Blount R, Corbin SM, Sturges JW, et al: The relationship between adults' behavior and child coping and distress during BMA/LP procedures: a sequential analysis. Behav Ther 20(4):585–601, 1989

Compas BE, Jaser SS, Dunn MJ, et al: Coping with chronic illness in childhood and adolescence. Annu Rev Clin Psychol 8:455–480, 2012 22224836

Dahlquist LM, Gil KM, Armstrong FD, et al: Preparing children for medical examinations: the importance of previous medical experience. Health Psychol 5(3):249–259, 1986 3527692

DeMaso DR, Bujoreanu IS: Enhancing working relationships between parents and surgeons. Semin Pediatr Surg 22(3):139–143, 2013 23870207

DeMaso DR, Campis LK, Wypij D, et al: The impact of maternal perceptions and medical severity on the adjustment of children with congenital heart disease. J Pediatr Psychol 16(2):137–149, 1991 2061786

DeMaso DR, Spratt EG, Vaughan BL, et al: Psychological functioning in children and adolescents undergoing radiofrequency catheter ablation. Psychosomatics 41(2):134–139, 2000 10749951

DeMaso DR, Lauretti A, Spieth L, et al: Psychosocial factors and quality of life in children and adolescents with implantable cardioverter-defibrillators. Am J Cardiol 93(5):582–587, 2004a 14996583

DeMaso DR, Douglas Kelley S, Bastardi H, et al: The longitudinal impact of psychological functioning, medical severity, and family functioning in pediatric heart transplantation. J Heart Lung Transplant 23(4):473–480, 2004b 15063408

DeMaso DR, Labella M, Taylor GA, et al: Psychiatric disorders and function in adolescents with d-transposition of the great arteries. J Pediatr 165(4):760–766, 2014 25063716

DeMaso DR, Calderon J, Taylor GA, et al: Psychiatric disorders in adolescents with single ventricle congenital heart disease. Pediatrics 139:e20162241, 2017 28148729

Dolgin MJ, Katz ER: Conditioned aversions in pediatric cancer patients receiving chemotherapy. J Dev Behav Pediatr 9(2):82–85, 1988 3366914

Doupnik SK, Lawlor J, Zima BT, et al: Mental health conditions and medical and surgical hospital utilization. Pediatrics 138(6):20162361, 2016 27940716

Folkman S, Lazarus RS: The relationship between coping and emotion: implications for theory and research. Soc Sci Med 26(3):309–317, 1988 3279520

Gerteis J, Izrael D, Deitz D, et al: Multiple chronic conditions chartbook: 2010 medical expenditure panel survey data for Agency for Healthcare Research and Quality. April 2014. Available at: http://www.ahrq.gov/professionals/prevention-chronic-care/decision/mcc/mccchartbook.pdf. Accessed March 13, 2019.

Holland JE, Cassidy AR, Stopp C, et al: Psychiatric disorders and function in adolescents with tetralogy of Fallot. J Pediatr 187:165–173, 2017 28533034

Lerwick JL: Minimizing pediatric healthcare-induced anxiety and trauma. World J Clin Pediatr 5(2):143–150, 2016 27170924

Melamed BG: Putting the family back in the child. Behav Res Ther 31(3):239–247, 1993 8476398

Miller GF, Coffield E, Leroy Z, Wallin R: Prevalence and costs of five chronic conditions in children. J Sch Nurs 32(5):357–364, 2016 27044668

Mitchell RJ, Curtis K, Braithwaite J: Health outcomes and costs for injured young people hospitalised with and without chronic health conditions. Injury 48(8):1776–1783, 2017 28602181

Perrin JM, Anderson LE, Van Cleave J: The rise in chronic conditions among infants, children, and youth can be met with continued health system innovations. Health Aff (Millwood) 33(12):2099–2105, 2014 25489027

Perrin JM, Asarnow JR, Stancin T, et al: Mental health conditions and healthcare payments for children with chronic medical conditions. Acad Pediatr 19(1):44–50, 2019 30315948

Rudolph KD, Dennig MD, Weisz JR: Determinants and consequences of children's coping in the medical setting: conceptualization, review, and critique. Psychol Bull 118(3):328–357, 1995 7501740

Snell S, DeMaso DR: Adaptation and coping in chronic childhood physical illness, in Textbook of Pediatric Psychosomatic Medicine. Edited by Shaw RJ, DeMaso DR. Washington, DC, American Psychiatric Publishing, 2010, pp 21–31

Snell C, Marcus NE, Skitt KS, et al: Illness-related concerns in caregivers of psychiatrically hospitalized children with depression. Res Treat Child Youth 27:115–126, 2010

Szigethy E, Bujoreanu SI, Youk AO, et al: Randomized efficacy trial of two psychotherapies for depression in youth with inflammatory bowel disease. J Am Acad Child Adolesc Psychiatry 53(7):726–735, 2014 24954822

Thompson RJ Jr, Hodges K, Hamlett KW: A matched comparison of adjustment in children with cystic fibrosis and psychiatrically referred and nonreferred children. J Pediatr Psychol 15(6):745–759, 1990 2283579

van der Lee JH, Mokkink LB, Grootenhuis MA, et al: Definitions and measurement of chronic health conditions in childhood: a systematic review. JAMA 297(24):2741–2751, 2007 17595275

Van Horn M, Campis LB, DeMaso DR: Reducing distress and promoting coping for the pediatric patient, in OMS Knowledge Update: Self-Study Program, Vol 3; Pediatric Surgery Section. Edited by Piecuch JF. Alpharetta, GA, American Association of Oral and Maxillofacial Surgeons, 2001a, pp 5–18

Van Horn M, DeMaso DR, Gonzalez-Heydrich J, et al: Illness-related concerns of mothers of children with congenital heart disease. J Am Acad Child Adolesc Psychiatry 40(7):847–854, 2001b 11437024

Wallander JL, Thompson RJ, Alriksson-Schmidt A: Psychosocial adjustment of children with chronic physical conditions, in Handbook of Pediatric Psychology, 3rd Edition. Edited by Roberts MC. New York, Guilford, 2003, pp 141–158

White PH, Cooley WC; Transitions Clinical Report Authoring Group, et al: Supporting the health care transition from adolescence to adulthood in the medical home. Pediatrics 142(5):e20182587, 2018 30348754

3

Assessment in Pediatric Consultation-Liaison Psychiatry

The goals of the assessment in pediatric consultation-liaison psychiatry (CLP) are to develop a clinical biopsychosocial formulation and to determine whether a patient's presentation meets the diagnostic criteria for a psychiatric disorder. Together, these findings inform the development and implementation of a comprehensive evidence-based treatment approach for a patient and his or her family. The assessment determines where a patient's presentation falls along a continuum from the normal psychological processes common to human experience at one end to the symptoms, distress, and functional impairment of psychiatric disorders at the other end (Wolraich et al. 1996). The communication of the assessment findings to patients and families is helpful in supporting and strengthening working relationships between families and their pediatric health care providers and thereby enhances the approach to and management of patients' physical illnesses.

In this chapter we outline the critical steps in the psychiatric consultation process. The chapter serves as a guide to help consultants understand and approach assessment, particularly in the pediatric hospital setting (Table 3–1).

Table 3–1. The consultation process: critical steps in pediatric consultation-liaison psychiatry assessments

1. Set up a responsive intake system.

2. Establish the referral question.

3. Obtain multiple sources of information.

4. Consider screening.

5. Prepare the patient and family for the psychiatric assessment.

6. Meet initially with the parent(s) or caretaker(s).

7. Interview the child or adolescent patient.

8. Consider standardized assessment instruments

9. Observe behavior and play.

10. Be alert to developmental issues in the assessment.

11. Develop a biopsychosocial formulation.

12. Communicate findings and recommendations to the pediatric team and family.

The Consultation Process

Set Up a Responsive Intake System

Ideally, it is best to have an intake worker with a dedicated phone line and/or email address as the first point of contact with the referring pediatric team. This person should respond quickly to routine and emergency requests, as well as to contacts that occur after hours or on weekends. The intake worker should obtain the following information: patient's name, birth date, hospital record number, hospital location, referring physician contact information, reason for request, level of urgency, and insurance information. Importantly, the intake worker must also find out whether the patient and family have been informed of the consultation request.

Given the inherent time required by consultants for nonbillable liaison work (i.e., speaking with physicians or nurses), it is critical that billing for direct patient care be maximized. In this regard, the CLP service (or CLP providers, if not working for a formal service) should establish policies regarding billing uninsured or out-of-managed-care-network patients and obtaining medical co-payments. Finally, there should be clear policies regarding the assessments of adults hospitalized in the pediatric setting and parents of hospitalized children.

Establish the Referral Question

There is considerable variability across pediatric settings regarding the reasons and regularity with which consultations are requested as well as the expectations for these consultations (Shaw et al. 2006, 2016). Nevertheless, consultation requests generally fall into three overlapping categories: diagnostic, management, and disposition (see Chapter 1, "Pediatric Consultation-Liaison Psychiatry"). Effective consultants will identify which of these request types the referring physician or pediatric team is primarily seeking. Consultants often need to tolerate some level of ambiguity regarding the referral questions and may find they need to assist pediatric practitioners in more clearly identifying the problem (DeMaso et al. 2009). As part of this process, consultants should attempt to delineate the circumstances, frequency, intensity, and duration of the problematic behaviors, as well as factors that may precipitate, worsen, or ameliorate the problem.

While consultants should acknowledge the explicit referral concerns, they must also be attentive to potential unspoken issues that may need to be addressed. For example, the referring pediatric team may be unaware of conflicts between the patient and themselves or of underlying emotional stresses that may be directly influencing the patient's current behavior. It is generally helpful to be aware of the referring team's expectations based on previous consultations. Consultants should be alert to identifying unrealistic expectations and/or a lack of knowledge regarding their role that may also adversely affect the consultation process.

Obtain Multiple Sources of Information

Consultants should review the medical record prior to beginning the consultation; this review should include nursing notes, which can often be important sources of information. Consultants can supplement this review by obtaining additional information from available nurses and from ancillary team members (i.e., other medical consultants, social workers, or child life specialists) who have had significant contact with the patient and/or family. Records of relevant outside psychiatric, psychological, or special educational evaluations can be reviewed when available, and in some cases, information should be obtained from the school. When children are involved with child welfare agencies or the juvenile justice system or are in institutional care, it may be important to obtain information from those sources.

Consider Screening

Consultants can consider the use of screening instruments to systematically and efficiently gather information about presenting problems prior to the assessment. In the context of frequent time pressures and work demands, this information can be used in helping to focus the consultant's queries while ensuring that all problems are identified. One such broadband measure that can be used is the American Psychiatric Association's parent- and self-rated Level 1 Cross-Cutting Symptom Measures (available at: https://www.psychiatry.org/psychiatrists/practice/dsm/educational-resources/assessment-measures). These measures, which screen for multiple psychiatric disorders, demonstrated good reliability in the DSM-5 field trials conducted in pediatric clinical samples across the United States (Narrow et al. 2013). Depending on the clinical concerns, consultants may also consider using a standardized symptom rating scale to characterize the nature and breadth of the presenting symptoms, such as those scales used for anxiety (see Chapter 8, "Anxiety Symptoms and Trauma/Stress Reactions") and depression (see Chapter 7, "Depressive Symptoms and Disorders").

Prepare the Patient and Family for the Psychiatric Assessment

Ensuring the patient's and family's full participation in a psychiatric assessment can present special challenges. Assessment in the pediatric hospital setting is unique in that the referring physician is in fact the consultee, in contrast to the more typical outpatient assessment where the parents are the referring agents. Slightly over one-third of patients and families have been found not to know who initiated the referral or the reason for the consultation (Kitts et al. 2013). Under these circumstances, many families may interpret the consultation request as a communication from their physician and/or pediatric team that they are not coping adequately. The stress of the child's physical illness and/or its treatment may make the family much less receptive to meeting with a representative from a service that they do not perceive as necessary for their child's care.

As should occur with consultations from other pediatric specialties, the referring physician should always inform the patient and family about the referral and its purpose prior to the consultation. Most families will respond to the idea that hospitalizations are stressful and that their children may benefit from the added support provided by meeting with the consultant. Parents often respond positively to explanations that the purpose of the consultation is to understand the impact of an illness on their child's emotions, behavior, and cognitions, as well as to understand their own impact on the child's physical illness. Parents are usually open to concepts such as the use of relaxation techniques or biofeedback to reduce anticipatory anxiety or to assist with pain management. In pediatric specialty programs, such as renal dialysis, or with high-stress procedures, such as solid organ transplantation, it is useful to present consultation as a routine part of the program's efforts to maximize health and wellness for all patients. In those circumstances in which consultants find a family unreceptive to proceeding with a requested assessment, it is best to ask the pediatric team to explain (or reexplain) to the family the team's reasons for wanting the consultation.

Meet Initially With the Parent(s) or Caretaker(s)

In most cases, the initial meeting begins with the consultant speaking separately with the parents (or primary caretakers). Given the importance of establishing a working relationship with the family, consultants should begin by eliciting the family's understanding of the reason for the referral. The consultant should keep in mind that this may be the family's first experience with a mental health professional and that they may be focused solely on medical causes for their child's problem and may not have considered the potential impact of psychosocial factors. One approach that has proven helpful in engaging the family is to start by inquiring about the child's pediatric illness history and its impact in the different domains of the child's life. A psychoeducational approach may be used to explain to the parents the developmental issues and typical reactions of children to illness and hospitalization. It may also be necessary to explain some of the psychiatric concepts that may be unfamiliar to parents, such as the need to meet separately with the child and the importance of confidentiality regarding sensitive information. Parents may have suggestions as to how to introduce the consultant to the child, and they are important allies to enlist in the assessment. As indicated by the referral concerns, consultants may need to inform the family of situations in which confidentiality cannot be maintained beyond the hospital setting (e.g., when allegations of physical or sexual abuse arise).

Interview the Child or Adolescent Patient

The child or adolescent should be seen routinely as part of each consultation. It may be necessary to meet with the patient together with the parents if either the child or the parents are reluctant to meet alone. Subsequent meetings may then occur alone with the child when there is greater familiarity and comfort with the consultant. Attention should be paid to concerns about confidentiality, particularly if the child is sharing a room with another patient. If possible, younger children should be taken to a playroom, but if the child is too ill to leave the bed, the consultant should have a selection of toys and accessories to help engage the child in the assessment.

Establishing a working relationship with the patient is one of the keys to an effective consultation. This relationship is facilitated through the provision of a simple normalizing explanation by the consultant regarding the pediatric team's concerns. With the patient, as with the parents, it may be helpful to start with a review of the medical problems, because the patient will generally be more familiar with and comfortable about giving this history. After this background is presented, it is easier for patients to transition to queries about the emotional impact of their illness and its treatment. Inquiry about non-pediatric-illness issues, such as school and social functioning, strengths and interests, and life outside the hospital, is an alternative starting point for the interview.

The following specific techniques can be useful in establishing rapport, while gaining insight into patients' current perceptions and understandings of their illness (Hobday and Ollier 1999).

Draw-a-Person Test

When administered to a physically ill child, the draw-a-person test is modified from the standard projective test. The child is asked to draw a picture of himself or herself prior to the illness or injury and then, in a second drawing, a picture of himself or herself after the illness or hospitalization. This exercise can be expanded by asking the child to draw a picture of his or her family both before and after the illness or hospitalization to examine the impact of the illness on family relationships. The child can also be asked to comment on the feelings of the individuals represented in the artwork.

Feelings Pie Project

In the feelings pie exercise, the consultant draws a large circle representing a pie and divides the circle into sections of different sizes. The consultant then designates specific feelings for each section of the circle and labels each section (Figure 3–1). The consultant gives examples of things that make him or her have the feeling represented in each section. After completing this part of the exercise, the consultant asks the child to draw a similar circle and pick a number of feelings that they can discuss together. The size of each section may designate the relative importance of each feeling. If this exercise is too threatening, the child may be asked to comment on the feelings labeled in the consultant's pie rather than on his or her own feelings. In another variation of this exercise, the consultant tells the child that the pie is about to have an operation or procedure and that the consultant and child are going to come up with some of the feelings that the pie might have.

Feelings Mandala Project

For the feelings mandala exercise, the consultant draws a large circle on a piece of paper. He or she then chooses four or five feelings—maybe happy, sad, angry, worried, and excited—and matches each of the feelings with a crayon or different colored pattern. The consultant then colors or draws in the circle to designate each feeling (Figure 3–2). The consultant next asks the child to create a similar mandala and comment on the drawing after its completion and may also ask the child to talk about the absence of relevant or expected feelings.

Mood Scales

With mood scales, the child is asked to rate his or her feelings on a scale from 1 to 10 after the consultant has specified the feelings that are to be rated. This may be done verbally, as part of an interview, or by using a visual scale similar to that used to rate pain (Figure 3–3). The exercise may be modified using certain prompts, such as "This is the way I feel on my birthday" or "When I come into the hospital, this is how I feel." Feelings may need to be modified based on the child's age.

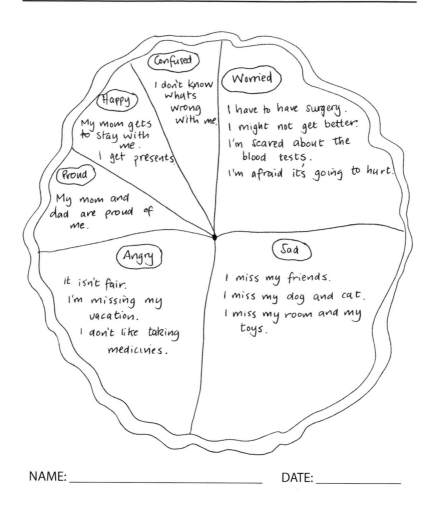

Figure 3–1.   Feelings pie.

Feelings Words Exercise

In the feelings words exercise, the consultant and child write a number of different feelings on small pieces of paper. These pieces of paper are placed in a "feelings box" or container, which can be created as an art project as part of the exercise. The consultant and child then take turns taking out pieces of paper

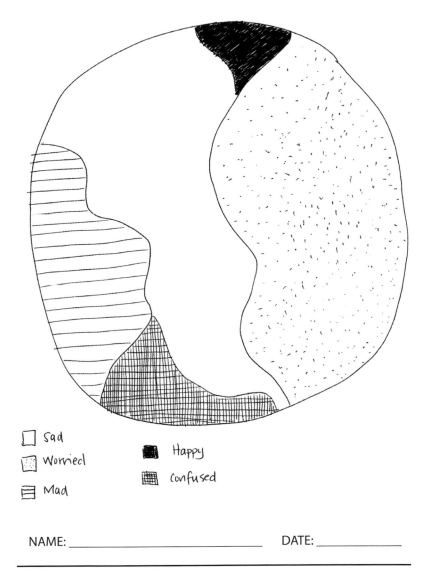

Figure 3–2.   Feelings mandala.

NAME: _____ DATE: _____									
These are my feelings when _____									
	Not at all									Most ever
Happy	1	2	3	4	5	6	7	8	9	10
Sad	1	2	3	4	5	6	7	8	9	10
Angry	1	2	3	4	5	6	7	8	9	10
Excited	1	2	3	4	5	6	7	8	9	10
Worried	1	2	3	4	5	6	7	8	9	10
Scared	1	2	3	4	5	6	7	8	9	10
Disappointed	1	2	3	4	5	6	7	8	9	10

Figure 3–3.   Mood scale.

and discussing the feeling that has been chosen. There are many variations in how questions may be asked. For example, the prompt can be, "I feel… (happy, sad, excited) whenever…" or "Whenever I feel…, I like to…." The consultant may need to model responses to the questions, depending on the child's age and ability.

Road Map of Life

For the road map of life technique, the consultant models how to draw a "road map" of his or her life (Figure 3–4). The map starts with birth and progresses through various stages of life, which are illustrated with pictures. When drawing his or her own road map, the child should be prompted to include the onset of his or her illness or injury. In a variation of this exercise, the child can be asked to draw a future road map that designates the important obstacles that have to be overcome for the child to get through a particular problem or difficulty.

Complete-a-Sentence Exercise

In the complete-a-sentence exercise, the consultant and child take turns completing sentences that start with simple, nonthreatening prompts, such as those listed in Figure 3–5. The consultant can then modify the task depending on the child's ability to engage in the discussion. It is also possible to introduce medical prompts toward the end of the exercise. To initiate this exercise, the consultant may want to introduce some humorous sentence completions.

Consider Standardized Assessment Instruments

The American Academy of Child and Adolescent Psychiatry's Practice Parameter for the Psychiatric Assessment and Management of Physically Ill Children and Adolescents provides standardized principles, outlined in Table 3–2, to guide consultants in the assessment and management of youth with physical illnesses (DeMaso et al. 2009). Consultants should use their patient and parent interviews and the medical chart review, supplemented by information from other sources when available, to generate a comprehensive biopsychosocial history that includes the chief complaint, history of presenting illness, current and past medications, and psychosocial stressors, as well as medical, psychiatric, developmental, social, and substance abuse histories. A full mental status examination should be completed whenever possible, though there may be times when a comprehensive and detailed examination is not possible. Serial mental status examinations may be indicated in consult requests such as for delirium.

In both the child and parent interviews, it is helpful for consultants to explore the following interrelated domains: illness factors, illness understanding, emotional impact on child, family functioning, impact on healthy siblings, social relationships, academic functioning, coping mechanisms, religion and spirituality, and the family's relationship with the medical team (Table 3–3). A list of questions that can help in gaining understanding into views and perceptions of physically ill children and adolescents regarding their medical conditions is provided in the appendix to this chapter.

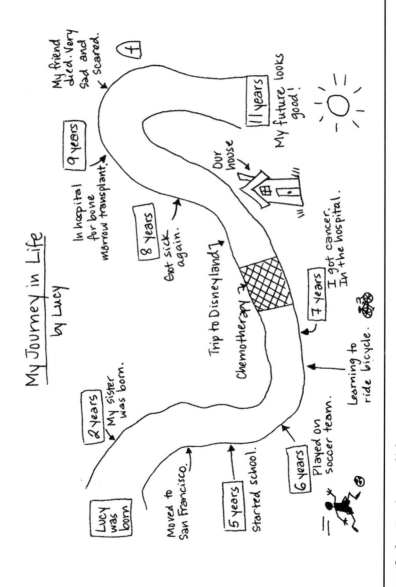

Figure 3–4.   Road map of life.

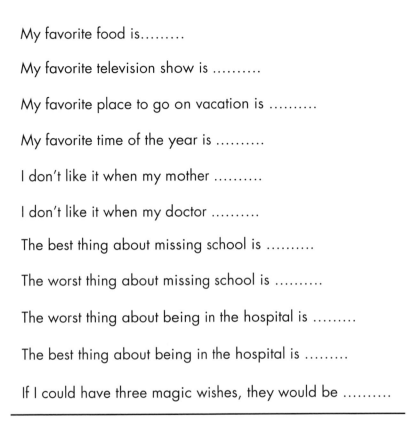

My favorite food is.........

My favorite television show is ....

My favorite place to go on vacation is ....

My favorite time of the year is ....

I don't like it when my mother ....

I don't like it when my doctor ....

The best thing about missing school is ....

The worst thing about missing school is ....

The worst thing about being in the hospital is ....

The best thing about being in the hospital is ....

If I could have three magic wishes, they would be ....

Figure 3–5.   Complete-a-sentence exercise.

Illness Factors

The impact of physical illness on children will vary depending on the stage of the illness. Reactions of a child receiving a new diagnosis of a life-threatening illness will differ from those of a patient who has been struggling with a chronic illness for many years or those of a child who has just relapsed after a period of remission. Also significant is the nature of the illness, in terms of whether it is a chronic progressive illness, an illness with the potential for normal functioning and recovery between episodes, or one with a terminal prognosis. It is important to collect information regarding the treatment history, including the frequency of hospitalizations, difficulties related to the treatment regimen, and experiences with traumatic and painful procedures.

Table 3–2.   American Academy of Child and Adolescent
Psychiatry principles for the psychiatric assessment
and management of physically ill children and
adolescents

1. Mental health clinicians should understand how to collaborate effectively with medical professionals to facilitate the health care of physically ill children.

2. The reason for and purpose of the mental health referral should be understood.

3. The assessment should integrate the impact of the child's physical illness into a developmentally informed biopsychosocial formulation.

4. General medical conditions and/or their treatments should be considered in the etiology of a child's psychological and behavioral symptoms.

5. Psychopharmacological management should consider a child's physical illness and its treatment.

6. Psychotherapeutic management should consider multiple treatment modalities.

7. The family context should be understood and addressed.

8. Adherence to the medical treatment regimen should be evaluated and optimized.

9. The use of complementary and alternative medicine should be explored.

10. Religious and cultural influences should be understood and considered.

11. Family contact with community-based agencies should be considered and facilitated where indicated.

12. Legal issues specific to physically ill children should be understood and considered.

13. The influence of the health care system on the care of a physically ill child should be considered.

Source.   Reprinted from DeMaso DR, Martini DR, Cahen LA; Work Group on Quality Issues: "Practice Parameter for the Psychiatric Assessment and Management of Physically Ill Children and Adolescents." *Journal of the American Academy of Child and Adolescent Psychiatry* 48(2):213–233, 2009. Copyright © 2009, American Academy of Child and Adolescent Psychiatry, with permission from Elsevier.

Table 3–3.   Protocol for the psychiatric assessment of the physically ill child or adolescent

What are the illness factors?

1. Stage of illness

    • New diagnosis of illness

    • Relapse following a period of recovery

    • Chronic phase of illness

2. Course of illness

    • Relapsing (e.g., cancer)

    • Single event with incomplete recovery (e.g., stroke, head trauma)

    • Inter-interval recovery with normal functioning between episodes (e.g., sickle cell disease)

    • Chronic deteriorating course (e.g., cystic fibrosis)

3. Prognosis

    • Preservation of functioning with adequate treatment (e.g., diabetes, organ transplant)

    • Decline in functioning over time (e.g., rheumatoid arthritis)

    • Terminal illness (e.g., cystic fibrosis)

4. Treatment history

    • Number of hospitalizations

    • Frequency of outpatient appointments

    • Treatment regimen

    • Medication side effects (e.g., cosmetic, cognitive, energy, nausea)

    • Difficulties with treatment adherence

    • History of traumatic procedures

    • Presence of pain

What is the understanding of the illness by the child and parent?

1. How was the illness explained to the child (e.g., full vs. partial explanation)?

2. Is there a realistic comprehension of the illness and its prognosis?

Table 3–3.   Protocol for the psychiatric assessment of the physically ill child or adolescent *(continued)*

What is the understanding of the illness by the child and parent? *(continued)*

3.   Is there an adequate understanding of the treatment?

4.   Are there cognitive factors affecting the comprehension of the illness and its treatment?

5.   Are there cultural issues affecting the assimilation of medical information?

What is the emotional impact of the illness on the child?

1.   How was the child's emotional functioning before the diagnosis of the illness?

2.   What are the child's current emotional reactions to the illness?

- Depression (e.g., understandable reaction vs. futility and hopelessness)

- Anxiety (e.g., fear of recurrence, posttraumatic stress disorder symptoms)

- Impact on self-esteem (e.g., body image, medication side effects, restriction on functioning)

- Anger (e.g., acting out, regressed behavior)

3.   What is the child's current degree of acceptance of the illness?

- Denial

- Acceptance and integration

What is the impact of the illness on family functioning?

1.   Family functioning

- What was the nature of the family functioning prior to the illness?

- What has been the impact of the illness on home life (e.g., demands of treatment, decreased time for recreational activities, lack of availability of parent, increased dependency of ill child, increased levels of family conflict)?

2.   Marital relationship

- Has the illness resulted in decreased time for the marital relationship?

- Have there been increased levels of conflict related to the illness (e.g., division of labor, disagreement regarding treatment, blaming of spouse)?

- What has been the impact of the illness on the quality of the marital relationship (e.g., estrangement vs. increased feelings of closeness)?

Table 3–3. Protocol for the psychiatric assessment of the physically ill child or adolescent *(continued)*

What is the impact of the illness on family functioning? *(continued)*

3. Occupational functioning

    •   Has there been a need to miss work for appointments, hospitalizations, or supervision of the treatment?

    •   Have parents had difficulties functioning at work due to emotional factors?

    •   Is there a need for one of the parents to work to maintain health insurance?

4. Financial issues

    •   What has been the financial burden of the treatment (e.g., lost income, transportation, increased need for child care, need for special home accommodations, medical expenses)?

What is the impact of the illness on the healthy siblings?

1. What has been the impact of the illness on the healthy siblings?

    •   Has there been decreased availability of parents (e.g., absence at important events and functions)?

    •   Has there been an inequitable distribution of parental and financial resources?

2. What have been the emotional reactions of the healthy siblings?

    •   Anger and resentment

    •   Anxiety about the health of affected sibling

    •   Embarrassment regarding affected sibling (e.g., physical appearance, stigma of illness)

What is the impact of the illness on social and peer relationships?

1. What has been the impact of the illness on peer relationships?

    •   Stigma of illness (e.g., teasing, exclusion from social group)

    •   Increased closeness with specific peers

2. Has there been a decreased ability for social and recreational activities?

3. What has been the impact of the illness on dating and sexuality?

    •   Insecurity about physical appearance

    •   Delays in growth and puberty

Table 3–3.   Protocol for the psychiatric assessment of the physically ill child or adolescent *(continued)*

What is the impact of the illness on academic functioning?

1.   What was the level of academic functioning prior to the illness?

2.   What has been the impact of the illness on academic functioning?

   •   Missed school days due to illness

   •   Academic difficulties due to illness or treatment

   •   Necessity for homeschooling

3.   Have there been difficulties with school reintegration?

4.   Are there appropriate educational resources, including special education services?

What are the child's habitual coping mechanisms?

1.   Turning to support from family members and friends

2.   Religious or spiritual resources

3.   Social withdrawal and isolation

4.   Denial and avoidance

5.   Maladaptive coping patterns (e.g., alcohol or substance abuse)

What is the role of religion and spirituality?

1.   What is the family's religious affiliation?

2.   What are the family's religious beliefs regarding illness and death?

3.   What is the role of religion and spirituality as a source of support for the family?

What is the relationship of the family with the medical team?

1.   Is the family able to trust members of the medical team?

2.   What is the quality of communication with the medical team?

3.   What is the family's desire for involvement in medical decision making?

Understanding of Illness

Both children and parents should be assessed regarding their understanding of the illness, including its prognosis and treatment. It is helpful to know how fully an illness was explained to the child at the time of diagnosis and whether the child has received age-appropriate explanations at his or her level of cognitive development. If there are cognitive issues that may affect the ability of a child or parents to understand the illness, the consultant should note these. Also, there may be cultural and religious factors that influence the way the family interprets and understands physical illness.

Emotional Impact

The assessment of emotional impact starts with an account of the patient's level of emotional functioning prior to the illness. This is followed by a review of the patient's reaction to the illness at the time of diagnosis and current psychological status. Symptoms of depression and anxiety may be appropriate reactions to the diagnosis of an illness or reflect a more serious underlying mood disorder (see Chapter 7, "Depressive Symptoms and Disorders," and Chapter 8, "Anxiety Symptoms and Trauma/Stress Reactions"). Self-esteem can be adversely affected because of limitations in the child's level of functioning and/or can be related to factors such as cosmetic side effects of medications and body image. Illness can interfere with important developmental milestones, including driving, dating, and leaving home. Adolescents are particularly prone to feelings of anger and resentment about their illness and its impact on their lives and may act out in several ways, including nonadherence with treatment (see Chapter 14, "Treatment Adherence").

Family Functioning

Pediatric illness may have a significant effect on family functioning. Demands of treatment may interfere with the normal family routine that had been established prior to the illness and may result in decreased time available for other activities. The illness may change the dynamics in the family. In addition to the logistical demands of treatment, previously healthy children may become more physically and emotionally dependent on their parents. The parents' marital relationship may be affected. An illness may result in there being less time for marital intimacy, and there is the potential for conflict related to such issues as how to divide labor related to the illness and how to manage the affected child.

Illness may have a significant effect on the parents' occupations. Parents may have to take additional time off work or put career aspirations on hold. Conversely, there may be pressure on one parent to maintain employment to continue necessary health insurance. Finally, there are often considerable financial implications, not only in terms of lost income if one parent has to miss work, but also because of the costs of additional child care and medical expenses.

It is common for consultants to receive requests to evaluate parents of physically ill children (Shaw et al. 2006). In these situations, it may be helpful to meet individually with the parent in question to conduct a more formal psychiatric assessment. In other situations, it may be more productive to conduct the assessment in the form of a family assessment. Parental reactions run the gamut from normative reactions of anxiety, anger, and depression to the more problematic symptoms of anxiety disorders and posttraumatic stress disorder (see Chapter 8, "Anxiety Symptoms and Trauma/Stress Reactions"). Specific instruments have been developed to assess parental stress in the hospital setting; for example, the Parental Stressor Scale is for use with parents who have children or infants hospitalized in pediatric or neonatal intensive care units (Carter and Miles 1989; Miles et al. 1993).

Siblings

Although often overlooked, siblings commonly experience symptoms of anxiety about the affected sibling as well as feelings of sadness and loss. Siblings may feel resentment about the lack of availability of their parents, whose attention is focused on the ill child, as well as the disruption to their daily routine. Parents may need to miss important school and social events in the healthy siblings' lives, and there may be a diversion of financial and other resources from siblings. Siblings may have feelings of embarrassment about the stigma of the illness and be reluctant to have friends over to their home.

Social Relationships

Physical illness and/or its treatment can have a significant impact on children's peer relationships. The illness may interfere with a child's ability to participate in desired social functions and activities, leading to isolation from the child's peer group. A child may experience feelings of being stigmatized by the illness, being teased at school, and even being further excluded from the peer group.

By contrast, and not infrequently, there may be a deepening of some close personal relationships as well as a reappraisal of other relationships. Adolescents face additional issues related to sexuality and dating. A number of illnesses, for example, result in delays in growth or delays in the onset of puberty, which can set patients further apart from their peers.

Academic Functioning

Physical illness may result in missed periods of schooling, which may result in difficulty keeping abreast of the academic work. In addition, many illnesses and their treatments have an adverse impact on cognitive functioning, resulting in lower academic performance (Bean Jaworski et al. 2018). There may need to be consideration as to whether a child needs referral for academic and/or neuropsychological assessment. Other considerations might be a planned school reintegration after treatment or periods of homeschooling during specific phases of an illness. It is important to ensure that children have adequate support from the school district, including (where appropriate) an up-to-date educational program to address specific health and learning disabilities.

Coping Mechanisms

It is helpful to understand the characteristic or habitual coping mechanisms used by the child at times of stress, including those used after the diagnosis of a major illness (see Chapter 2, "Coping and Adaptation in Physically Ill Children"). Knowledge of these mechanisms may assist in formulating an effective treatment plan. Children who are helped by talking about their illness may benefit from a referral for psychotherapy. However, it is more common for children to have periods of denial, especially during periods of remission from their illness, when they are quite reluctant to engage in any discussion about potential future implications. It is important to know about potential maladaptive coping mechanisms, including alcohol and substance abuse and risk-taking behaviors.

Spirituality and Religion

An assessment of the family's religious and faith traditions may identify potential sources of support. There may also be specific religious factors that interfere with the treatment of the illness, such as when a family has strong religious or cultural beliefs that are at odds with the treatment recommendations being made by the medical team. Table 3–4 outlines a list of questions that may be relevant in the assessment of the child's religion and spirituality (Barnes et al. 2000; Moncher and Josephson 2004; Sexson 2004).

Relationship With the Medical Team

It is important for consultants to explore the feelings of the patient and family in relation to the pediatric team. Although it is more common to find collaborative working relationships between families and the pediatric teams, the identification of problematic working relationships is important given their potential to adversely impact a child's treatment (DeMaso and Bujoreanu 2013; see also Chapter 16, "Family Interventions").

Observe Behavior and Play

After the initial assessment, it can be helpful to collect additional data based on observations of the child and family members both informally and, for younger children, in the format of a structured play assessment.

Hospital Behavior

It is important to assess children's behavioral changes in different hospital contexts—for example, during visits or absences of family members or during participation in hospital-based activities with physical therapists or child life specialists. For example, in children with somatic symptom disorders, the consultant may observe changes in symptoms that reflect aspects of the children's relationships with their parents or pediatric team. For instance, after observing inadvertent reinforcement by family members or the pediatric team of a child's somatic behaviors and symptoms, the consultant might suggest potential treatment interventions.

Play Observation

For preverbal toddlers and many younger children, play is the primary instrument to assess the mental status. Consultants can make direct observations of children's interactions with their parents and discover, for example, issues involving parenting, feeding disorders, or disorders of attachment. Observation can be used to assess the developmental stage of the child's play and whether it is chronologically age appropriate (King and American Academy of Child and Adolescent Psychiatry 1997). Consultants can invite the parents to interact with their child as they usually would at home for approximately 15–20 min-

Table 3–4. Questions related to religious and spiritual assessment

1. Is the family affiliated with a specific faith background?

2. What is the level of activity within the family's religious community?

3. To what extent does the family receive support from their religious community?

4. What are the particular religious rituals that are important to the family?

5. To what degree is the child involved in these religious activities?

6. What is the family's approach to religious or spiritual questions that arise in the context of a serious medical illness?

   • How does the family understand life's purpose and meaning?

   • How does the family explain illness and suffering?

   • What are the family's beliefs regarding the afterlife?

   • How do religious beliefs intersect with feelings of fairness and blame?

   • How does the family view the person in the context of body, mind, soul, and spirit?

Source. Adapted from Barnes et al. 2000; Moncher and Josephson 2004; Sexson 2004.

utes. Unstructured parent-child or family play provides the best opportunity for observation of the interaction. The role of the consultant during the family play session should be clearly explained to the family, including the degree to which the consultant will be involved in the interaction. It is important to observe a parent's ability to attend to and read the child's cues as well as the child's response to separation from the parent. Observations should also be made regarding the child's ability to engage in symbolic and age-appropriate play and the child's reactions to the ending of the session.

Specific issues observed during play include the parents' level of affection expressed toward the child, their willingness and ability to engage the child both verbally and nonverbally, their level of attunement, and their ability to both regulate the child's emotional responses and set appropriate limits. Consultants should assess the child's capacity for and interest in interpersonal relatedness, the amount and extent of physical and eye contact, the degree to which the child engages in or initiates play with the parents, and the quality and quantity of verbal exchange. Observations should be made regarding the child's capacity for affective involvement with the parents, their capacity for imaginative play, and the thematic content of the play.

Develop a Diagnosis

A DSM-5 mental disorder is defined as "a syndrome characterized by clinically significant disturbance in an individual's cognition, emotion regulation, or behavior that reflects a dysfunction in the psychological, biological, or developmental processes underlying mental functioning" (American Psychiatric Association 2013, p. 20). In the assessment, consultants aim to acquire information regarding symptom frequency, onset, duration, distress, and functional impairment as well as characterization of previous symptom presentations and response to prior treatment. Consultants will often find themselves in clinical situations where they have inadequate information to make a disorder diagnosis and/or the patient does not appear to have all of the required diagnostic criteria for a disorder, yet consultants are faced with clinically significant symptoms. Under these circumstances, the "unspecified" diagnosis within a specific DSM-5 disorder category can be used at the clinical judgment of the consultant (American Psychiatric Association 2013).

Develop a Biopsychosocial Formulation

The biopsychosocial formulation is a summary of what the consultant "thinks is going on" from a model that makes meaning of the patient's current circumstances. In this model, biological, psychiatric, and social dimensions need to be evaluated both separately and in relation to each other (Richtsmeier and Aschkenasy 1988). The formulation prioritizes and integrates the information gained in the assessment into a concise summary that describes the patient's problems and places them in the context of his or her current life situation and developmental history. An effective formulation organizes the clinical material into a format that is pragmatic and understandable to the patient, family, and referring medical team.

Predisposing, precipitating, perpetuating, and protective factors (the 4 Ps) that influence the patient's overall functioning can be used to organize the formulation (Kline and Cameron 1978; Winters et al. 2007). *Predisposing factors* involve areas of vulnerability and generally encompass biological factors in the formulation. *Precipitating factors* are the stressors faced by the patient, such as the onset of a physical illness or its treatment, and each should be interpreted based on its specific meaning to the patient. These could encompass a variety of issues, including the loss of omnipotence regarding the child's physical health, concerns about abandonment and loss, or reenactments of past traumatic medical events. *Perpetuating factors* are any aspects of the patient, family, community, or medical environment that serve to perpetuate the problem. *Protective factors* include special strengths of the child and family and related factors.

This biopsychosocial formulation is carefully integrated with the diagnosis in such a manner that a comprehensive treatment plan logically emerges. The biopsychosocial approach has the advantage of being more accessible to the family and the pediatric team, who commonly approach the problem solely from a medical model understanding, which does not account for psychosocial contributors. The three components of the biopsychosocial model are described in the following subsections.

Biological Factors

Biological factors in the biopsychosocial formulation include the child's family and genetic history; inborn temperament; physical developmental stage, including height, weight, physical ability, age, and stage of maturity; and intelligence. Physical health and intrauterine drug exposure, as well as family psychiatric histories of anxiety, depression, substance use, and other disorders, are also relevant.

Psychological Factors

Psychological factors in the biopsychosocial formulation include the child and family's emotional development, personality styles, primary defenses and weaknesses, and history of emotional trauma. The child's developmental stage and relevant developmental issues should be highlighted. Noted psychological issues should include self-esteem, habitual ways of managing anger, reaction to loss, and functioning in the major areas of daily life (see Chapter 2, "Adaptation and Coping in Physically Ill Children").

Social Factors

Social factors in the biopsychosocial formulation include an assessment of the child's functioning within the larger social unit. Relevant factors include community, ethnic background, economic status, and spiritual and cultural traditions. It is important to comment on the presence of social isolation or support in the context of the family and to consider the concept of the child as the *identified patient*, or the individual who is expressing the conflicts of the family and bringing the family into treatment (see Chapter 16, "Family Interventions").

Communicate Findings and Recommendations to the Medical Team and Family

Referring Physician or Pediatric Team

The consultant should first communicate their biopsychosocial formulation and diagnoses to the referring physician or pediatric team. Generally, the consultant presents findings in a *direct conversation with the referring physician* or at a *pediatric team meeting* that is focused on gathering pediatric information used to make a diagnosis and formulate the treatment plan and that usually does not include the family. As noted in the previous subsection, the consultant formulates the referral problem within a biopsychosocial framework as opposed to the limited (and common) medical model framework in which psychosocial factors have been thought to have little or no role in a patient's clinical presentation. In so doing, the consultant should be attuned to the frustration that is commonly engendered in the pediatric team in caring for patients with emotional and behavior presentations that they find hard to understand or manage. Communication of the formulation generally goes a long way in lessening this frustration and increasing the empathy for the patient.

Patient and Family

Following the conveyance of the consultant's findings to the referring physician or pediatric team, a *family conference* is scheduled to provide medical and psychosocial information to the family in order to establish a consensus with the family about the treatment plan (Williams and DeMaso 2000). The family conference typically includes referring physician(s) and family as well as other important pediatric team members, such as the primary nurse. Consultants may or may not attend this meeting, depending on the comfort and expertise

Table 3–5. Consultation intervention recommendations based on the type of consultation requests in the pediatric hospital setting

Consultation request type	Potential intervention recommendations by consultant
Diagnostic	Continued psychiatric assessment
	Obtaining outside information; involving other medical or psychiatry medical providers
	Further medical assessment as indicated, including laboratory and/or radiographic tests
	Other subspecialty pediatric consultation
	Neuropsychological testing consultation
Management	Behavioral management strategies for medical team, including nurses
	Behavioral management strategies for parents
	Individual therapy, including support, cognitive-behavioral therapy, behavioral modification, relaxation, hypnosis
	Family interventions
	Psychopharmacology recommendations for target symptoms (anxiety, agitation, etc.)
	Social work to support family
	Child life specialist involvement to support patient
	Physical and/or occupational therapy referrals as part of rehabilitation intervention
	Chaplain involvement as indicated for family spiritual support
	Legal and/or child protection consultation, as indicated
	Transfer to intensive psychiatric services, such as inpatient/partial hospitalizations

Table 3–5. Consultation intervention recommendations based on the type of consultation requests in the pediatric hospital setting *(continued)*

Consultation request type	Potential intervention recommendations by consultant
Disposition	Referral to outpatient services; individual, family, and/or psychopharmacology services
	Educational assessment through patient's school district, as indicated
	Referral to child welfare services, as indicated
	Referral to social services, as indicated
	Coordination of follow-up treatment with patient's medical home

of the referring physician and pediatric team as well as the strength of the working relationship with the family. In a supportive and nonjudgmental manner, the referring physician should present the patient and family with both the pediatric and psychosocial findings. Even if the consultant is present, the referring physician should ideally lead the presentation, given the importance of reframing the clinical concerns from a medical model approach to a biopsychosocial one.

The importance of consultants conveying their clinical impressions and recommendations, communicating effectively, and providing helpful recommendations to families has been associated with high satisfaction with the consultations. In one study, nearly 90% of families reported that they would recommend a psychiatry consultation to a friend (Kitts et al. 2013). Generally, the family accepts the biopsychosocial formulation and diagnoses, and then the team can develop and implement effective psychiatric treatment recommendations that are responsive to the presenting problem(s) (Table 3–5).

Other Teams and Staff

In addition to the aforementioned *pediatric team* and *family conference meetings*, other types of team meetings commonly occur in the pediatric setting (Williams and DeMaso 2000). The *psychosocial team meeting* predominantly assesses psychosocial issues, such as treatment adherence or child abuse, and has the goal of reviewing psychosocial issues and formulating a treatment plan that addresses coping and emotional adjustment. The *staff-centered meeting* commonly addresses ethical issues that may arise in the context of the child's treatment. The role of consultants across these respective meeting formats involves giving advice to the pediatric team, advocating for the family, providing psychosocial support for team members, and educating the pediatric team about the developmental and mental health needs of the child.

Writing the Report

The consultant's assessment must be documented in the medical record (Garrick and Stotland 1982). While the consultation note serves to document the assessment for medical-legal and billing purposes, it also functions as an official document for clinician-to-clinician communication. Although the note contains treatment recommendations, it does not constitute an official order for the pediatric team. It is important always to leave a note after every contact with the patient or family, even if it is not possible to give a full, definitive report. Short notes that indicate that the consultation is in process are helpful to the pediatric team. It is important for consultants to remember that their notes are available to the patient and family for review. Also, the report should be clear and concise and should generally avoid including personal details that are inappropriate or not required by the pediatric team. The components of each written report are discussed below.

Title, date, and time.   Today's ubiquitous electronic medical records (EMRs) nearly always indicate the involvement of the psychiatry service/division/ department and the title or position of the individual consultant providing the service as well as the service provided (e.g., initial evaluation, individual psychotherapy, family therapy, team conference, discharge note), date, and time. The frequency of contact and the time of each session should also be recorded to facilitate billing and insurance issues. These items should be included in the written note should the EMR not include these items or if an EMR is unavailable.

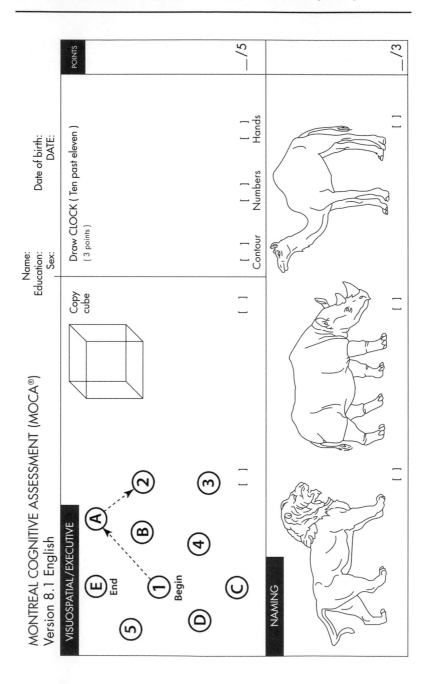

MEMORY		FACE	VELVET	CHURCH	DAISY	RED	
Read list of words; subject must repeat them. Do 2 trials, even if 1st trial is successful. Do a recall after 5 minutes.	1ST TRIAL						NO POINTS
	2ND TRIAL						

ATTENTION	Read list of digits (1 digit/sec.). Subject has to repeat them in the forward order. [ ] 2 1 8 5 4 Subject has to repeat them in the backward order. [ ] 7 4 2	__/2
	Read list of letters. The subject must tap with his hand at each letter A. No points if ≥ 2 errors [ ] F B A C M N A A J K L B A F A K D E A A A J A M O F A A B	__/1
	Serial 7 subtraction starting at 100. [ ] 93 [ ] 86 [ ] 79 [ ] 72 [ ] 65 4 or 5 correct subtractions: **3pts.**, 2 or 3 correct: **2 pts.**, 1 correct: **1pt.**, 0 correct: **0pt.**	__/3
LANGUAGE	Repeat: I only know that John is the one to help today. [ ] The cat always hid under the couch when dogs were in the room. [ ]	__/2
	Fluency / Name maximum number of words in one minute that begin with the letter F. [ ] ____ (N≥11 words)	__/1
ABSTRACTION	Similarity between e.g. banana–orange = fruit [ ] train–bicycle [ ] watch–ruler	__/2

DELAYED RECALL	(MIS)		FACE	VELVET	CHURCH	DAISY	RED		
Memory Index Score (MIS)	X3	Has to recall words WITH NO CUE	[ ]	[ ]	[ ]	[ ]	[ ]	Points for UNCUED recall only	__/5
	X2	Category cue						MIS = ____ /15	
	X1	Multiple choice cue							

ORIENTATION	[ ] Date [ ] Month [ ] Year [ ] Day [ ] Place [ ] City	__/6

© Z. Nasreddine MD www.mocatest.org MIS: /15

Administered by: ____________

(Normal ≥ 26/30) TOTAL __/30

Add 1 point if ≤ 12 yr edu

Training and Certification are required to ensure accuracy

Figure 3–6. Montreal Cognitive Assessment.

Source. Copyright © Z. Nasreddine, M.D. Used with permission. Copies are available at https://www.mocatest.org.

Reason for consultation.   The consultation note should include a brief summary of the original consultation request, in addition to any clarification or amplification obtained after further discussion with the pediatric team. Including a summary helps focus the perception of the patient's problems. The note's opening sentence should attempt to distill the information into a succinctly worded summary of the presenting condition as well as help clarify the reason(s) for the consultation. The sources of information for the report should be included so that the database used in the preparation of the report is known.

History of presenting illness.   Symptom onset, frequency and duration of symptoms, distress, and functional impairment should be concisely presented, without unnecessary duplication of history that is already available elsewhere in the medical record. The written history should include chronologically organized presentation of the medical, social, developmental, and interpersonal issues that have led to the consultation request. The history should also include a review of relevant stresses; academic, family, and social issues; habitual coping mechanisms; and previous psychiatric treatment, including psychopharmacology. Summary statements that do not include potentially sensitive information are useful for sections of the history in which issues of confidentiality are important.

Mental status examination.   The mental status examination should be comprehensive and include significant negative findings, particularly with regard to suicidality and other risk behaviors. The initial mental status examination provides a clinical baseline for comparison in subsequent serial evaluations, which can help in documenting changes in the patient's clinical course. It is important to delineate any specific tests that are carried out in the examination, such as the Montreal Cognitive Assessment (MoCA) questionnaire, which is used as a brief cognitive screening tool (Figure 3–6).

Biopsychosocial formulation and diagnoses.   As discussed previously, the written report should include a clearly worded biopsychosocial formulation that presents the biological, psychological, and social factors that are involved in the symptom presentation. Standardized psychiatric diagnoses should be included to facilitate communication with subsequent mental health care providers, to help determine the most effective treatment interventions, and to assist with patient billing. The formulation can be used to outline the differential diagnosis that is being considered as well as the steps that are needed before a definitive diagnosis can be made.

Treatment recommendations. Detailed, practical recommendations should be made, organized in terms of priority, and should indicate whether further evaluation is necessary prior to the implementation of specific recommendations, such as those for pharmacological interventions. There should be details of who will be responsible for specific interventions.

Electronic signature. Electronic signatures are commonplace in today's hospital setting, and reports must be signed in a timely manner. If there is a written report, consultants must make sure their signatures are clear and legible and provide a pager or telephone number so that the referring medical team can easily contact the consultant.

References

American Psychiatric Association: Diagnostic and Statistical Manual for Mental Disorders, 5th Edition. Arlington, VA, American Psychiatric Association, 2013

Barnes LL, Plotnikoff GA, Fox K, et al: Spirituality, religion, and pediatrics: intersecting worlds of healing. Pediatrics 106(4)(Suppl):899–908, 2000 11044142

Bean Jaworski JL, White MT, DeMaso DR, et al: Visuospatial processing in adolescents with critical congenital heart disease: organization, integration, and implications for academic achievement. Child Neuropsychol 24(4):451–468, 2018 28277152

Carter MC, Miles MS: The Parental Stressor Scale: Pediatric Intensive Care Unit. Matern Child Nurs J 18(3):187–198, 1989 2491508

DeMaso DR, Bujoreanu IS: Enhancing working relationships between parents and surgeons. Semin Pediatr Surg 22(3):139–143, 2013 23870207

DeMaso DR, Martini DR, Cahen LA, et al; Work Group on Quality Issues: Practice parameter for the psychiatric assessment and management of physically ill children and adolescents. J Am Acad Child Adolesc Psychiatry 48(2):213–233, 2009 20040826

Garrick TR, Stotland NL: How to write a psychiatric consultation. Am J Psychiatry 139(7):849–855, 1982 6979943

Hobday A, Ollier K: Creative Therapy With Children and Adolescents. Atascadero, CA, Impact Publishers, 1999

King RA; American Academy of Child and Adolescent Psychiatry: Practice parameters for the psychiatric assessment of children and adolescents. J Am Acad Child Adolesc Psychiatry 36(10)(Suppl):4S–20S, 1997 9606102

Kitts RL, Gallagher K, Ibeziako P, et al: Parent and young adult satisfaction with psychiatry consultation services in a children's hospital. Psychosomatics 54(6):575–584, 2013 23453126

Kline S, Cameron PM: I. Formulation. Can Psychiatr Assoc J 23(1):39–42, 1978 638931

Miles MS, Funk SG, Carlson J: Parental Stressor Scale: neonatal intensive care unit. Nurs Res 42(3):148–152, 1993 8506163

Moncher FJ, Josephson AM: Religious and spiritual aspects of family assessment. Child Adolesc Psychiatr Clin N Am 13(1):49–70, vi, 2004 14723300

Narrow WE, Clarke DE, Kuramoto SJ, et al: DSM-5 field trials in the United States and Canada, Part III: development and reliability testing of a cross-cutting symptom assessment for DSM-5. Am J Psychiatry 170(1):71–82, 2013 23111499

Richtsmeier AJ, Aschkenasy JR: Psychological consultation and psychosomatic diagnosis. Psychosomatics 29(3):338–341, 1988 3406351

Sexson SB: Religious and spiritual assessment of the child and adolescent. Child Adolesc Psychiatr Clin N Am 13(1):35–47, vi, 2004 14723299

Shaw RJ, Wamboldt M, Bursch B, et al: Practice patterns in pediatric consultation-liaison psychiatry: a national survey. Psychosomatics 47(1):43–49, 2006 16384806

Shaw RJ, Pao M, Holland JE, et al: Practice patterns revisited in pediatric psychosomatic medicine. Psychosomatics 57(6):576–585, 2016 27393387

Williams J, DeMaso DR: Pediatric team meetings: the mental health consultant's role. Clin Child Psychol Psychiatry 5:105–113, 2000

Winters NC, Hanson G, Stoyanova V: The case formulation in child and adolescent psychiatry. Child Adolesc Psychiatric Clin N Am 16:111–132, 2007 17141121

Wolraich ML, Felice ME, Drotar D (eds): The Classification of Child and Adolescent Mental Diagnoses in Primary Care: Child and Adolescent Version. Elk Grove Village, IL, American Academy of Pediatrics, 1996

Appendix: Questions to Consider Asking Children and Adolescents Facing a Physical Illness

The following questions are useful for consultants to consider in their assessment to gain understanding into views and perceptions of children and adolescents regarding their physical illnesses.

1. Description of Illness

- Tell me about your illness. When were you diagnosed?
- What is the name of your illness?
- What did the doctors tell you when you first became ill?
- How did you feel when you first found out you were ill?
- Do you know what is going to happen with your illness when you get older?
- What do you have to do to stay healthy in terms of your illness?
- Have you had to go to the hospital? How often?
- Have you had any surgeries?
- What has it been like when you have had to go into the hospital?
- What are the hardest things about being in the hospital?
- Do you have a hard time with blood tests or procedures?
- How many medications do you have to take every day?
- Is it hard to swallow the pills? Do any of them taste bad?
- How often do you forget your medications each week? Do you ever skip doses?
- Do you have to follow any special diet or restrict how much you drink each day?

2. Emotional Impact of Illness on Child

- Since getting sick, with the stress of having this illness, have you noticed yourself getting sad or down?
- Since getting sick, have you found yourself worrying more about things? Feeling nervous or anxious?
- A lot of kids who get sick feel frustrated about it or feel that it isn't fair. Have you noticed yourself getting frustrated or angry more easily?
- Has your illness changed the way you feel about yourself?
- Do you feel less confident?
- Do you worry about getting sick again? About your illness coming back?
- Have you found yourself worrying that you might die earlier than other kids your age?
- Have you told anyone about these worries?

3. Impact of Illness on Child's Social Relationships

- How did people at school react when they heard you were ill?
- Did you feel that your school supported you when you were in the hospital?
- Did any of your friends have a hard time when you got sick?
- Have some of your friends been avoiding you?
- Do you get left out of activities because of your illness?
- Are there things you used to do with friends that are more difficult since you got sick?
- Do you get teased about your illness?
- Do you feel embarrassed about people at school learning that you're ill?
- Do you try to cover up the fact that you have an illness? How come?

4. Impact of Illness on Education

- Do you have to miss a lot of school because of your illness? How often?
- Have these absences made it harder for you at school?
- Have you fallen behind at school?
- Have your grades been affected by your illness?
- Have you found it harder to concentrate or focus on your work since getting sick? Why do you think this is?

5. Impact of Illness on Family

- How has your illness affected your family?
- Are there things your family does not get to do anymore because of your being ill?
- Do you think your parents have had a hard time with your being ill?
- Do they worry about you?
- Do you think they have been more down or sad?
- Do you feel bad about all the things they have to do for your illness? Are there times when you feel guilty? How come?
- Do your parents argue about your illness?
- Do you feel that your parents support you enough?

- Do you think that your parents are overprotective or do not let you do things you think you should be able to do?
- Do you feel you have gotten closer to anyone in your family since getting sick?

6. Impact of Illness on Siblings (in Families With More Than One Child)

- Has your illness affected your siblings? How so?
- Do your siblings get less attention from your parents because of your illness?
- Do your siblings complain that you get more attention?
- Do your siblings worry about you?
- Do your siblings seem to be angrier since you have gotten sick? Sadder?

7. Relationship With the Medical Team

- Do you like your doctors?
- Do you trust your doctors?
- Do your doctors listen to your concerns?
- Have there been experiences with your doctors that have upset you? What happened?

8. Coping

- What has helped you get through this experience?
- Have you had support from your family? From your friends? From your religious community?

4

Legal and Forensic Issues

Psychiatry consultants face a number of challenging legal and forensic issues in the pediatric setting. It is critical that they have a solid understanding of these issues and that they are knowledgeable about the specific statutes in their particular jurisdictions because these rules have a significant impact on patients, pediatric teams, and even the consultants themselves. Consultants must be open to looking for legal assistance if they have questions. It is advisable that consultants establish an ongoing working relationship with the lawyer or legal service responsible for and/or knowledgeable about the pediatric setting in which they practice; together they can effectively advise and coach pediatric practitioners in their responses to the legal and forensic issues presented by patients and their families. This chapter offers a general orientation to treatment consent and confidentiality with children and adolescents and an overview regarding the role of consultants in the assessment of parental capacity and medical neglect in the pediatric setting.

Consent for Treatment

Consent is required for all pediatric medical treatments except in unusual circumstances. Any health care provider who provides treatment without proper consent would be open to a charge of battery and could be subject to a civil action for damages for performing a procedure or investigation without the consent of the individual(s) concerned (Sankaran and Macbeth 2010).

Informed consent requires that the patient or legal guardian (if the patient is a minor) receive information regarding 1) the nature of the illness or condition; 2) the proposed diagnostic steps and treatments along with the probability of their success; and 3) the potential risks, benefits, and uncertainties of the proposed treatment and alternative treatments, including the option of no treatment other than comfort measures (Committee on Bioethics 2016; Katz and Webb 2016). There should also be an assessment of the patient's and/or guardians' understanding and medical decision-making capacity, including assurance of time for questions by the patient and/or legal guardians. The consent must be voluntary; it must also be volitional and not reflect mere acquiescence to consequence (Committee on Bioethics 2016; Katz and Webb 2016). Physicians should obtain written consent, particularly for complicated treatments, even though statutes may not always require this.

Issues regarding consent are more complicated with children and adolescents because the doctrine of informed consent has only a limited direct application in pediatrics. Only those patients with legal entitlement and decisional capacity can give informed consent. If a patient does not meet these criteria, a parent or guardian must provide permission. Minors (in most states, under age 18 years) are generally considered to be incompetent to make decisions regarding their medical treatment. Instead, consent must be obtained from the parent or legal guardian, who historically has been assumed to act in the best interest of the child.

In relation to guardian decision making in pediatrics, several standards have emerged: 1) *best-interest standard*, where the guardian, using a holistic view of the patient's interest, aims to maximize benefits and minimize harms to the patient; 2) *harm principle*, where a harm threshold is identified below which parental decisions will not be tolerated; 3) *constrained parental autonomy*, where parents balance the best interest of the patient with the family's best interests; and 4) *shared, family-centered decision making*, which is a process that builds on collaborative mechanism between families and clinicians (Committee on Bioethics 2016).

There is increasing recognition that most adolescents have the capacity to participate in decisions about their health care, which is reflected in the greater willingness of parent and health care providers to include them in decision making (Ibeziako et al. 2010; Katz and Webb 2016). The American Academy of Pediatrics Committee on Bioethics (2016) has taken a developmental perspective toward informed consent and recognizes that as minors approach and progress through adolescence, they need a more independent relationship with their health care givers. Physicians should recognize that some pediatric patients, especially older adolescents and those with medical experience because of chronic illness, may possess adequate capacity, cognitive ability, and judgment to engage effectively in the informed consent or refusal process for the proposed goals of their care (Committee on Bioethics 2016).

At the same time, in approaching the adolescent as decision maker, consultants should keep in mind emerging neuropsychological research on maturation of the brain. The research to date indicates that, in general, adolescents make decisions differently than adults do, and although adolescents may have cognitive skills, they are more likely to underutilize these skills (Katz and Webb 2016). In the midst of a stressful health care environment, an adolescent may rely more on the mature limbic system (socioemotional) than on the less developed and impulse-controlling prefrontal cognitive system (Katz and Webb 2016).

Assent is a means of involving minors in treatment decisions. The commonly accepted definition of *assent*—a minor's agreement to participate—sets a lower standard of competence than informed consent because assent does not require the depth of understanding or the demonstration of reasoning ability required for informed consent. It is an interactive process between a minor and a health care provider that involves developmentally appropriate disclosure about the illness and solicitation of the minor's willingness and preferences regarding treatment (Committee on Bioethics 2016).

Consultants can serve an invaluable role in helping the pediatric team navigate the developmental issues involved in medical decision making. Assent is a means of empowering children and adolescents to their full abilities and may promote adherence to a treatment plan (Katz and Webb 2016).

Treatment Without Parental Consent: Exceptions

There are important exceptions to the rule requiring parental consent prior to treatment. These include emergency treatment, treatment of emancipated minors, treatment of mature minors, reproductive health (sexually transmitted disease; pregnancy prevention, treatment, and termination); sexual abuse; substance-related disorder treatment; and mental health treatment.

Emergency Treatment

Consent is generally not required when the child needs emergency treatment, but consultants (when involved) should make every attempt to contact and inform the parent or legal guardian and should document such efforts in the patient's medical record. This exception is based on the assumption that the parent or legal guardian would agree to allow emergency treatment if there were sufficient time to obtain consent. Courts are especially willing to allow this exception if delay in treatment caused by efforts to obtain legal consent would endanger the child's health. Physicians are also generally permitted to carry out diagnostic tests, including skeletal X-rays, to diagnose child abuse or neglect without parental consent. Consultants must be aware of the statutes and their legal implications in the jurisdictions in which they practice.

Treatment of a patient who is acutely agitated or having a panic attack may not be considered an emergency unless there is an associated threat of harm to self or others (Ibeziako et al. 2010). Administering an antipsychotic medication or benzodiazepine to an acutely agitated patient in the emergency department or on medical floors would generally be considered a medical necessity because there is a significant risk of harm to self or others if untreated. In a patient with an eating disorder and acute food refusal, administering intravenous fluids for dehydration might be considered emergent (depending on the clinical findings and duration of food refusal), whereas placement of a nasogastric tube as part of an eating disorder protocol would not. Table 4–1 outlines considerations in the assessment of children and adolescents for emergency medication treatment.

Treatment of Emancipated Minors

Emancipated minors have the authority to make their own decisions regarding treatment, and parental consent is not required to treat these patients. Youth become emancipated minors through marriage, military service, parenthood, or by demonstrating their ability to financially manage their own affairs. Homeless minors, defined as children under age 18 years who are living apart from their parents in a supervised shelter or temporary accommodation, also have

Table 4–1. Considerations in assessment of children and adolescents for emergency medication treatment

1. Benefits of treatment and risks of withholding treatment.

2. Benefits and potential risks of proposed medication.

3. Route of medication administration: Is oral administration possible? If not, is alternative route already in place (e.g., intravenous access or gastric tube), or would medication have to be administered rectally or intramuscularly and potentially be more traumatic?

4. Necessity of physical restraint to administer medication

5. Patient age: A mature minor may be able to consent to treatment. Efforts should be made to document that physician has communicated with patient before giving medication. The younger the child, the less input he or she would have regarding treatment.

6. Level of anxiety: Mild panic attack episodes characterized by hyperventilation and tremors may not require any immediate intervention, whereas severe attacks associated with acute agitation (e.g., pulling out intravenous or nasogastric tubes or removal of oxygen mask) would constitute a higher level of urgency.

7. Level of agitation: Mild episodes characterized by restlessness may not require immediate intervention, whereas severe agitation associated with significant threat of harm to self of others would constitute a higher level of urgency.

Source. Adapted from Ibeziako P, Bourne R, Shaw RJ, et al: "Legal and Forensic Issues," in *Textbook of Pediatric Psychosomatic Medicine.* Edited by Shaw RJ, DeMaso DM. Washington, DC, American Psychiatric Publishing, 2010, p. 49. Copyright © 2010, American Psychiatric Publishing, Inc. Used with permission.

authority to give consent. Although financial independence is an important issue, an adolescent may be an emancipated minor even if he or she is still obtaining financial support from his or her parents, provided the minor is independently managing his or her own financial affairs. Youth under age 18 may also receive a declaration of emancipation through the courts.

Treatment of Mature Minors

Older children who do not meet the criteria for being emancipated minors may still have authority to give consent for treatment in limited situations. One such situation is when the child is capable of appreciating the nature, extent, and consequences of the pediatric treatment. This exception is designed to cover situations in which the parents are not available to give consent for low-risk treatments. This exception requires an assessment by the pediatric team of the child's maturity and judgment and the nature of the treatment in question. For example, treatments that involve psychiatric medications may be of higher risk than treatments with psychotherapy. It is important to document the rationale used to justify the belief that the child is competent to give his or her own consent.

Reproductive Health

Sexually Transmitted Diseases

Under the statutes of some jurisdictions, parental consent is not required for treatment of sexually transmitted diseases in minors. Similarly, minors may be able to give consent for HIV testing without notification of their parents or legal guardians.

Pregnancy Prevention, Treatment, and Termination

Minors can generally consent to medical care related to the prevention (contraceptives) or treatment of pregnancy, including prenatal care, but not sterilization. Children of any age are usually entitled to free contraception services without parental consent. Obviously, the age of the patient and his or her partner and the nature of the activity and relationship may trigger other clinical and legal obligations. Consent issues regarding abortion are complex, with individual jurisdictions having different laws governing the authorization for an abortion without parental consent (Ibeziako et al. 2010). Emancipated (married, widowed, or divorced) minors may generally consent to an abortion. In some states an unmarried minor younger than 18 years cannot have an abortion unless the physician first gets written consent of the pregnant woman and of her parents or legal guardian or a court order authorizing the procedure. If the minor does not want to tell her parent or guardian that she is pregnant or if the parent or legal guardian does not consent to an abortion, the minor can apply to a court to ask permission for an abortion. Parents cannot provide consent for an abortion if the minor does not want to go through with the procedure.

Sexual Abuse

Victims of sexual assault can be evaluated and treated without parental consent, but local statutes may require the physician to inform the parent or legal guardian unless it is believed that the parent or legal guardian committed the assault. The younger the minor, the more caution clinicians should exercise before making a choice not to notify the parent of a child who has been sexually molested (Ibeziako et al. 2010).

Substance-Related Disorder Treatment

Many jurisdictions allow emergency treatment of intoxicated minors or minors at risk of complications from withdrawal from alcohol or substances without parental consent. Minors can often consent to medical care and counseling related to the diagnosis and treatment of alcohol and other substance abuse–related disorders. However, minors cannot receive replacement opioid abuse treatment without parental consent. Federally funded substance abuse treatment programs are bound by federal confidentiality laws that prohibit disclosure of any information to the parents unless the consultant believes that the minor's situation poses a substantial threat to the life or physical well-being of the minor or another person and that the threat may be reduced by communicating with the minor's parents or guardian.

Mental Health Treatment

In some jurisdictions, minors can give consent for mental health treatment or for residential shelter services if a doctor or clinician decides that they are mature enough to participate in these treatment services and that there is potential risk of physical or mental harm without the treatment. If a minor who is admitted to the emergency department or on a medical/surgical floor asks for a psychiatric consult but requests that his or her parents not be informed, the minor may be granted the consultation (Ibeziako et al. 2010).

In general, there is greater reluctance to override the request of a minor age 16 or 17 than to override such a request from a younger minor (Ibeziako et al. 2010). The threshold to obtain consent for a consultation should be different from that required for ongoing treatment. When performing the assessment, however, the consultant should try to understand the motivation behind the request not to have parents involved in the consult as well as the possible consequences. The treating therapist should try to open lines of communication between the child and the parents or to involve the parents in treatment unless the provider decides that such involvement is inappropriate.

In some states, a voluntary application for psychiatric hospitalization can be made by the parent or guardian of a child under age 18 years or by a child who is 16 years or older (Ibeziako et al. 2010). If a minor is unwilling to be hospitalized, a voluntary application for hospitalization can be made by parents without a court hearing. In some jurisdictions minors age 16 years or older can sign themselves out after 72 hours' written notice unless they are involuntarily committed. Two standards must be met for such a commitment to occur: the child must 1) be determined to be mentally ill and 2) be either a danger to self or to others or show an inability to care for self.

Limits of Parental Authority

In certain situations, such as those involving intellectual disability and minors in state custody, parents or legal guardians have limited authority.

Intellectual Disability

In many states, parents of a patient with an intellectual disability who has reached the age of majority do not automatically become the legal guardians and therefore have no legal authority to consent to their child's treatment until they have been appointed guardians by the court (Ibeziako et al. 2010). This appointment depends on the degree of intellectual disability because an adult with a mild disability may not need a guardian. Even after being appointed, parents or legal guardians cannot provide consent for psychiatric hospitalization and/or treatment with antipsychotic medications without a court order. Parents or legal guardians of a minor with an intellectual disability in need of psychiatric admission can provide consent for hospitalization. A patient over age 16 years with mild intellectual disability who has the capacity to consent to psychiatric admission and treatment may do so even if parents or legal guardians object. If the patient refuses the admission and is thought to be in need of such after evaluation by a clinician, then a court order must be obtained.

Minors in State Custody

When a minor is in state custody, the consultant should clarify whether it is a voluntary custody arrangement or whether the state obtained legal guardianship by judicial order (Ibeziako et al. 2010). In the former situation, parents still retain legal rights and can authorize most treatments, including psychiatric hospitalization and administration of antipsychotic medications. In the latter situation, the state will need to obtain a further court order to authorize such psychiatric treatment as well as to give or withhold life-prolonging treatment.

Refusal of Treatment by an Adolescent

Situations can arise in which a child wishes to refuse a treatment that the parent or legal guardian has requested. In most cases, depending on age and maturity, courts do not allow a child to refuse medical treatment if the treatment is necessary to save the child's life or preserve the child's health (Katz and Webb 2016). Some jurisdictions have similar stipulations regarding substance-related disorder treatment. These issues may be pertinent when a child has religious beliefs that influence his or her opinions about medical treatment or when a child with an eating disorder wants to refuse food and yet is at acute medical risk. As always, consultants must be aware of the relevant statutes in their jurisdiction.

Consent for Children of Divorced or Separated Parents

Consultants should be aware that one of a child's parents may not have the legal right to make decisions regarding the child's treatment. Health care providers are not obligated to raise this question unless there are reasonable grounds that suggest that a parent may not have legal custody. If the physician becomes aware of questions regarding legal guardianship or if parents with equal legal rights differ on treatment options, he or she must take immediate steps to clarify the custody situation, including obtaining a copy of the custody decree. It may then be necessary to get legal informed consent from the authorized parent or for the parents to return to court for judicial clarification.

In general, communication with both parents is recommended when there is a disagreement between parents with joint legal custody even if the parent who has physical custody brought the child for treatment (Ibeziako et al. 2010). After becoming aware that parents with equal legal authority disagree, the consultant should attempt direct communication with the opposing parent to better understand his or her position. If disagreement continues, the consultant can consider two alternatives: advising the consenting parent to consult with an attorney to attempt resolution of differences either informally or formally (through a court) or, if medication is immediately necessary and the benefits exceed risks, obtaining authorization for treatment from the consenting parent and notifying the opposing parent that these steps are being taken based on the belief that medications are imminently necessary and appropriate (Ibeziako et al. 2010). Attempts should be made to continue a dialogue with the opposing parent and welcome his or her involvement, but treatment may be initiated with the focus on the child's "best interest."

Payment for Treatment

There are complications regarding payment for treatment for minors who can legally give their own consent for treatment. In emergency situations the health care providers may look to the parent or legal guardian for payment, but in situations in which the purpose of allowing the minor to give consent is to protect confidentiality, the physician must look to the minor for payment. However, most jurisdictions do not allow health care providers to demand payment from the minor until he or she turns age 18, and minors cannot be held liable for payment until they do so. Minors who do not have the financial means to pay for health care services may be eligible for free or low-cost programs that reimburse confidential health services provided to the young. Providers may have to be enrolled in these programs to be reimbursed.

Confidentiality and Privilege

Privilege is a legal term used to describe the protection afforded certain types of relationships (e.g., physician-patient, therapist-client) during legal and administrative proceedings. Information revealed to a mental health clinician in the course of treatment is regarded as privileged, which means that no one else is generally entitled to see the information shared between clinician and patient. *Confidentiality* rules are broader and govern the disclosure of personal information to anyone not involved in the patient's care. Physicians and health care providers are legally and ethically mandated to protect the confidentiality of information they obtain through their clinical work.

Confidentiality

Elements of confidentiality that are taken for granted in work with adult patients are more complicated in work with children. A child's parents or legal guardians are entitled to access some personal information to help them make treatment decisions, but the child has some independent rights to confidentiality that must be considered. Many jurisdictions have statutes that govern the handling and protection of medical information and records. Violations of these rules place the treating clinician and institution at risk of lawsuits or fines. Parents or legal guardians who authorize treatment are generally also authorized to waive confidentiality and to give permission for release of information.

In the pediatric setting, issues are further complicated by the fact that a consultant has a professional relationship with the pediatric team and is expected to share information and opinions with other individuals involved in the patient's care. This relationship should be explicitly defined so that there is a clear understanding of how information obtained in the psychiatric consultation will be used, including potential limits on confidentiality in the hospital setting. The team relationship does not exempt the consultant from protecting confidential information that does not need to be disclosed and that is not immediately relevant to the patient's medical care.

Release of Information

Parent access.   Parents often expect full access to information regarding their child's treatment. This expectation is usually met with regard to pediatric treatment except in cases where there is investigation of possible child abuse. Information obtained by consultants may be of a delicate nature, and disclosure to parents may complicate the relationship between the child and the consultant and potentially jeopardize the child's treatment. Consultants should discuss these issues with both the child and the parents prior to any intervention and stipulate which types of information may be released and which will be protected. This type of conversation can clarify expectations and inform all parties about the terms of the treatment.

Adolescents have greater authority regarding the release of information, particularly regarding issues of their sexual behavior and substance abuse. Many jurisdictions link the ability to consent to treatment with the authority to release information, so that the adolescent who is competent to consent to treatment has the right to protect information that emerges in treatment. Other jurisdictions require the consent of both the parent and the adolescent to disclose confidential information once the adolescent has reached a certain age. If the adolescent cannot consent to treatment, it is important to discuss the disclosure rules with both the patient and the parents.

Issues can arise when a patient's parents are divorced or separated. Generally, the parent with legal custody retains the legal rights regarding access to information and authority to disclose this information. However, many jurisdictions have granted similar rights to the noncustodial parent. In situations in which the noncustodial parent has visitation rights, it is important that the physician provide this parent with any information regarding the treatment necessary to ensure the child's safety. The physician may have to obtain consent for the release of this information from the parent who has legal custody.

Consultants are bound by legal and ethical codes. Consultants who fail to disclose information that would allow the parents to protect the child may be held liable if the child is harmed. Some jurisdictions require disclosure if the child's safety is at risk. Consultants should always attempt to work therapeutically to encourage the child to disclose relevant information to his or her parents.

Third-party access.   Authority for release of information to schools, insurance companies, and researchers normally lies with the custodial parents, but each jurisdiction has its own statutes that may be relevant. Certain jurisdictions permit the disclosure of information for the purposes of continuity of care. Consultants should carefully monitor the information that is released to ensure that any disclosure does not harm the child.

Consultants must ensure that the consent form qualifies the extent of the information that may be released and that it complies with state statutes. Specific sections of the consent form may describe how the information can be used and may allow the consenting party to examine any disclosed information. Before information is released, consultants should establish that the patient and the parents have given fully informed consent by describing the nature of information that has been requested and specifying what information will be released. If the consultant believes that the patient or parents would not have consented to the release of information to third parties (e.g., schools or insurance companies) had they been aware of the nature of information involved, it may be necessary for the consultant to obtain a new consent from the family.

Exceptions to Confidentiality

Child abuse reporting. Consultants who identify or have reasonable cause to suspect child abuse are mandated to report this information to the appropriate child protection agencies. Each jurisdiction has a list of professionals (e.g., physicians, mental health practitioners) who must disclose child abuse. Child abuse reports from "mandated reporters" usually need to be made within 24–48 hours of learning about the abuse. All jurisdictions have statutes in place to provide immunity from civil liability for clinicians who are required to report concerns.

Before starting an assessment or treatment, consultants should inform patients and families that they have a mandate to report child abuse. Consultants must be familiar with the definition of abuse or neglect in their jurisdiction. Reporting obligations may vary based on who perpetrated the abuse. Although some jurisdictions require the report only if a parent, legal guardian, or person with caretaking authority perpetrated or tolerated the abuse, most states require reporting when there is any suspicion or reasonable belief of abuse or neglect. The reporting obligation can be limited to those health care providers who have had clinical interactions with the child. If abuse is suspected but a report is not made, the reasons for this decision must be documented. Because most jurisdictions have a sanction for not reporting and immunity for a false allegation, consultants should take the legally prudent action and report to protective services if in doubt about the mandate to do so.

Consultants may report consensual sexual activity if they learn that there is a significant age disparity between the two individuals concerned or if the minor is below the legal age of consent (Ibeziako et al. 2010). Each jurisdiction has specific laws regarding permissible age disparities, statutory rape, and circumstances that trigger a mandatory report to the child abuse authorities. Sexual activity by a minor may need to be reported if the consultant believes that the patient was coerced or intimidated into the activity, regardless of whether the minor describes the activity as consensual. In many states, a minor under age 16 cannot legally consent to sexual activity. Regardless of legal requirements, consultants must consider the nature and extent of harm to the patient and consider what interventions might potentially benefit his or her health and safety.

Health-related statutes. Jurisdictions may have reporting requirements that include notification regarding infectious diseases or disorders that could impair driving. These statutes may cover emotional disorders and substance abuse that can potentially impair motor skills. Some laws authorize or require health care providers to breach confidentiality to issue warnings about certain dangers posed by a patient. Physicians may be required to disclose information that suggests that a patient may endanger the life or safety of another person and can be held legally liable for failure to do so. Similarly, patients who disclose thoughts or plans regarding suicidality lose their right to confidentiality and may face civil commitment procedures.

Custody disputes.   When the parents of a patient separate or divorce during the child's treatment, one or both parents may request a consultant's assistance in the custody hearing as well as access to confidential or privileged information. Legal rules may prevent this testimony from being admitted in court, but even when such testimony is legally allowable, it is advisable for consultants to avoid allying with one of the parents because doing so could jeopardize the child's mental health treatment. Independent custody evaluations are preferable in these situations.

Privilege

Privilege Rules Between Physician or Psychotherapist and Patient

Privilege rules govern the disclosure of confidential information in judicial and administrative proceedings. Statutes protect certain types of relationships at the expense of full disclosure to encourage open communication in these relationships. One type of privilege exists between a physician or psychotherapist and a patient, including a child or adolescent patient. Federal regulations protect information disclosed in the course of psychotherapy based on the assumption that effective treatment would be impossible without patient confidence in a confidential discourse. In work with children and adolescents, some important issues of privilege may arise. Information disclosed in the presence of a third person such as a parent has traditionally not been regarded as privileged, but this rule is under review in many jurisdictions. Another issue is whether information that a physician receives from family members or other third parties about a child's treatment is protected by privilege. Consultants need to be aware of the specific rulings on these questions in their jurisdictions.

Exceptions to and Waiver of Privilege

There are several exceptions to the general rule of privilege that apply to commitment proceedings, will contests, and criminal matters. In work with minors, exceptions are also made regarding information about child abuse or neglect. In some jurisdictions, privilege can be lost in child custody cases, even if the child and parents object.

Physician-patient privileges may be waived at the discretion of the patient or the person authorized to act on the patient's behalf. In some court hearings, a guardian *ad litem* is appointed to decide whether an incompetent child would choose to waive privilege if he or she were competent to do so. Children and adolescents may decline to exercise their right to privilege, and in some jurisdictions, parents or legal guardians can waive privilege on behalf of their child. When parents are divorced or separated, the consultant must establish whether this authorization to waive privilege needs to be obtained from both parents. In custody disputes there is often disagreement between the parents about disclosure of confidential information. Privilege may also be waived when the patient has already testified about his or her treatment. The consultant should be particularly cautious about releasing information to lawyers or legal representatives unless he or she has a signed release from the patient or parents. This caution extends to subpoenaed requests for information.

Assessment for Parenting Capacity and Medical Neglect

Issues of parental competence arise in the pediatric setting, often with regard to the parents' ability to manage their child's treatment regimen. It is not uncommon for consultants to receive consultations asking for the assessment of parental neglect and abuse. Child protective service agencies can become involved during the inpatient admission and are ultimately responsible for decisions regarding placement, although consultants can be asked to give an opinion about parental capacity.

Parental Capacity

Effective parents support the cognitive development of their child by imparting knowledge and fostering the development of abilities such as language, self-care, academic functioning, and social skills. They promote positive and social behavior by providing adequate and consistent supervision and by setting developmentally appropriate limits on negative or antisocial behavior. It is important for parents to foster the emotional development of the child by providing support, guidance, and direction. Parents whose coping styles are characterized by anger, conflict, or criticism are likely to undermine their child's development, whereas overly protective parental behavior may result in insecurity and lack of confidence in the child.

Parents are expected to provide a safe and secure environment and protection from physical harm or exposure to emotional trauma, including domestic violence and sexual or emotional abuse. This expectation includes the parental responsibilities to provide appropriate medical care for children with physical illnesses and to ensure that their child maintains satisfactory school attendance. Parents must recognize and assist children with mental or physical disabilities. Parents who cannot provide these basic functions may be guilty of medical, emotional, or educational neglect.

Medical Neglect

Medical neglect is the failure of parents or legal guardians to provide appropriate health care, including psychological treatment, for their child even though they have the financial means to do so. Medical neglect can result in adverse health consequences, such as the worsening of the child's existing physical illness. According to 2016 data, medical neglect affected 14,028 U.S. children, accounting for 2.1% of substantiated cases of child maltreatment (U.S. Department of Health and Human Services 2018).

Concern is warranted when a parent refuses pediatric care for a child in an emergency or for a child with an acute illness and when a parent ignores pediatric recommendations for a child who has a treatable chronic disease, resulting in frequent hospitalizations or significant physical illness deterioration. Cases in which parents withhold pediatric care based on their religious beliefs do not fall under the definition of medical neglect, but most jurisdictions are moving toward eliminating these religious exemptions. Parents may also fail to provide pediatric care because of cultural norms, insufficient information, or lack of financial resources.

Child protective service agencies generally will intervene when a child needs emergency medical treatment or when a child has a life-threatening or chronic illness that may result in disability or disfigurement if left untreated. Most jurisdictions issue court orders to permit appropriate medical treatment in these situations. Social and financial assistance may be available when poverty rather than neglect limits parents' resources to provide adequate medical treatment for their child.

Assessment

In helping assess parenting capacity and medical neglect, consultants need to clarify the expectations underlying the request. Consultants must be clear that they can provide a psychiatric assessment that includes parental psychopathology and a sense of the parent-child relationship but that they are not "detectives" who are able to determine if abuse or neglect actually took place. In the hospital setting, the source of these referrals may be a child abuse protection team that generally consults with the pediatric team on all cases of suspected neglect or abuse. Consultants should not begin an assessment until the patient and family have been told of the consultation and its purposes. If the parents refuse appropriate assessment, the refusal itself may constitute neglect. Consultants should explicitly state to the family that the information and findings obtained in this assessment are not confidential or privileged and must be communicated to the pediatric team.

In the assessment, consultants should consider a number of parental strengths, including cognitive understanding of the child's physical, medical, and emotional needs; presence of adequate organizational skills and ability to supervise the child's treatment; consistency; presence of extended family and social support; and capacity for emotional warmth and nurturance (Barnum 2002). Parental vulnerabilities to consider include cognitive limitations interfering with their understanding of the child's needs; inadequate financial resources to support the child's needs; inability to enforce discipline or set limits in an appropriate manner; parental psychopathology; parental substance-related disorders; and parental history of abuse or neglect (Barnum 2002).

Transfer of Custody and Termination of Parental Rights

Depending on the jurisdiction, transfer of a child's legal and/or physical custody from the parents is usually a temporary arrangement (Ibeziako et al. 2010). In a voluntary transfer of custody, parents retain legal rights but voluntarily request the assistance of state agencies when a child is unable to function at home and sign over physical custody for placement in an appropriate setting. Alternatively, child protective service agencies can file a petition with the court for involuntary transfer of custody if the parents are found to be unfit, unwilling, or unable to competently manage their child's medical care.

An involuntary custody transfer occurs when there is evidence that the child is at risk of significant harm as a result of the parents' behavior. In some instances the child may remain within physical custody of the parents while all legal decisions are made by court-appointed persons on the child's behalf (e.g., guardians ad litem, state protective agencies, the court itself). When there is concern about ongoing risk of harm to a child while living with the parents, the child is removed from the home and may be placed in the physical care of extended family members, foster parents, or state residential facilities. This arrangement is usually temporary, with the goal of reunification after treatment if possible.

The mere presence of parental psychopathology does not automatically result in loss of custody unless there is evidence that the child is at significant risk of harm as a result of the parental illness. When parents with severe neurocognitive impairments have a child with complex health issues and are unable to provide sufficient care despite external supports, there may be sufficient basis for transfer of custody. On the other hand, parents who are cognitively competent and high functioning may be found unfit in certain situations by contributing to their child's deterioration by forming an alliance with the illness, resisting treatment recommendations, and pulling their child out of treatment facilities.

Children may be placed in temporary foster care or other substitute care to give parents the opportunity to correct issues that are interfering with their ability to support appropriate medical treatment. Children who are removed from their parents may experience the separation as unexpected and traumatic because removal frequently occurs without preparation or adequate explanation to the child. Placement may disrupt the child's social support network and may entail a change in schools.

Consultants may be asked to assist in these evaluations and to make recommendations regarding the mental health needs of children placed in foster care. In making these decisions, it is important for consultants to consider data suggesting that foster children are at greater risk for maltreatment and physical abuse than the general population (Biehal 2014). Despite the deficiencies of foster care and out-of-home placement, placement may be necessary to lessen the likelihood of reinjury by parents or legal guardians.

Conclusion

Consultants must have a solid foundation in legal and forensic issues in the pediatric setting. They need to understand the specific statutes in their own jurisdictions that are most germane to their work setting. Consultants should establish a working relationship with a lawyer familiar with the pediatric setting in which they work. This partnership can have enormous impact on advancing patient care. Consultants should never hesitate to call for legal assistance.

References

Barnum R: Parenting assessment in cases of neglect and abuse, in Principles and Practice of Child and Adolescent Forensic Psychiatry. Edited by Schetky DH, Benedek EP. Washington, DC, American Psychiatric Publishing, 2002, pp 81–96

Biehal N: Maltreatment in foster care: a review of the evidence. Child Abuse Review 23(1):48–60, 2014

Committee on Bioethics: Informed consent in decision-making in pediatric practice [policy statement]. Pediatrics 138(2):e20161484, 2016 27456514

Ibeziako P, Bourne R, Shaw RJ, et al: Legal and forensic issues, in Textbook of Pediatric Psychosomatic Medicine. Edited by Shaw RJ, DeMaso MD. Washington, DC, American Psychiatric Publishing, 2010, pp 47–59

Katz A, Webb SA; Committee on Bioethics: Informed consent in decision-making in pediatric practice [technical report]. Pediatrics 138:e2016148, 2016 27456510

Sankaran VS, Macbeth JE: Legal issues in the treatment of minors, in Principles and Practice of Child and Adolescent Forensic Psychiatry. Edited by Benedek EP, Ash P, Scott CL. Washington, DC, American Psychiatric Publishing, 2010, pp 109–1303

U.S. Department of Health and Human Services; Administration for Children and Families, Administration on Children, Youth, and Families; Children's Bureau: Child Maltreatment 2016. February 1, 2018. Available at: https://www.acf.hhs.gov/cb/resource/child-maltreatment-2016. Accessed March 15, 2019.

PART II

Specific Psychiatric Symptoms and Disorders

5

Delirium

Delirium is a neurocognitive disorder that results from the direct physiological consequences of a medical condition, substance intoxication or withdrawal, exposure to a toxin, or multiple etiologies (see Box 5–1) (American Psychiatric Association 2013). This clinical syndrome is characterized by a fluctuating disturbance in attention and awareness that is accompanied by a change in baseline cognition. Delirium is associated with increased rates of morbidity and mortality in youth with critical illnesses (Hatherill and Flisher 2010; Patel et al. 2017a; Smith et al. 2009; Traube et al. 2017a; Turkel 2010).

Box 5–1.   DSM-5 Diagnostic Criteria for Delirium

A. A disturbance in attention (i.e., reduced ability to direct, focus, sustain, and shift attention) and awareness (reduced orientation to the environment).
B. The disturbance develops over a short period of time (usually hours to a few days), represents a change from baseline attention and awareness, and tends to fluctuate in severity during the course of a day.

C. An additional disturbance in cognition (e.g., memory deficit, disorientation, language, visuospatial ability, or perception).

D. The disturbances in Criteria A and C are not better explained by another preexisting, established, or evolving neurocognitive disorder and do not occur in the context of a severely reduced level of arousal, such as coma.

E. There is evidence from the history, physical examination, or laboratory findings that the disturbance is a direct physiological consequence of another medical condition, substance intoxication or withdrawal (i.e., due to a drug of abuse or to a medication), or exposure to a toxin, or is due to multiple etiologies.

Specify whether:

Substance intoxication delirium: This diagnosis should be made instead of substance intoxication when the symptoms in Criteria A and C predominate in the clinical picture and when they are sufficiently severe to warrant clinical attention.

Substance withdrawal delirium: This diagnosis should be made instead of substance withdrawal when the symptoms in Criteria A and C predominate in the clinical picture and when they are sufficiently severe to warrant clinical attention.

Medication-induced delirium: This diagnosis applies when the symptoms in Criteria A and C arise as a side effect of a medication taken as prescribed.

Delirium due to another medical condition: There is evidence from the history, physical examination, or laboratory findings that the disturbance is attributable to the physiological consequences of another medical condition.

Delirium due to multiple etiologies: There is evidence from the history, physical examination, or laboratory findings that the delirium has more than one etiology (e.g., more than one etiological medical condition; another medical condition plus substance intoxication or medication side effect).

Specify if:

Acute: Lasting a few hours or days.
Persistent: Lasting weeks or months.

Specify if:

Hyperactive: The individual has a hyperactive level of psychomotor activity that may be accompanied by mood lability, agitation, and/or refusal to cooperate with medical care.

Hypoactive: The individual has a hypoactive level of psychomotor activity that may be accompanied by sluggishness and lethargy that approaches stupor.

Mixed level of activity: The individual has a normal level of psychomotor activity even though attention and awareness are disturbed. Also includes individuals whose activity level rapidly fluctuates.

Source. Reprinted from American Psychiatric Association: *Diagnostic and Statistical Manual of Mental Disorders*, 5th Edition. Arlington, VA, American Psychiatric Association, 2013. Copyright © 2013 American Psychiatric Association. Used with permission.

With the continued use of many different labels, including acute brain syndrome, encephalopathy, confusional state, and intensive care unit (ICU) psychosis, across medical disciplines, it is important for psychiatric consultants to be knowledgeable regarding the clinical characteristics, epidemiology, pathophysiology, differential diagnosis, assessment, and management of pediatric delirium.

Clinical Characteristics

Patients with delirium have characteristic changes in several neurocognitive domains of functioning, reflective of the diffuse nature of the underlying central nervous system (CNS) pathology. A disturbance in attention and awareness that cannot be better explained by a preexisting or evolving neurocognitive disorder and that does not occur in the context of a severely reduced level of awareness is the essential feature of delirium (American Psychiatric Association 2013). Reductions in the ability to direct, focus, sustain, and shift attention along with reduced orientation toward the patient's environment are central features. The diagnosis includes a requirement for at least one additional disturbance in memory, disorientation, language, visuospatial ability, or perception. There must also be evidence from history, physical examination, or laboratory findings that the delirium is a direct physiological consequence of a medical condition, medication or drug, toxin, or multiple etiologies (American Psychiatric Association 2013).

Sleep-wake disturbance, fluctuating symptoms, impaired attention, irritability, agitation, affective lability, and confusion have been noted more often in younger children, whereas impaired memory, depressed mood, speech disturbance, delusions, and paranoia are more common in adolescents and adults (Turkel 2010; Turkel et al. 2006). Impaired alertness, apathy, anxiety, disorientation, and illusions/hallucinations are equally common across all ages (Turkel 2010; Turkel et al. 2006).

Temporal Course

Delirium can have an abrupt or acute onset, particularly after surgery or when sedative and hypnotic medications are being withdrawn. Delirium can also present with early nonspecific symptoms, such as restlessness, anxiety, irritability, and sleep disturbances (i.e., nightmares), in the hours to days prior to the more florid manifestations of an acute delirium. There is often a stepwise decline or alteration in behavior associated with a characteristic waxing and waning of symptoms with lucid intervals and fluctuating levels of consciousness. However, if closely examined, cognitive impairment persists even during the apparent lucid intervals. Symptoms are often worse at night, a phenomenon referred to as *sundowning*.

Pediatric studies have found that delirium generally occurs early in the ICU course of children with critical illnesses, with a median onset time of 1–3 days and a relatively brief duration of 2 days (Alvarez et al. 2018; Patel et al. 2017b). Up to one-third of patients who remain in the ICU may go on to demonstrate a recurrent episode. In a study following elective surgery requiring an ICU stay, those patients who developed a delirium had longer hospital stays, required more mechanical ventilation, and had increased utilization of health care resources than those without delirium (Meyburg et al. 2017).

Patients may make a full recovery if the underlying etiology is identified and found to be reversible, but a significant number of patients may progress to stupor, coma, or even death. Delirium and delusional or traumatic memory (frightening and/or psychotic experiences about the ICU stay), along with younger age, female gender, previous psychiatric history, and the use of mechanical restraint, have been found to be risk factors for the later development of posttraumatic stress disorder (Morrissey and Collier 2016). There may be an association between delirium and subsequent symptoms of anxiety and depression (Davydow 2009). There are no available long-term studies on the association between delirium and cognitive outcomes after discharge or on long-term psychological health (Patel et al. 2017a).

Cognitive Impairment

Attention

Patients with delirium characteristically present with difficulties in sustained attention. Indeed, a review of delirium studies found inattention in nearly 100% of cases (Turkel and Tavaré 2003). In young children, impaired attention may be most apparent in the inability to interpersonally engage with the consultant, pediatric care providers, and family members, whereas in older children and adolescents, the attention difficulties are more similar to those in adults (i.e., difficulties in concentration and focus) (Turkel 2010; Turkel et al. 2006).

Memory

Immediate and recent event memory is frequently impaired. Patients have trouble with registration, retention, and recall. Although their long-term declarative (or explicit) memory of facts, data, and events is generally intact, patients may have problems with procedural (or implicit) memory of "knowing how to do things." After successful recovery, patients often have amnesia for the entire delirium episode or limited recollection of events (generally recall of the negative ones). Problems with memory in younger children are not as common as those experienced by adolescents (Turkel 2010; Turkel et al. 2006).

Disorientation

Patients are usually disoriented with regard to time and place but rarely to person. There may be some fluctuation in levels of orientation during lucid periods. Although disorientation may be difficult to assess in younger children, who may have a developmentally limited conception of time, a review of pediatric delirium suggested that disorientation is present in approximately 77% of cases (Turkel et al. 2004). Children who have developed verbal skills are usually able to cooperate with questions regarding orientation.

Executive Functions

Delirium is often associated with an impaired ability to process information, reason, plan, make decisions, solve problems, anticipate consequences of actions, and grasp the meanings of abstract words. These deficits are thought to develop as a result of impaired functioning in the prefrontal cortex and thalamus (Turkel 2010).

Visuospatial Impairment

Patients with delirium may be unable to copy simple geometric designs or complex figures (dysgraphia and constructional apraxia). The ability to draw a clock face is a useful test because it assesses functioning in three different neuroanatomical regions: the nondominant parietal cortex (overall spatial proportions and relations), the dominant parietal cortex (details such as numbers and hands), and the prefrontal cortex (understanding the concept of time).

Thought and Language Disturbance

Thought processes of patients with delirium may become disorganized and inaccurate, with tangentiality and loosening of associations. Patients may develop poorly systematized and mood-incongruent paranoid delusions that can lead to violent behavior. Speech can be characterized by incoherence, rambling, mild dysarthria, mumbling, muteness, and/or word-finding difficulties.

Perceptual Disturbance

Illusions (misperceptions of real objects) and hallucinations (false perceptions) are common. Visual hallucinations or visual combined with auditory hallucinations occur in up to 43% of cases, whereas tactile, gustatory, and olfactory hallucinations occur less frequently (Turkel et al. 2004). Organized delusions are rare. Patients have a reduced ability to discriminate and integrate perceptions, resulting in their confusion of images, dreams, and hallucinations. Confusion and misidentification are present in delirium, as opposed to the perceptional disturbances of derealization and depersonalization. Younger children may be less likely to report perceptual disturbances.

Psychomotor Disturbance: Subtype Classification

Impaired psychomotor activity is common in patients with delirium. This has led to the classification of delirium based on the nature of the psychomotor disturbance (American Psychiatric Association 2013). A *hyperactive* delirium classically presents with confusion, psychosis, disorientation, psychomotor agitation, hypervigilance, hyperalertness, fast or loud speech, combativeness, and/or behavioral problems (e.g., pulling out catheters and lines). A *hypoactive*, or silent, delirium presents with somnolence, decreased activity, slow or decreased speech, psychomotor slowing, apathy, and/or confusion. Patients with this latter presentation are less likely to be diagnosed or may be misdiagnosed with depression. *Mixed-type* delirium describes fluctuation between hyperactive and hypoactive states. Hypoactive (46%) and mixed (45%) subtypes were most common in children with critical illnesses, with the hyperactive subtype (8%) occurring much less often (Traube et al. 2017b).

Sleep-Wake Cycle Disruptions

Delirium classically presents with disruptions to the sleep-wake cycle. There is often a reversal in the diurnal rhythm, with lethargy during the day and arousal, disorientation, and agitation at night.

Affective Lability

Patients with delirium may have rapid fluctuations in their emotional state, with symptoms of anxiety, fear, anger, sadness, apathy, and less commonly euphoria (e.g., steroid-induced delirium). Affective lability, anxiety, and irritability are found in the majority of children with delirium (Turkel 2010; Turkel and Tavaré 2003).

Neurological Abnormalities

Physical Examination

In patients with delirium, findings on physical examination may include tremor, myoclonus, and asterixis, particularly in those patients with metabolic uremia and hepatic insufficiency. The nature of the tremor varies according to etiology but is more commonly an intention tremor. Symmetric reflex and muscle tone changes may be seen in myxedema, carbon monoxide poisoning, and neuroleptic malignant syndrome (see Chapter 6, "Neurocognitive Disturbances"). Nystagmus and ataxia may occur in patients with drug intoxications.

Electroencephalograms

Patients with delirium classically have a generalized nonspecific slowing on their electroencephalogram, with the degree of slowing correlating with delirium severity (American Psychiatric Association 2013). Less typically, there may be excess activity (i.e., alcohol withdrawal delirium). The electroencephalogram is insufficiently sensitive and specific for diagnostic purposes (American Psychiatric Association 2013).

Epidemiology

With reported prevalence rates between 12% and 65%, pediatric delirium is common (Patel et al. 2017a; Silver et al. 2010, 2012, 2015b). In a large multi-institutional point prevalence study of 994 critically ill children in 25 different ICUs, the overall prevalence of delirium was 25% (Traube et al. 2017b). The highest delirium rates were found in children admitted for infectious or inflammatory disorders. An incidence of delirium of 49%–57% has been found in the pediatric cardiac ICU, where patients with delirium were found to be younger, have cyanotic disease, undergo longer periods of mechanical ventilations, and have longer cardiopulmonary bypass times (Alvarez et al. 2018; Patel et al. 2017b).

Predisposing risk factors for delirium in pediatric patients include age younger than 5 years, preexisting neurodevelopmental delay, high severity of acute pediatric illness, presence of a preexisting pediatric condition, low serum albumen resulting in reduced protein-bound drug carrying capacity (i.e., malnutrition, nephrotic syndrome, and hepatic insufficiency), and/or medical ventilation. Precipitating modifiable risk factors include anticholinergic medications, benzodiazepines, opioids, immobilization, and/or restraints (Alvarez et al. 2018; Mody et al. 2018; Patel et al. 2017a). After controlling for age, gender, severity of illness, and length of stay, Traube et al. (2016) found that delirium was associated with an 85% increase in pediatric ICU costs.

Pathophysiology

Three pathophysiological pathways are hypothesized to play important roles in the evolution of pediatric delirium: 1) neuroinflammatory changes compromising the integrity of the blood-brain barrier and/or de novo inflammatory productions within the brain (systemic inflammation and enhanced cytokine activity); 2) neurotransmitter dysregulation related to medications that change acetylcholine, dopamine, glutamine, γ-aminobutyric acid, and/or serotonin neurotransmitter function; and 3) oxidative stress related to reduced oxygen delivery, which reduces oxidative metabolism required to convert toxic chemicals (i.e., oxygen free radicals, arachidonic acid metabolites, and cytokines) (Patel et al. 2017a). Regardless of the pathophysiology, the final common pathway to delirium appears to be an alteration in neurotransmission that leads to failure of integration and processing of sensory information and motor response (Patel et al. 2017a).

Differential Diagnosis

Virtually any pediatric condition or its treatment has the ability to induce the disabling neurocognitive disturbances of delirium. It is important to remember that delirium is often multifactorial in nature. Table 5–1 outlines a differential diagnosis of pediatric delirium that uses the mnemonic "I WATCH DEATH." The most common medical etiologies for pediatric delirium (and frequencies with which they occur) are infection with CNS involvement (i.e., meningitis or sepsis) (33%) and medication (i.e., steroid, benzodiazepine, or narcotic) (19%), followed by head trauma, autoimmune conditions, post-transplant sequela, postoperative condition, neoplasm, and organ failure (each 7%–9%) (Turkel and Tavaré 2003).

Steroids have long been known to contribute to the development of delirium, although they may also be used in the treatment of the underlying disease (e.g., autoimmune disease) that itself causes acute mental status changes. Opioids and analgesic medications, which are frequently used to treat anxiety and pain in critically ill children, are also well known to have an adverse impact on a patient's mental status. A causal link between delirium and benzodiazepine use in the ICU for sedation or anxiety, either alone or in combination with opioids (e.g., midazolam and fentanyl), has been reported, with recommendations being made to limit use of the medication(s) (Mody et al. 2018; Turkel 2010).

Anticholinergic medications or medications with anticholinergic side effects can contribute to the development of delirium. The following well-known medications have potential for anticholinergic side effects: codeine, oxycodone, fentanyl, ampicillin, carbamazepine, bupropion, citalopram, escitalopram, mirtazapine, sertraline, trazodone, venlafaxine, risperidone, aripiprazole, ziprasidone, captopril, cimetidine, digoxin, furosemide, azathioprine, cyclosporine, prednisolone, prednisone, and warfarin.

Delirium may prove difficult to separate from and in fact may co-occur with a catatonic disorder due to another medical condition (see Chapter 6, "Neurocognitive Disturbances"); the two may share features such as excitement, stupor, mutism, and/or negativism or may present with similar psycho-

Table 5–1.   Potential physiological etiologies for pediatric delirium: the "I WATCH DEATH" mnemonic

Infection	Encephalitis*, meningitis*, syphilis, HIV, or sepsis*
Withdrawal	Alcohol, barbiturates, or sedative-hypnotics*
Acute metabolic conditions	Acidosis, alkalosis, electrolyte disturbance*, hepatic failure, or renal failure
Trauma	Closed-head injury*, heatstroke, postoperative*, or severe burns*
Central nervous system pathology	Abscess, hemorrhage, hydrocephalus, subdural hematoma, infection*, seizures*, stroke, tumors, metastases, or vasculitis*
Hypoxia	Anemia, carbon monoxide poisoning, hypotension, pulmonary failure, or cardiac failure
Deficiencies	Vitamin B_{12}, folate, niacin, or thiamine
Endocrinopathies	Hyper/hypoadrenocorticism, hyper/hypoglycemia, myxedema, or hyperparathyroidism
Acute vascular conditions	Hypertensive encephalopathy, stroke, arrhythmia, or shock*
Toxins or drugs	Medications*, illicit drugs, pesticides, or solvents
Heavy metals	Lead, manganese, or mercury*

*More commonly seen in pediatric delirium.
Source.   Reprinted from Wise MG, Brandt G: "Delirium," in *American Psychiatry Press Textbook of Neuropsychiatry,* 2nd Edition. Edited by Hales RE, Yudofsky SC. Washington, DC, American Psychiatric Press, 1992, p. 302. Copyright © American Psychiatric Press, Inc. Used with permission.

motor subtypes (American Psychiatric Association 2013; Grover et al. 2014; Oldham and Lee 2015). This is an important consideration because the treatment of one disorder has the potential to exacerbate the other disorder (i.e., antipsychotics may worsen catatonia and help delirium, whereas benzodiazepines may help catatonia and worsen delirium) (Rosebush and Mazurek 2010; Zaal et al. 2015). Currently, close clinical observation for pathognomonic psychomotor findings of catatonia is most useful in targeting the direction of intervention.

The hypoactive and hyperactive symptoms of delirium may mimic the symptoms of anxiety and depression. The latter are more responsive to interpersonal support and intervention because they lack the level of impairment in attention and awareness.

Assessment

Medical History and Laboratory and Imaging Tests

The pediatric assessment for delirium includes an interview with parents to obtain a thorough medical history. Consultants should review the patient's medical record, including laboratory and imaging test results (Table 5–2). Nursing staff observations should be obtained at different points in time to capture fluctuations in level of consciousness.

Direct Examination

The direct examination is dictated by the nature of the cognitive disturbances, as described earlier in this chapter (see section "Clinical Characteristics"). Depending on the patient's mental status functioning, questioning can range from basic orientation questions (i.e., time, person, place, and circumstances) to specific questions about cognitive and perceptual disturbances (i.e., hearing and seeing things). In moments of lucidity, patients will often acknowledge that their thinking is "confused" or "mixed up." Consultants can often spend a few minutes outside a patient's bed space and readily observe the presence or absence of psychomotor agitation.

Assessment Instruments

Vanderbilt Assessment for Delirium in Infants and Children

The Vanderbilt Assessment for Delirium in Infants and Children (VADIC; also available at: https://www.icudelirium.org/medical-professionals/pediatric-care) (Figure 5–1) was developed to provide consultants with a comprehensive framework within which to standardize pediatric delirium assessment (Gangopadhyay et al. 2017). With demonstrated high content validity, the VADIC provides a standardized framework for the consultant to use DSM-5 delirium criteria (American Psychiatric Association 2013) and integrate behavioral observations and patient reactions to developmentally appropriate interactive tasks as part of the assessment for delirium.

Table 5–2.   Selected laboratory and imaging tests to be considered in the pediatric assessment of delirium

Basic hematological and chemistry tests

Complete blood cell count	Creatinine level
Electrolyte levels	Glucose level
Calcium level	Liver function tests
Serum urea nitrogen	Urinary analysis

Other laboratory test considerations based on clinical presentation

Ammonia level	Magnesium level
Antinuclear antibody titers	NMDA receptor antibody titer
Arterial blood gas analysis	Phosphorus level
B_{12} and folate level	Serum alcohol/drug concentrations
C-reactive protein test	Thyroid function tests
Erythrocyte sedimentation rate	Urinary toxicology screen
Lupus erythematosus cell test	Urinary porphyrin concentrations

Radiographic and other tests

Chest radiography	Lumbar puncture
Computed tomography	Electroencephalography
Magnetic resonance imaging	Electrocardiography

Note.   NMDA = *N*-methyl-D-aspartate.

Delirium Screening Tools

Because consultants are most commonly called regarding extreme cases of delirium, milder and/or hypoactive delirium may be left undiagnosed and untreated. Therefore, delirium screening tools have been designed that the pediatric team can use at bedside to monitor delirium in critically ill children and adolescents. These screening tools are increasingly becoming used in the pediatric ICU setting for earlier detection of delirium, which might improve outcomes.

Richmond Agitation Sedation Scale.   The Richmond Agitation Sedation Scale (RASS) is a measure used to determine a patient's level of arousal or consciousness (available at: https://www.icudelirium.org/medical-professionals/pediatric-care). Arousal assessment with the RASS is shown in Table 5–3. The RASS allows physicians and nursing staff to delineate patient arousal along a continuum ranging from *unarousable/deep sedation* at one end to *combative* at the other end with *alert and calm* in the middle (Sessler et al. 2002).

Assuming that the patient as assessed by the RAAS is at least responsive to voice, either the Pediatric Confusion Assessment Method for the ICU Series or the Cornell Assessment of Pediatric Delirium, which are discussed next, can then be used by physicians and nurses in the intensive care setting to screen for delirium.

Pediatric Confusion Assessment Method for the ICU Series.   Developed by Vanderbilt University, the Pediatric Confusion Assessment Method for the ICU (pCAM-ICU) (for children ages 5 years and older) and the Preschool Confusion Assessment Method for the ICU (psCAM-ICU) (for children younger than 5 years) are reliable and valid measures that assess delirium in critically ill youth (Smith et al. 2009, 2011, 2016). The pCAM-ICU and the psCAM-ICU (Figure 5–2; also available at: https://www.icudelirium.org/medical-professionals/pediatric-care) can be used to assess the patient for inattention, altered level of consciousness, and disorganized thinking. These measures are to be used across nursing shifts or more frequently as indicated.

Cornell Assessment of Pediatric Delirium.   The Cornell Assessment of Pediatric Delirium (CAPD) (available at: https://www.icudelirium.org/medical-professionals/pediatric-care) (Figure 5–3) is an observational screen that can provide a longitudinal snapshot over the course of two nursing observations covering 24 hours (Patel et al. 2017a; Silver et al. 2015a; Traube et al. 2014). Suitable for ages 0–21 years, the CAPD has been validated by experienced nurses in both developmentally typical and atypical patients. Development anchor points are available to guide use of the tool in young patients from birth through age 2 years (Silver et al. 2015a). Similar to the pCAM-ICU and the psCAM-ICU, the CAPD is most useful when used to screen all patients in pediatric ICU settings, with its results included in the clinical bedside discussion of the patient, in essence as a vital sign.

Vanderbilt Assessment for Delirium in Infants and Children

			Clinician:
Age:	**Patient Intubated?** □ YES □ NO	Date/Time:	

Pertinent medication exposure ≤ 24 hrs prior to assessment (DRUG / DOSE)

1.	4.
2.	5.
3.	6.

MENTAL STATUS

State of current mental status – *Check one option*

LEVEL OF CONSCIOUSNESS (check one)

Combative	□ YES	State of current mental status		□ Chronic Change			
Agitated	□ YES	□ At Baseline	□ Acute Change				
Restless	□ YES	**Pattern of mental status** – *past 24 hours*		□ Stable	□ Fluctuating		
Alert and Calm	□ YES						

PERCEPTION

Drowsy: Not fully alert but easily demonstrates sustained awakening with stimulation only from voice	□ YES	**Hallucinations:** □ *auditory* □ *visual*	□ N/A	□ NO	□ YES
Lethargy: Arouses to **voice** but difficult to <u>maintain</u> the aroused state	□ YES	**Hyperacusis** present? *Comments:*	□ N/A	□ NO	□ YES
Obtundation: Responds to stimulation other than pain. May briefly open eyes or have movement; doesn't <u>interact</u> with person or environment	□ YES	**Atypical response** to normal stimuli? *(stuffed animals, familiar toys)*	□ N/A	□ NO	□ YES
Stupor: Responsive **only** to pain	□ YES	**Unable to soothe** when fearful stimuli removed?	□ N/A	□ NO	□ YES
Coma: Unresponsive to pain	□ YES	*Comments:*			

ATTENTION and COGNITION

DECREASED ability to:	**Focus attention:**	□ NO	□ YES	**ORIENTATION:**	□ Person	□ Place □ N/A
	Sustain attention:	□ NO	□ YES	*Comments:*		
	Shift attention:	□ NO	□ YES			

DECREASED indication of **consistent preference** for objects such as toys, rattle, stuffed animals, blankie, Ipad?	□ NO	□ YES
DECREASED ability to **screen out** extraneous stimuli? (Easily distracted by noise, people)	□ NO	□ YES
DECREASED ability to **interact** with toys/objects appropriately? (No interaction/recognition, uses toy inappropriately)	□ NO	□ YES
DECREASED **social smile** in response to toys or stuffed animals?	□ NO	□ YES
Object permanence present? (interacts while playing Peek-a-boo, hide-and-seek)	□ NO	□ YES

SLEEP-WAKE CYCLE

Naps: (Q2-4h infant, Q6h toddler, QD preschool) □ NO □ YES
Day-Night Reversal present: □ NO □ YES
- *More difficult to recognize in infants*
Nocturnal Disturbance □ NO □ YES
- *Consider initial, middle, terminal insomnia, phase shift*
Comments:

AFFECT

Excessive energy for age and context/environment? □ NO □ YES
Irritability or anger □ NO □ YES
Inconsolability □ NO □ YES
Inappropriate Affect □ NO □ YES
Describe Affect:

Confounders present? □ Anxiety □ Pain □ Volitional □ None

LANGUAGE and THOUGHT

□ **Not Present** (*immature development or developmental delay*)
□ **Present**

Receptive Language: **One** - Step Command □ NO □ YES
Two - Step Command □ NO □ YES
Three - Step Command □ NO □ YES

Does not follow commands (check reason below):
□ Unable due to immaturity/illness (intubated)
□ Inappropriately not following commands

Describe baseline speech and language per parent/nurse if available:
□ Appropriate
□ Decreased amount
□ Decreased spontaneity
□ Increased latency
□ Change from baseline
□ Circumstantial
□ Tangential
□ Obstructed due to disease or device

IS ACUTE DELIRIUM PRESENT?

UTA	When LOC severely depressed, unable to directly clinically assess patient, and prior clinical assessment not available.
NO	If NO consider → **Subsyndromal delirium (SS)** (Delirium probable but NOT all criteria met): □ **NO** □ **YES**
YES	If YES then choose type → □ **HYPOACTIVE** □ **HYPERACTIVE** □ **MIXED** Drug Withdrawal? □ **N/A** □ **NO** □ **YES**

24-HOUR assessment → **IS DELIRIUM PRESENT?** □ **PRESENT** □ **ABSENT** □ **SUBSYNDROMAL** □ **UTA**

□ 1. Acute Change in Mental Status	□ 3. Inattention Present	□ 5. Change in Cognition	□ 7. Change in Affect
□ 2. Fluctuating Course	□ 4. Inconsolability	□ 6. Change in Language/Thought	□ 8. Change in Sleep/Wake Cycle

DELIRIUM = 1+2+3+5+7 AND 4 OR 6 OR 8
SUBSYNDROMAL = 1+2 AND 3 OR 5 OR 7

Figure 5–1. Vanderbilt Assessment of Delirium in Infants and Children (VADIC).

Source. Developed by Vanderbilt University. Copyright © 2017, Vanderbilt University. Used with permission. Reprinted from Gangopadhyay M, Smith H, Pao M, et al.: "Development of the Vanderbilt Assessment for Delirium in Infants and Children to Standardize Pediatric Delirium Assessment by Psychiatrists." *Psychosomatics* 58(4):357–358, 2017. Copyright © 2017, with permission from Elsevier.

Table 5–3. Arousal assessment with the Richmond Agitation-Sedation Scale (RASS)

Scale	Label	Description
+4	Combative	Combative/VIOLENT/immediate danger to staff
+3	Very agitated	Pulls to remove tubes or catheters/AGGRESSIVE
+2	Agitated	Frequent nonpurposeful movement/FIGHTS VENTILATOR
+1	RESTLESS	ANXIOUS/apprehensive/movement not aggressive
+0	ALERT and CALM	SPONTANEOUS ATTENTION to caregiver
−1	DROWSY	Not fully alert but has SUSTAINED AWAKENING TO VOICE; eye opening and eye contact > 10 sec
−2	LIGHT SEDATION	BRIEFLY awakens to VOICE; eyes open but contact < 10 secs
−3	MODERATE SEDATION	Movement or eye opening to VOICE/NO eye contact

If RASS score is ≥ (−3), proceed to STEP 2 (give pCAM-ICU or CAPD)

Scale	Label	Description
−4	DEEP SEDATION	NO RESPONSE to VOICE Some movement or eye opening to TOUCH (physical stimuli)
−5	UNAROUSEABLE	NO REPONSE to NOXIOUS stimuli

If RASS score is (−4) OR (−5), STOP and REASSESS patient later

Note. pCAM-ICU = Pediatric Confusion Assessment Method for the ICU Series; CAPD = Cornell Assessment of Pediatric Delirium.

Source. Used with permission of the American Thoracic Society. Copyright © 2019 American Thoracic Society. Sessler CN, Gosnell MD, Grap MJ, et al.: "The Richmond Agitation-Sedation Scale: Validity and Reliability in Adult Intensive Care Unit Patients." *The American Journal of Respiratory and Critical Care Medicine* 166:1338–1344, 2002. *The American Journal of Respiratory and Critical Care Medicine* is an official journal of the American Thoracic Society.

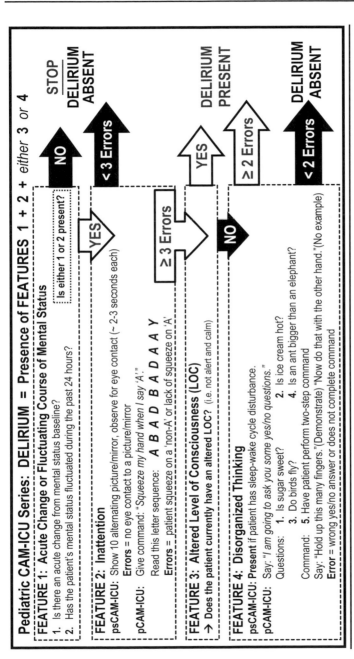

Figure 5–2.   Pediatric Confusion Assessment Method for the ICU Series.

Note.   pCAM-ICU=Pediatric Confusion Assessment Method for the Intensive Care Unit (5 years and older); psCAM-ICU=Preschool Confusion Assessment Method for the ICU (younger than 5 years).

Source.   Reprinted from Pediatric Care for Medical Professionals. Vanderbilt University. Available at: https://www.icudelirium.org/medical-professionals/pediatric-care. Used with permission.

RASS Score _____ (if –4 or –5, do not proceed)

Please answer the following questions based on your interactions with patient over the course of your shift:

	Never 4	Rarely 3	Sometimes 2	Often 1	Always 0	Score
1. Does the child make eye contact with the caregiver?						
2. Are the child's actions purposeful?						
3. Is the child aware of his/her surroundings?						
4. Does the child communicate needs and wants?						

	Never 0	Rarely 1	Sometimes 2	Often 3	Always 4	Score
5. Is the child restless?						
6. Is the child inconsolable?						
7. Is the child underactive—very little movement while awake?						
8. Does it take the child a long time to respond to interactions?						
					TOTAL	

Figure 5–3.   Delirium assessment using the revised Cornell Assessment of Pediatric Delirium (CAPD).

Note.   Although not diagnostic, a score of 9 or higher is consistent with delirium; RASS = Richmond Agitation-Sedation Scale.

Source.   Reprinted from Silver G, Kearney J, Traube C, et al.: "Delirium Screening Anchored in Child Development: The Cornell Assessment of Pediatric Delirium." *Palliative and Supportive Care* 13(4):1005–1011, 2015. Copyright © 2015, Cambridge University Press. Used with permission.

Management

Efforts should be made wherever possible to prevent the onset of delirium by identifying those patients at high risk and proactively treating their underlying pediatric conditions. Prevention of perioperative hypotension and hypoxemia, as well as attention to the choice of anesthetic and pain agents, may help reduce the incidence of delirium. Appropriate tapering of sedative-hypnotic agents used in the intensive care setting to prevent withdrawal delirium is important and frequently overlooked. Steps to reduce the anticholinergic load of medications may be helpful.

When called about a mental status change consistent with delirium, consultants must remember that the neurocognitive dysfunction is due to the direct physiological consequences of a pediatric condition or its treatment as well as potential substance intoxication or withdrawal. Consultants may need to advocate for the pediatric team to continue investigating and treating potential delirium etiologies.

Environmental Interventions

Nonpharmacological interventions include placing the patient near the nursing station, preferably in a private room, with a family member or staff person present to provide one-to-one observation to ensure the patient's safety. Repeated reorientation and reassurance of the patient combined with a predictable schedule, including rest periods, and minimization of noise are helpful (Crawford et al. 2017; Turkel 2017). Efforts to restore the normal sleep-wake cycle should be made by having room lights on during the day and off at night, but with sufficient nighttime illumination to decrease the likelihood of illusions (Crawford et al. 2017; Patel et al. 2014; Turkel 2017). The presence of familiar objects from home, pictures of family, a calendar, and a clock may help to reassure and reorient the patient. The use of physical and occupational therapy, even with mechanically ventilated patients, can prove helpful (Schweickert et al. 2009).

It is important to ensure good oxygenation and fluid intake. Although minimization of immobilizing lines, catheters, and restraints can be helpful, some patients may require physical restraint to keep them from harming themselves or others and to prevent them from inadvertently pulling out intravenous lines and catheters. In these situations, established hospital protocols for the use of mechanical restraints should be closely followed.

Consultants can be helpful to family members by providing psychoeducation and support for the acute mental status changes that they are witnessing. Helping parents understand the confusion that their child is experiencing may allow parents to more effectively implement supportive interpersonal techniques with their child (e.g., use simple and repeated words of reassurance and reorientation). The American Academy of Child and Adolescent Psychiatry (2017) has created a brochure on delirium in children and adolescents that can be given to parents and family members.

Pharmacological Interventions

Consultants should conduct a thorough review of all of a patient's current and recent medications. This review may suggest that the patient is overmedicated or is responding adversely to the current regimen, leading to suggestions to discontinue rather than add medications.

Opioids are particularly notorious for their adverse impact on a patient's mental status, whereas benzodiazepines may disinhibit the child rather than relieve anxiety. Consultants also may identify situations in which medications (e.g., opioids or benzodiazepines) are being withdrawn too rapidly, resulting in a withdrawal syndrome. The latter likely will involve reinstitution of the medication with design of a more gradual taper or addition of other medication (e.g., methadone).

There are situations in the pediatric setting in which a patient's agitation and distress cannot await resolution of the physical illness or a change in its treatment. At these junctures, it is critical to the patient's care and safety that these behaviors be rapidly contained through pharmacological therapy.

Use of Antipsychotics

Although antipsychotics have not been approved by the U.S. Food and Drug Administration (FDA) for the treatment of pediatric delirium, clinical consensus continues to support this use (Patel et al. 2017a; Smith et al. 2009; Turkel 2010, 2017; Turkel and Hanft 2014; Turkel et al. 2012). Table 5–4 provides suggested dosing for haloperidol, risperidone, and olanzapine for children and adolescents. Consultants are advised to utilize medication on a daily basis, given the transient nature of delirium, and to help titrate the dosage as well as monitor for medication side effects (e.g., QT_c prolongation, dysrhythmias, extrapyramidal signs).

Table 5–4. Pharmacological management guidelines for pediatric delirium

Clinical scenario: agitated or NPO
Medication: Haloperidol IV
Dosing: 0.01–0.02 mg/kg Q1H PRN agitation or psychotic symptoms × 3 days, then reassess

Age	Weight	Low end of range (per dose)	High end of range (per dose)	Maximum daily dose
1–3 years	10–20 kg	0.1 mg	0.4 mg	1 mg
>3–6 years	20–30 kg	0.2 mg	0.6 mg	2 mg
>6–10 years	30–40 kg	0.3 mg	0.8 mg	4 mg
>10–18 years	>40 kg	0.4 mg	1.0 mg	7 mg

Clinical scenario: not agitated and taking PO
Medication: Risperidone
Dosing: 0.0125–0.025 mg/kg Q6H PRN psychotic symptoms × 3 days, then reassess

Age	Weight	Low end of range (per dose)	High end of range (per dose)	Maximum daily dose
1–3 years	10–20 kg	0.125 mg	0.5 mg	1 mg
>3–6 years	20–30 kg	0.25 mg	0.75 mg	2 mg
>6–10 years	30–40 kg	0.375 mg	1.0 mg	3 mg
>10–18 years	>40 kg	0.5 mg	1.0 mg	4 mg

Clinical scenario: agitated with insomnia and taking PO
Medication: Olanzapine
Dosing: QHS for delirium with insomnia × 3 days, then reassess

Age	Weight	Low end of range (per dose)	High end of range (per dose)	Maximum daily dose
7–10 years	30–40 kg	1.25 mg	2.5 mg	2.5 mg
10–18 years	>40 kg	2.5 mg	5 mg	5 mg

Note. IV=intravenous; NPO=nothing by mouth; PO=by mouth; PRN=as needed; Q1H=every hour; QHS=every night.

Source. Reprinted from Goldsmith M, Ortiz-Rubio P, Staveski S, et al.: "Delirium," in *Textbook of Interdisciplinary Pediatric Palliative Care.* Edited by Wolfe J, Hinds P, Sourkes B. Philadelphia, PA, Elsevier Saunders, 2011, p. 261. Copyright © 2011, Elsevier. With permission from Elsevier.

The dopamine D_2 receptor antagonist haloperidol is the most commonly used typical antipsychotic. In many cases, patients with delirium, particularly hyperactive delirium, will respond to even low dosages of haloperidol given once or twice a day. For those with hypoactive symptoms, haloperidol may exacerbate symptoms of delirium (Smith et al. 2009).

Although not FDA approved for intravenous use, haloperidol can be given either by bolus injection or by continuous infusion. Intravenous use results in more reliable absorption and a decreased incidence of extrapyramidal reactions along with minimal effect on blood pressure, respiration, and heart rate (Beliles 2000; Menza et al. 1987). Intravenous administration is twice as potent as oral administration. The incidence of *torsades de pointes*, a specific form of ventricular tachycardia, is less than 0.01%, although there may be an elevated risk in cardiomyopathy (Hunt and Stern 1995). Cardiac monitoring is recommended, and if the QT_c is greater than 450 msec or greater than 25% over baseline, it is prudent to obtain a cardiology consultation and consider stopping the medication.

Atypical antipsychotics such as risperidone, olanzapine, and quetiapine are also used to manage pediatric delirium symptoms (Han and Kim 2004; Turkel 2010; Turkel et al. 2012). In contrast to haloperidol, given their impact as dopamine D_2, serotonin 5-HT_2, and norepinephrine NE α_2 receptor antagonists, the atypical antipsychotics may have positive impact on both hyperactive and hypoactive symptoms of delirium (Smith et al. 2009).

Use of Benzodiazepines, Dexmedetomidine, and Melatonin

Benzodiazepines.   As receptor agonists, benzodiazepines are generally not recommended in the treatment of delirium except in cases of withdrawal delirium. There is concern about the potential for disinhibition in children treated with benzodiazepines as well as a temporal relationship suggesting causality between benzodiazepine exposure and delirium, which supports limiting their use (Mody et al. 2018). Slow benzodiazepine tapers are considered the best preventive measure for a benzodiazepine withdrawal delirium, as determined by each patient's duration of use (e.g., following continuous benzodiazepine infusion for 1–3 days, wean by 20% daily; for 4–7 days, by 13%–20%; for 8–14 days, by 13%; for 15–21 days, by 8%; and for more than 21 days, by 2%–4%) (Ducharme et al. 2005).

Dexmedetomidine.   The highly selective α_2-adrenergic receptor agonist dexmedetomidine has been used for sedation, anxiety reduction, and pain medication with critically ill pediatric patients (Mason and Lerman 2011). Although not FDA approved for pediatric patients, it may offer an alternative to benzodiazepine sedation and has been reported to potentially prevent and/or treat delirium (Carrasco et al. 2016; Pandharipande et al. 2007; Patel et al. 2017a; Reade et al. 2016).

Melatonin.   Supporting the regular sleep-wake cycle through use of exogenous melatonin or ramelteon (Mel_1 and Mel_2 receptor agonists) may have promise in preventing and decreasing duration of delirium (Luther and McLeod 2018; Turkel and Hanft 2014). There are randomized controlled trials of exogenous melatonin targeting delirium prevention that have found reductions in pediatric delirium incidence in hospitalized patients as well as studies suggesting that melatonin given preoperatively may decrease emergence delirium (Chen et al. 2016; Kain et al. 2009).

Substance Withdrawal

Consultants must be alert to delirium resulting from substance withdrawal from alcohol and/or illicit drugs, such as opioids, stimulants, bath salts (synthetic cathinones), cocaine, cannabis preparations, and/or ecstasy (MDMA, or 3,4-methylenedioxymethamphetamine). A careful history from both patient and family is critical in combination with basic laboratory tests, a urinary drug screen, and a blood alcohol level (see Table 5–2). The CRAFFT Screening Questionnaire (Center for Adolescent Substance Abuse Research 2018; Knight et al. 2002) can be used to screen for substance-related problems in adolescents; the Alcohol Use Disorder Identification Test (AUDIT) (Barbor et al. 2001; World Health Organization 2001) can serve a similar function specifically for alcohol use disorder.

Medical stabilization is determined on the basis of the identified and/or suspected substance(s) and the expected clinical symptom time course beginning with the patient's last substance usage. Baseline management involves abstinence from the substance(s), adequate nutrition, maintenance of the correct fluid and electrolyte balance, and careful monitoring of vital signs, with more severe symptoms requiring inpatient medical and/or psychiatric management.

Patient: _____ Date: _____ Time: _____ (24-hour clock, midnight = 00:00)

Pulse or heart rate, taken for one minute: _____ Blood pressure: _____

NAUSEA AND VOMITING—Ask "Do you feel sick to your stomach? Have you vomited?" Observation.

0 no nausea and no vomiting
1 mild nausea with no vomiting
2
3
4 intermittent nausea with dry heaves
5
6
7 constant nausea, frequent dry heaves and vomiting

TREMOR—Arms extended and fingers spread apart. Observation.

0 no tremor
1 not visible, but can be felt fingertip to fingertip
2
3
4 moderate, with patient's arms extended
5
6
7 severe, even with arms not extended

PAROXYSMAL SWEATS—Observation.

0 no sweat visible
1 barely perceptible sweating, palms moist
2
3
4 beads of sweat obvious on forehead
5
6
7 drenching sweats

TACTILE DISTURBANCES—Ask "Have you any itching, pins and needles sensations, any burning, any numbness, or do you feel bugs crawling on or under your skin?" Observation.

0 none
1 very mild itching, pins and needles, burnng or numbness
2 mild itching, pins and needles, burning or numbness
3 moderate itching, pins and needles, burning or numbness
4 moderately severe hallucinations
5 severe hallucinations
6 extremely severe hallucinations
7 continuous hallucinations

AUDITORY DISTURBANCES—Ask "Are you more aware of sounds around you? Are they harsh? Do they frighten you? Are you hearing anything that is disturbing to you? Are you hearing things you know are not there?" Observation.

0 not present
1 very mild harshness or ability to frighten
2 mild harshness or ability to frighten
3 moderate harshness or ability to frighten
4 moderately severe hallucinations
5 severe hallucinations
6 extremely severe hallucinations
7 continuous hallucinations

VISUAL DISTURBANCES—Ask "Does the light appear to be too bright? Is its color different? Does it hurt your eyes? Are you seeing anything that is disturbing to you? Are you seeing things you know are not there?" Observation.

0 not present
1 very mild sensitivity
2 mild sensitivity
3 moderate sensitivity
4 moderately severe hallucinations
5 severe hallucinations
6 extremely severe hallucinations
7 continuous hallucinations

ANXIETY—Ask "Do you feel nervous?"
Observation.
0 no anxiety, at ease
1 mildly anxious
2
3
4 moderately anxious, or guarded,
   so anxiety is inferred
5
6
7 equivalent to acute panic states as seen in severe
   delirium or acute schizophrenic reactions

AGITATION—Observation.
0 normal activity
1 somewhat more than normal acitvity
2
3
4 moderately fidgety and restless
5
6
7 paces back and forth during most of the interview,
   or constantly thrashes about

HEADACHE, FULLNESS IN HEAD—Ask "Does your
head feel different? Does it feel like there is a band around
your head?" Do not rate for dizziness or lightheadedness.
Otherwise, rate severity.
0 not present
1 very mild
2 mild
3 moderate
4 moderately severe
5 severe
6 very severe
7 extremely severe

ORIENTATION AND CLOUDING OF SENSORIUM—
Ask "What day is this? Where are you? Who am I?"
0 oriented and can do serial additions
1 cannot do serial additions or is uncertain about date
2 disoriented for date by no more than 2 calendar days
3 disoriented for date by more than 2 calendar days
4 disoriented for place or person

Total **CIWA-Ar** Score _____
Rater's Initials _____
Maximum Possible Score: 67

Figure 5–4.   Clinical Institute Withdrawal Assessment for Alcohol, Revised (CIWA-Ar).

Note.   Scale for scoring: 0–9: absent or minimal withdrawal; 10–19: mild to moderate withdrawal; >20: severe withdrawal.

Source.   Reprinted from Sullivan JT, Sykora K, Schneiderman J, et al.: "Assessment of Alcohol Withdrawal: The Revised Clinical Institute Withdrawal Assessment for Alcohol Scale (CIWA-Ar)." *British Journal of Addiction* 84(11):1353–1357, 1989. Copyright © 1989, Society for the Study of Addiction. Used with permission from Wiley.

Clinical Opiate Withdrawal Scale

For each item, circle the number that best describes the patient's signs or symptom. Rate on just the apparent relationship to opiate withdrawal. For example, if heart rate is increased because the patient was jogging just prior to assessment, the increase pulse rate would not add to the score

Patient's Name: _____   Date and Time _____ / _____ / _____ _____ : _____

Reason for This Assessment: _____

Resting Pulse Rate: _____ beats/minute
Measure after patient is sitting or lying for one minute
0 pulse rate 80 or below
1 pulse rate 81–100
2 pulse rate 101–120
4 pulse rate greater than 120

Sweating: *over the past half hour not accounted for by room temperature or patient activity*
0 no report of chills or flushing
1 subjective report of chills or flushing
2 flushed or observable moisture on face
3 beads of sweat on brow or face
4 sweat streaming off face

Restlessness: *observation during assessment*
0 able to sit still
1 reports difficulty sitting still, but is able to do so
3 frequent shifting or extraneous movements of legs/arms
5 unable to sit still for more than a few seconds

GI Upset: *over last half hour*
0 no GI symptoms
1 stomach cramps
2 nausea or loose stool
3 vomiting or diarrhea
5 multiple episodes of diarrhea or vomiting

Tremor: *observation of outstretched hands*
0 no tremor
1 tremor can be felt but not observed
2 slight tremor observable
4 gross tremor or muscle twitching

Yawning: *observation during assessment*
0 no yawning
1 yawning once or twice during assessment
2 yawning three or more times during assessment
4 yawning several times/minute

Pupil Size:

0 pupils pinned or normal size for room light
1 pupils possibly larger than normal for room light
2 pupils moderately dilated
5 pupils so dilated that only the rim of the iris is visible

Bone or Joint Aches: *if patient was having pain previously, only the additional component attributed to opiate withdrawal is scored*

0 not present
1 mild diffuse discomfort
2 patient reports severe diffuse aching of joints/muscles
4 patient is rubbing joints or muscles and is unable to sit still because of discomfort

Runny Nose or Tearing: *not accounted for by cold symptoms or allergies*

0 not present
1 nasal stuffiness or unusually moist eyes
2 nose running or tearing
4 nose constantly running or tears streaming down cheeks

Anxiety or Irritability:

0 none
1 patient reports increasing irritability or anxiousness
2 patient obviously irritable or anxious
4 patient so irritable or anxious that participation in the assessment is difficult

Gooseflesh Skin:

0 skin is smooth
3 piloerection of skin can be felt or hairs standing up on arms
5 prominent piloerection

Total Score _____
The total score is the sum of all 11 items

Initials of person completing assessment: _____

Score: 5–12 = mild; 13–24 = moderate; 25–36 = moderately severe; more than 36 = severe withdrawal
This version may be copied and used clinically.

Figure 5–5. Clinical Opiate Withdrawal Scale.

Source. Reprinted from Wesson DR, Ling W: "The Clinical Opiate Withdrawal Scale (COWS)." *Journal of Psychoactive Drugs* 35(2):253–259, 2003. Copyright © 2003, Taylor & Francis, Ltd. (http://www.tandfonline.com). Used with permission.

The pharmacological management of alcohol withdrawal involves the use of long-acting benzodiazepines, which results in reduced severity of withdrawal, incidence of delirium, and incidence of seizures (Mayo-Smith 1997). In practice, diazepam and chlordiazepoxide are the most widely used benzodiazepines, although it may be necessary to add haloperidol for severe agitation. The patient is given a loading dose of benzodiazepines to achieve a reduction in vital signs, although dosing is stopped if the patient becomes somnolent or difficult to rouse or has signs of respiratory depression with a respiratory rate of less than 10 per minute. The Clinical Institute Withdrawal Assessment for Alcohol, Revised (CIWA-Ar; Figure 5–4), can be used to assess and monitor the severity of withdrawal and guide management (Sullivan et al. 1989).

The management of opiate withdrawal may require medication-assisted treatment. Buprenorphine may be a consideration if the patient is experiencing at least moderate signs of withdrawal not less than 6 hours after last use, whereas methadone can only be used in the outpatient management of withdrawal in patients 18 years or older with opiate disorder or in the inpatient management of withdrawal related to narcotic treatment of pain in patients of any age without a substance use disorder. The consultant can use the Clinical Opiate Withdrawal Scale (COWS; Figure 5–5) to help monitor symptom severity in opiate withdrawal (Wesson and Ling 2003). Medication management of other illicit substances may involve use of benzodiazepines for disabling acute situation anxiety and/or antipsychotics for severe agitation or psychotic symptoms; these treatments are beyond the scope of this text.

Conclusion

Pediatric delirium is a common neurocognitive disorder associated with increased rates of morbidity and mortality in children and adolescents. It is crucial that consultants be knowledgeable about and vigilant for the clinical presentation of this troubling problem because early identification and intervention can significantly improve the patient's and family's experience while enhancing patient care quality and improving health care utilization.

References

Alvarez RV, Palmer C, Czaja AS, et al: Delirium is a common and early finding in patients in the pediatric cardiac intensive care unit. J Pediatr 195:206–212, 2018 29395177

American Academy of Child and Adolescent Psychiatry: In the pediatric hospital: delirium in children and adolescents. 2017. Available at: https://uploads-ssl.webflow.com/5b0849daec50243a0a1e5e0c/5bb3799ac6dad8fe76ea72b0_DeliriumFlyer-AA-CAP.pdf. Accessed March 15, 2019.

American Psychiatric Association: Diagnostic and Statistical Manual of Mental Disorders, 5th Edition. Arlington, VA, American Psychiatric Association, 2013

Barbor TF, Higgins-Biddle JC, Saunders JB, et al: AUDIT the Alcohol Use Disorders Identification Test: Guidelines for Use in Primary Health Care, 2nd Edition. Geneva, World Health Organization, 2001

Beliles KE: Alternative routes of administration of psychotropic medications, in Psychiatric Care of the Medical Patient, 2nd Edition. Edited by Stoudemire A, Fogel BS, Greenberg DB. New York, Oxford University Press, 2000, pp 395–405

Carrasco G, Baeza N, Cabré L, et al: Dexmedetomidine for the treatment of hyperactive delirium refractory to haloperidol in nonintubated ICU patients: a nonrandomized controlled trial. Crit Care Med 44(7):1295–1306, 2016 26925523

Center for Adolescent Substance Abuse Research (CeASAR): The CRAFFT Questionnaire, Version 2.1. 2018. Available at: https://ceasar.childrenshospital.org/wp-content/uploads/2018/04/CRAFFT-2.1_Selfadministered_2018-04-23.pdf. Accessed March 15, 2019.

Chen S, Shi L, Liang F, et al: Exogenous melatonin for delirium prevention: a meta-analysis of randomized controlled trials. Mol Neurobiol 53(6):4046–4053, 2016 26189834

Crawford JL, Wortzel JR, Goldsmith M, Shaw RJ: Pediatric delirium in complex disorders, in Pediatric Psychiatry: A Clinician's Guide. Edited by Driver DI, Thomas SS. Philadephia, PA, Elsevier Saunders, 2017, pp 135–154

Davydow DS: Symptoms of depression and anxiety after delirium. Psychosomatics 50(4):309–316, 2009 19687169

Ducharme C, Carnevale FA, Clermont M-S, et al: A prospective study of adverse reactions to the weaning of opioids and benzodiazepines among critically ill children. Intensive Crit Care Nurs 21(3):179–186, 2005 15907670

Gangopadhyay M, Smith H, Pao M, et al: Development of the Vanderbilt Assessment for Delirium in Infants and Children to standardize pediatric delirium assessment by psychiatrists. Psychosomatics 58(4):355–363, 2017 28506544

Goldsmith M, Ortiz-Rubio P, Staveski S, et al: Delirium, in Textbook of Interdisciplinary Pediatric Palliative Care, 1st Edition. Edited by Wolfe J, Hinds P, Sourkes B. Philadelphia, PA, Elsevier Saunders, 2011, pp 251–265

Grover S, Ghosh A, Ghormode D: Do patients of delirium have catatonic features? An exploratory study. Psychiatry Clin Neurosci 68(8):644–651, 2014 24521083

Han C-S, Kim Y-K: A double-blind trial of risperidone and haloperidol for the treatment of delirium. Psychosomatics 45(4):297–301, 2004 15232043

Hatherill S, Flisher AJ: Delirium in children and adolescents: A systematic review of the literature. J Psychosom Res 68(4):337–344, 2010 20307700

Hunt N, Stern TA: The association between intravenous haloperidol and Torsades de Pointes. Three cases and a literature review. Psychosomatics 36(6):541–549, 1995 7501784

Kain ZN, MacLaren JE, Herrmann L, et al: Preoperative melatonin and its effects on induction and emergence in children undergoing anesthesia and surgery. Anesthesiology 111(1):44–49, 2009 19546692

Knight JR, Sherritt L, Shrier LA, et al: Validity of the CRAFFT substance abuse screening test among adolescent clinic patients. Arch Pediatr Adolesc Med 156(6):607–614, 2002 12038895

Luther R, McLeod A: The effect of chronotherapy on delirium in critical care—a systematic review. Nurs Crit Care 23(6):283–290, 2018 28508438

Mason KP, Lerman J: Review article: Dexmedetomidine in children: current knowledge and future applications. Anesth Analg 113(5):1129–1142, 2011 21821507

Mayo-Smith MF; American Society of Addiction Medicine Working Group on Pharmacological Management of Alcohol Withdrawal: Pharmacological management of alcohol withdrawal. A meta-analysis and evidence-based practice guideline. JAMA 278(2):144–151, 1997 9214531

Menza MA, Murray GB, Holmes VF, et al: Decreased extrapyramidal symptoms with intravenous haloperidol. J Clin Psychiatry 48(7):278–280, 1987 3597329

Meyburg J, Dill ML, Traube C, et al: Patterns of postoperative delirium in children. Pediatr Crit Care Med 18(2):128–133, 2017 27776085

Mody K, Kaur S, Mauer EA, et al: Benzodiazepines and development of delirium in critically ill children: estimating the causal effect. Crit Care Med 46(9):1486–1491, 2018 29727363

Morrissey M, Collier E: Literature review of post-traumatic stress disorder in the critical care population. J Clin Nurs 25(11–12):1501–1514, 2016 27108662

Oldham MA, Lee HB: Catatonia vis-à-vis delirium: the significance of recognizing catatonia in altered mental status. Gen Hosp Psychiatry 37(6):554–559, 2015 26162545

Pandharipande PP, Pun BT, Herr DL, et al: Effect of sedation with dexmedetomidine vs lorazepam on acute brain dysfunction in mechanically ventilated patients: the MENDS randomized controlled trial. JAMA 298(22):2644–2653, 2007 18073360

Patel AK, Bell MJ, Traube C: Delirium in pediatric critical care. Pediatr Clin North Am 64(5):1117–1132, 2017a 28941539

Patel AK, Biagas KV, Clarke EC, et al: Delirium in children after cardiac bypass surgery. Pediatr Crit Care Med 18(2):165–171, 2017b 27977539

Patel J, Baldwin J, Bunting P, et al: The effect of a multicomponent multidisciplinary bundle of interventions on sleep and delirium in medical and surgical intensive care patients. Anaesthesia 69(6):540–549, 2014 24813132

Reade MC, Eastwood GM, Bellomo R, et al; DahLIA Investigators; Australian and New Zealand Intensive Care Society Clinical Trials Group: Effect of dexmedetomidine added to standard care in ventilator-free time in patients with agitated delirium: a randomized clinical trial. JAMA 315(14):1460–1468, 2016 26975647

Rosebush PI, Mazurek MF: Catatonia and its treatment. Schizophr Bull 36(2):239–242, 2010 19969591

Schweickert WD, Pohlman MC, Pohlman AS, et al: Early physical and occupational therapy in mechanically ventilated, critically ill patients: a randomised controlled trial. Lancet 373(9678):1874–1882, 2009 19446324

Sessler CN, Gosnell MS, Grap MJ, et al: The Richmond Agitation-Sedation Scale: validity and reliability in adult intensive care unit patients. Am J Respir Crit Care Med 166(10):1338–1344, 2002 12421743

Silver G, Kearney JA, Kutko MC, et al: Infant delirium in pediatric critical care settings. Am J Psychiatry 167(10):1172–1177, 2010 20889664

Silver G, Traube C, Kearney J, et al: Detecting pediatric delirium: development of a rapid observational assessment tool. Intensive Care Med 38(6):1025–1031, 2012 22407142

Silver G, Kearney J, Traube C, et al: Delirium screening anchored in child development: The Cornell Assessment for Pediatric Delirium. Palliat Support Care 13(4):1005–1011, 2015a 25127028

Silver G, Traube C, Gerber LM, et al: Pediatric delirium and associated risk factors: a single-center prospective observational study. Pediatr Crit Care Med 16(4):303–309, 2015b 25647240

Smith HA, Fuchs DC, Pandharipande PP, et al: Delirium: an emerging frontier in the management of critically ill children. Crit Care Clin 25(3):593–614, 2009 19576533

Smith HA, Boyd J, Fuchs DC, et al: Diagnosing delirium in critically ill children: validity and reliability of the Pediatric Confusion Assessment Method for the Intensive Care Unit. Crit Care Med 39(1):150–157, 2011 20959783

Smith HA, Gangopadhyay M, Goben CM, et al: The Preschool Confusion Assessment Method for the ICU: valid and reliable delirium monitoring for critically ill infants and children. Crit Care Med 44(3):592–600, 2016 26565631

Sullivan JT, Sykora K, Schneiderman J, et al: Assessment of alcohol withdrawal: the revised clinical institute withdrawal assessment for alcohol scale (CIWA-Ar). Br J Addict 84(11):1353–1357, 1989 2597811

Traube C, Silver G, Kearney J, et al: Cornell Assessment of Pediatric Delirium: a valid, rapid, observational tool for screening delirium in the PICU. Crit Care Med 42(3):656–663, 2014 24145848

Traube C, Mauer EA, Gerber LM, et al: Cost associated with pediatric delirium in the ICU. Crit Care Med 44(12):e1175–e1179, 2016 27518377

Traube C, Silver G, Gerber LM, et al: Delirium and mortality in critically ill children: epidemiology and outcomes of pediatric delirium. Crit Care Med 45(5):891–898, 2017a 28288026

Traube C, Silver G, Reeder RW, et al: Delirium in critically ill children: an international point prevalence study. Crit Care Med 45(4):584–590, 2017b 28079605

Turkel SB: Delirium, in Textbook of Pediatric Psychosomatic Medicine. Edited by Shaw RJ, DeMaso DR. Arlington, VA, American Psychiatric Publishing, 2010, pp 63–75

Turkel SB: Pediatric delirium: recognition, management, and outcome. Curr Psychiatry Rep 19(12):101, 2017 29110102

Turkel SB, Hanft A: The pharmacologic management of delirium in children and adolescents. Paediatr Drugs 16(4):267–274, 2014 24898718

Turkel SB, Tavaré CJ: Delirium in children and adolescents. J Neuropsychiatry Clin Neurosci 15(4):431–435, 2003 14627769

Turkel SB, Trzepacz PT, Tavaré CJ: Comparison of delirium symptoms across the life cycle. Psychosomatics 45:162, 2004

Turkel SB, Trzepacz PT, Tavaré CJ: Comparing symptoms of delirium in adults and children. Psychosomatics 47(4):320–324, 2006 16844890

Turkel SB, Jacobson J, Munzig E, et al: Atypical antipsychotic medications to control the symptoms of delirium in children and adolescents. J Child Adolesc Psychopharm 22(2):126–130, 2012 22364403

Wesson DR, Ling W: The clinical opiate withdrawal scale (COWS). J Psychoactive Drugs 35(2):253–259, 2003 12924748

World Health Organization: Adolescent Use Disorders Test (AUDIT). 2001. Available at: https://www.drugabuse.gov/sites/default/files/files/AUDIT.pdf. Accessed March 15, 2019.

Zaal IJ, Devlin JW, Hazelbag M, et al: Benzodiazepine-associated delirium in critically ill adults. Intensive Care Med 41(12):2130–2137, 2015 26404392

6

Neurocognitive Disturbances

Although delirium is the most common neurocognitive disorder in the pediatric setting (see Chapter 5, "Delirium"), there are other important neurocognitive disturbances that may precipitate consultation for assistance in assessment and management. As is the case with delirium, the underlying pathophysiology and etiology of these disturbances are generally known. In these disturbances, the potentially affected neurocognitive domains include complex attention, executive function, learning and memory, language, perceptual-motor function, and social cognition (American Psychiatric Association 2013). Catatonia, neuroleptic malignant syndrome (NMS), serotonin syndrome, autoimmune encephalitis (AIE), and pediatric acute-onset neuropsychiatric syndrome (PANS) are reviewed in this chapter.

Catatonia

First reported in the early 1900s, catatonia continues to be seen in the pediatric setting. Early recognition, differential diagnosis, and treatment of catatonia are essential given the high rates of mortality. Although catatonia was originally conceptualized as a psychiatric condition commonly associated with autism spectrum, schizophrenia, and mood disorders, up to 20% of cases have been found to be secondary to an underlying medical condition, including autoimmune disorders or encephalitis, or to have drug-related etiologies (Consoli et al. 2012; Hauptman and Benjamin, 2016).

Epidemiology

Epidemiological studies have suggested that catatonia prevalence rates vary between 0.6% and 17% in child psychiatric inpatients; these rates are somewhat lower than the 10% reported in adult psychiatric inpatient facilities (Cohen et al. 1999). Catatonia is more common in boys (in adults, women are more affected) and is more prevalent in cases of early-onset schizophrenia. The morbidity and mortality rates associated with catatonia are high, and rates of suicide are increased.

Clinical Presentation

Whether catatonia is associated with another mental disorder or due to another medical condition, the DSM-5 diagnosis of catatonia requires the presence of three or more of the following 12 symptoms: stupor, catalepsy, waxy flexibility, mutism, negativism, posturing, mannerism, stereotypy, agitation, grimacing, echolalia, and echopraxia (see definitions in Table 6–1) (American Psychiatric Association 2013). Weiss et al. (2012) have grouped catatonia cases into three categories based on psychomotor activity: retarded (stupor and repetitive movements), excited (agitation and delirium), and malignant (autonomic instability including hypertension, elevated heart rate, and rise in temperature). Patients generally present with an acute onset, with symptoms of refusal to eat or drink and intermittent motor rigidity (Weiss et al. 2012). There is some evidence that younger children are more likely to present with ambiguous symptoms, including agitation, tantrums, and vague behavior changes, whereas adolescents present with more classic adult symptoms (Florance et al. 2009).

Pathophysiology

Although a wide range of theories have been proposed to explain the phenomenon of catatonia, dysfunction in the γ-aminobutyric acid (GABA), dopamine,

Table 6–1.   DSM-5 criterion A symptoms for catatonia

Stupor: no psychomotor activity; not actively relating to environment

Catalepsy: passive induction of a posture held against gravity

Waxy flexibility: slight, even resistance to positioning by examiner

Mutism: no, or very little, verbal response (exclude if known aphasia)

Negativism: opposition or no response to instructions or external stimuli

Posturing: spontaneous and active maintenance of a posture
  against gravity

Mannerism: odd, circumstantial caricature of normal actions

Stereotypy: repetitive, abnormally frequent, non-goal-directed
  movements

Agitation, not influenced by external stimuli

Grimacing

Echolalia: mimicking another's speech

Echopraxia: mimicking another's movements

Source.   American Psychiatric Association: *Diagnostic and Statistical Manual of Mental Disorders,*
5th Edition. Arlington, VA, American Psychiatric Association, 2013. Copyright © 2013, American Psychiatric Association. Used with permission.

and glutamine circuits between the prefrontal cortex and the hypothalamus appears to play a central role (Hauptman and Benjamin 2016). However, given the multiple etiologies of catatonia, which include infectious, autoimmune, inflammatory, and paraneoplastic conditions, it is likely that the underlying pathophysiology is complex.

Differential Diagnosis

Pediatric Conditions

Table 6–2 lists many of the potential psychiatric and pediatric etiologies for malignant catatonia or for NMS (reviewed later in this chapter). Early recognition and a search for underlying pathophysiological etiologies are essential given the high rates of morbidity and mortality associated with many of the underlying pediatric conditions. For example, autoimmune encephalitis, paraneoplastic conditions, malignant catatonia, NMS, serotonin syndrome, substance-induced catatonia, and complex partial status epilepticus are serious conditions that are amenable to treatment (Hauptman and Benjamin 2016).

Psychiatric Disorders

Catatonia has been reported in a wide range of patients with a number of psychiatric disorders, including major depressive, schizophrenia spectrum, and bipolar disorders. There is an association with neurodevelopmental disorders, including autism spectrum disorder and intellectual disability. Over 30% of adolescent inpatients with catatonia have a history of developmental disorders, and 12%–17% of adolescents diagnosed with autism have catatonia (Hauptman and Benjamin 2016; Wing and Shah 2000). DSM-5 recognizes the presence of catatonia as a subtype of autism spectrum disorder. Catatonia has also been reported in several genetic disorders, including Prader-Willi, Kleine-Levin, fragile X, velocardiofacial, and Down syndromes.

Assessment

The Bush-Francis Catatonia Rating Scale (Bush et al. 1996; Fink 1990) was developed to help evaluate the severity of catatonia as well as track the responses of patients to treatment (available at: http://www.psychtools.info/bfcrs/, accessed January 29, 2019). More recently, Benarous et al. (2016) have validated the use of the Pediatric Catatonia Rating Scale. Factor analysis of the scale generated four factors in line with previous findings in adults: negative withdrawal, catalepsy, abnormal movements, and echo phenomenon (see Table 6–3).

Treatment

Treatment of catatonia should always include a response to the underlying pediatric condition (e.g., immunomodulatory treatment for encephalitis, antiviral treatment for viral infections, tumor resection) and/or psychiatric disorder (e.g., antipsychotic for schizophrenia). It may also be necessary to provide supportive interventions, which include ventilation, management of hyperthermia, and vasopressors in the setting of the intensive care unit (Hauptman and Benjamin 2016).

Table 6–2. Differential diagnosis for malignant catatonia or neuroleptic malignant syndrome

Primary psychiatric disorders

Acute psychosis

Conversion disorder

Dissociative disorder

Schizophrenia

Neurodevelopmental disorder

Autoimmune disorder

Systemic lupus erythematosus

Infectious disorders

Bacterial sepsis

Borrelia

Brain abscess

Encephalitis (idiopathic and anti–NMDA receptor encephalitis)

Glioma

Hepatic amebiasis

HIV encephalopathy

Malaria

Meningitis

Rabies

Tertiary syphilis

Tetanus

Typhoid fever

Viral hepatitis

Cerebrovascular conditions

Angioma

Basilar artery thrombosis

Bilateral infarction of the anterior cingulate gyrus

Bilateral infarction of the temporal lobes

CNS vasculitis (e.g., systemic lupus erythematosus)

CNS disorders

Cerebral anoxia

Closed head injury

Delirium

Lethal catatonia

Normal pressure hydrocephalus

Nonconvulsive status epilepticus

Parkinsonism hyperthermia syndrome in Parkinson's disease

Seizure disorder

Stroke involving brain stem or basal ganglia

Surgery involving the hypothalamus

Nutritional disorder

Vitamin B_{12} deficiency

Table 6–2.   Differential diagnosis for malignant catatonia or neuroleptic malignant syndrome *(continued)*

Drug-induced disorders

Anticholinergic delirium

Anticonvulsants

Antipsychotic agents

Corticosteroids

Disulfiram

Drug-drug interaction

Extrapyramidal side effects

Lithium

Metoclopramide

Malignant hyperthermia (in surgical settings following anesthesia)

3,4-Methylenedioxymethamphetamine (MDMA, or ecstasy)

Sedative-hypnotic withdrawal

Tetrabenazine

Toxicities

Amphetamines

Hallucinogens

Heavy metals (lead, arsenic)

Salicylates

Serotonin syndrome

Stimulants (amphetamines, methylphenidate)

Metabolic disorders

Acute intermittent porphyria

Addison's disease

Cushing's disease

Uremia

Endocrine disorders

Addison's disease

Cushing's disease

Diabetic ketoacidosis

Hyperthyroidism

Pheochromocytoma

Thyrotoxicosis

Environmental condition

Heatstroke

Note.   CNS = central nervous system; NMDA = *N*-methyl-D-aspartate.
Source.   Adapted from Freudenreich et al. 2019, pp. 270–271; Ghaziuddin et al. 2017; Pileggi and Cook 2016; Velamoor 2017.

Table 6–3. Pediatric Catatonia Rating Scale

1. **Catalepsy:** Passive induction of a posture held against gravity
    0 = Absent
    1 = Less than 1 minute
    2 = Greater than 1 minute, less than 15 minutes
    3 = More than 15 minutes

2. **Stupor:** Extreme hypoactivity, immobile, minimally responsive to stimuli
    0 = Absent
    1 = Sits abnormally still, may interact briefly
    2 = Virtually no interaction with external world
    3 = Nonreactive to painful stimuli

3. **Posturing:** Active and/or spontaneous maintenance of a posture against gravity
    0 = Absent
    1 = Less than 1 minute
    2 = Greater than 1 minute, less than 15 minutes
    3 = More than 15 minutes

4. **Waxy flexibility:** Slight and even resistance to positioning by examiner
    0 = Absent
    3 = Present

5. **Staring:** Fixed gaze, little visual scanning of environment, decreased blinking
    0 = Absent
    1 = Poor eye contact, decreased blinking
    2 = Gaze held longer than 20 seconds, occasionally shifts attention
    3 = Fixed gaze, nonreactive

6. **Negativism:** Opposing or not responding to instructions or external stimuli
    0 = Absent
    1 = Mild resistance and/or occasionally contrary
    2 = Moderate resistance and/or frequently contrary
    3 = Severe resistance and/or continually contrary

7. **Stereotypes:** Repetitive, abnormally frequent, non-goal-directed movements
    0 = Absent
    1 = Occasional
    2 = Frequent
    3 = Constant

Table 6–3.   Pediatric Catatonia Rating Scale *(continued)*

8. **Excitement:** Extreme hyperactivity, constant motor unrest which is apparently nonpurposeful. Not to be attributed to akathisia or goal-directed agitation
    0 = Absent
    1 = Excessive motion
    2 = Constant motion, hyperkinetic without rest periods
    3 = Full-blown catatonic excitements, endless frenzied motor activity

9. **Automatic compulsive movements:** Involuntary muscle activity exhibited in posture, attitudes, mimic, or gesture due to inhibition or forced motor action
    0 = Absent
    1 = Occasional
    2 = Frequent
    3 = Constant

10. **Rigidity:** Maintenance of a rigid position despite efforts to be moved, exclude if cogwheeling or tremor present
    0 = Absent
    1 = Mild resistance
    2 = Moderate
    3 = Severe, cannot be repostured

11. **Withdrawal:** Refusal to make eye contact and not responding to nonverbal communication
    0 = Absent
    1 = Occasional
    2 = Frequent
    3 = Constant

12. **Mutism:** No, or very little, verbal response; not applicable if there is an established aphasia
    0 = Absent
    1 = Verbally unresponsive to majority of questions, incomprehensible whispers
    2 = Speaks less than 20 words/5 minutes
    3 = No speech

13. **Mannerisms:** Odd caricature of normal actions
    0 = Absent
    1 = Occasional
    2 = Frequent
    3 = Constant

Table 6–3.   Pediatric Catatonia Rating Scale *(continued)*

14. **Echopraxia:** Mimicking another's movements
    0 = Absent
    1 = Occasional
    2 = Frequent
    3 = Constant

15. **Echolalia:** Mimicking another's speech
    0 = Absent
    1 = Occasional
    2 = Frequent
    3 = Constant

16. **Incontinence:** Nocturnal enuresis, daytime urinary incontinence, or fecal
    incontinence
    0 = Absent (or no recent worsening)
    1 = Nocturnal and/or occasionally diurnal
    2 = Frequently diurnal
    3 = Constant

17. **Verbigeration:** Repetition of phrases or sentences, like a scratched record
    0 = Absent
    1 = Occasional
    2 = Frequent
    3 = Constant

18. **Schizophasia:** Scrambled speech, word salad, seemingly random words and
    phrases linked
    0 = Absent
    1 = Occasional
    2 = Frequent
    3 = Constant

19. **Acrocyanosis:** Cyanosis of the extremities
    0 = Absent
    1 = Occasional
    2 = Frequent
    3 = Constant

20. **Refusal to eat, drink:** Severe decrease of daily food or drink intake
    0 = Absent
    1 = Minimal po intake for less than 1 day
    2 = Minimal po intake for more than 1 day
    3 = No po intake for 1 day or more

Source. Reprinted from Benarous et al. Copyright © 2016, Schizophrenia International Research Society. Used with permission from Elsevier.

Benzodiazepines

Benzodiazepines are the first-line treatment of catatonia. In the inpatient setting, intravenous administration of lorazepam, often in high doses, can ameliorate the symptoms while the pediatric workup is in progress (Hauptman and Benjamin 2016). It is common to administer a test dose of lorazepam as a "challenge test" to help determine whether the patient is likely to respond and to help differentiate symptoms from other conditions, such as delirium (Dhossche and Wachtel 2010). Treatment may need to be prolonged, especially in complex pediatric conditions such as autoimmune encephalitis, because premature withdrawal of benzodiazepines may result in a recurrence of symptoms. There are limited data on the use of zolpidem to treat catatonia in adult patients when lorazepam is not well tolerated (Peglow et al. 2013).

Electroconvulsive Therapy

The American Psychiatric Association Task Force on Electroconvulsive Therapy (ECT) (1990) has recommended the use of ECT in children and adolescents in whom other treatments either have been ineffective or cannot be safely administered. Studies suggest a response rate of 80%–100% for all patients, with pediatric patients often responding well to lower thresholds (Hauptman and Benjamin 2016). ECT can be a lifesaving and relatively safe treatment for catatonia in the context of underlying complex medical conditions, including anti–N-methyl-D-aspartate (NMDA) receptor encephalopathy, lupus cerebritis, and status epilepticus, as well as in children with developmental disabilities. ECT side effects include immediate confusion, headache, and memory loss. Knowledge of restrictions on the use of ECT in certain states or countries is necessary; sometimes families pursue out-of-state treatment for refractory catatonia.

N-Methyl-D-Aspartate Blockade

NMDA antagonists, such as amantadine and memantine, are second-line agents used for catatonia that is not responsive to benzodiazepines or ECT (Sani et al. 2012).

Neuroleptics

Atypical antipsychotics have been used to treat catatonia in pediatric patients in the context of schizophrenia, persistent major depression, and bipolar disorder (Lima et al. 2013). However, caution needs to be exercised because neuroleptics have the potential to worsen catatonia or even lead to the development of NMS (see below). Therefore, the use of neuroleptics is recommended only after benzodiazepines and ECT have been tried.

Immunomodulation

Catatonia in the context of anti–NMDA receptor encephalitis may require treatment with immunomodulatory treatment, including corticosteroids, immunoglobulin, rituximab, cyclophosphamide, and plasmapheresis.

Neuroleptic Malignant Syndrome

First recognized in the 1960s, NMS is a rare and potentially fatal reaction that may occur during treatment with antipsychotic agents (Pileggi and Cook 2016). Two-thirds of patients developing NMS have symptoms within the first week of treatment, and in most cases symptoms start within the first month (Velamoor 2017); however, some patients can develop NMS after months or years of treatment with the same antipsychotic agent. Although the syndrome was named with reference to the neuroleptic, or first-generation, antipsychotic agents, it also occurs during treatment with atypical, or second-generation, antipsychotic agents.

Epidemiology

NMS has been estimated to occur in 0.2%–1% of patients treated with dopamine antagonists. A study of second-generation antipsychotics found an incidence of 0.02%–0.03% (Sahlholm et al. 2016). Malnutrition and dehydration may increase the risk of NMS in the context of neurocognitive disorders (e.g., delirium or dementia) that are being treated with lithium and antipsychotic agents. Mortality rates are elevated, often because of respiratory failure, cardiovascular collapse, renal failure, arrhythmias, and thromboembolism. Although early recognition has improved outcomes, a mortality rate of 5.6% has been estimated (Ghaziuddin et al. 2017; Modi et al. 2016).

Clinical Presentation

NMS symptoms include hyperthermia, lead pipe muscle rigidity, altered mental status (reduced or fluctuating level of consciousness), and autonomic instability (Velamoor 2017). Other symptoms include tremor, incontinence, and profuse diaphoresis, along with changes in heart rate and blood pressure. Accepted consensus diagnostic criteria developed by a panel of experts are shown in Table 6–4. However, diagnosis can be delayed because the presentation does not follow a predictable sequence and because other pediatric issues, such as fever, may obscure the clinical diagnosis early on (Pileggi and Cook 2016). Hyperthermia on at least two occasions associated with profuse diaphoresis is a distinguishing feature of NMS, setting it apart from the other neurological side effects of antipsychotic medications (American Psychiatric Association 2013).

Characteristic laboratory findings include elevated serum creatine kinase levels, often above 1,000 $\mu g/L^2$, and leukocytosis. Complications include rhabdomyolysis with acute renal injury, cardiac failure, respiratory failure requiring ventilatory support, aspiration and pneumonia, dehydration, disseminated intravascular coagulation, sepsis, and/or long-term cognitive sequelae due to hypoxia and prolonged hyperthermia (Velamoor 2017). Common risk factors for NMS are listed in Table 6–5.

Pathophysiology

Common hypotheses regarding NMS pathophysiology include blockage of dopamine D_2 receptors in the nigrostriatal, hypothalamic, and mesolimbic/cortical pathways, which may explain the symptoms of rigidity, hyperthermia, and altered mental status (Pileggi and Cook 2016). However, other theories include sympathoadrenal dysfunction, imbalance in norepinephrine, GABA and serotonin syndromes, and a direct toxic effect on musculoskeletal fibers (Mann et al. 2000).

Differential Diagnosis

The differentiation of NMS from catatonia can prove difficult because they may well be variants of the same disorder sharing a common pathophysiological pathway (Lang et al. 2015; Velamoor 2017). Further evidence of this assumption is the fact that NMS and catatonia share the same list of potential etiologies (see Table 6–2). The manifestations of NMS must also be differentiated from serotonin and anticholinergic syndromes (Table 6–6). NMS has been reported in other neurological disorders (e.g., Wilson's disease; Parkinson's disease treated with dopamine-blocking agents). It may occur in patients treated with dopamine antagonists given for nausea (i.e., metoclopramide and prochlorperazine).

Table 6–4. Consensus diagnostic criteria for neuroleptic malignant syndrome

Exposure to dopamine antagonist or dopamine antagonist withdrawal within past 72 hours

Hyperthermia (>100.4°F or >38.0°C on at least two occasions measured orally)

Rigidity

Mental status alteration (reduced or fluctuating level of consciousness)

Creatine kinase elevations at least four times the upper limit of normal

Sympathetic nervous system lability defined as at least two of the following:

Blood pressure elevation ≥20 mmHg above baseline

Blood pressure fluctuation ≥20 mmHg diastolic change or ≥25 mmHg systolic change within 24 hours

Diaphoresis

Urinary incontinence

Hypermetabolism defined as heart rate increase (≥25% above baseline)

Respiratory rate increase (≥50% above baseline)

Negative workup for infectious, toxic, metabolic, or neurological causes

Source. American Psychiatric Association 2013; Gurrera et al. 2017; Velamoor 2017. Adapted from Gurrera RJ, Mortillaro G, Velamoor V, et al.: "A Validation Study of the International Consensus Diagnostic Criteria for Neuroleptic Malignant Syndrome." *Journal of Clinical Psychopharmacology* 37(1):67–71, 2017. Copyright © 2017, Wolters Kluwer/Lippincott Williams & Wilkins. Used with permission.

Assessment

In the assessment of a patient for NMS, investigations should include a complete blood cell count (leukocytosis), electrolyte levels (metabolic disturbance due to acidosis or renal impairment), arterial blood gas analysis (acid base balance), liver function tests (lactic dehydrogenase), creatine kinase, urine analysis (myoglobin), coagulations studies, blood culture (to rule out sepsis), and urine toxicology screen, as well as computed tomography imaging and electroencephalography studies (Velamoor 2017).

Table 6–5.   Risk factors for neuroleptic malignant syndrome (NMS)

Environmental

Prolonged heat exposure

Use of patient restraints

Dehydration

Surgical intervention

Patient specific

Alcohol intoxication and withdrawal

Electrolyte imbalance (vomiting, diarrhea)

Exhaustion

Family history of NMS or dystonic reactions

Increased age

Organic brain syndrome

Malnutrition

Medical comorbidity

Mood disorders

Postpartum women

Prior history of NMS

Pharmacological

Antipsychotic treatment

Rapid dose escalation or high doses of antipsychotics

Intravenous administration of antipsychotics

Polypharmacy, especially in combination with lithium and anticholinergic agents

Rapid withdrawal of antipsychotics

Withdrawal of medications (Parkinson's disease)

Source.   Pileggi and Cook 2016; Velamoor 2017.

Table 6–6. Manifestations of severe serotonin, neuroleptic malignant, and anticholinergic syndromes

	Serotonin syndrome	Neuroleptic malignant syndrome	Anticholinergic syndrome
Medication	Serotonin agents	Dopamine antagonist	Anticholinergic agent
Time for condition to develop	< 12 hours	1–3 days	< 12 hours
Mental status	Agitation, coma	Stupor, alert, mutism, coma	Agitated delirium
Vital signs	Hypertension	Hypertension	Hypertension
	Tachycardia	Tachycardia	Tachycardia
	Tachypnea	Tachypnea	Tachypnea
	>41.1°C	>41.1°C	<38.8°C
Pupils	Mydriasis	Normal	Mydriasis
Mucosa	Sialorrhea	Sialorrhea	Dry
Skin	Diaphoresis	Diaphoresis, pallor	Erythema
Neuromuscular tone	Increased (lower extremities)	"Lead-pipe" rigidity (all muscle groups)	Normal

Source. Reprinted from Boyer EW, Shannon M: "The Serotonin Syndrome." *New England Journal of Medicine* 352:1112–1120, 2005. Copyright © 2005, Massachusetts Medical Society. All rights reserved. Used with permission.

Treatment

Early recognition, discontinuation of antipsychotic agents, and supportive treatment are the foundation of NMS treatment (Pileggi and Cook 2016). Intravenous hydration, correction of electrolyte abnormalities, cooling of the body (including through cooling blanket and use of antipyretics), protection of the airway, treatment of infections, and intubation in an intensive care unit can all be required. Calcium channel blockers can be helpful for labile hypertension (Tse et al. 2015).

Dantrolene

Dantrolene, a skeletal muscle relaxant that blocks calcium efflux from the sarcoplasmic reticulum, has been used for malignant hyperthermia and is commonly used in the treatment of NMS at an intravenous dose of 8–10 mg/kg body weight (Pileggi and Cook 2016). It is also used in combination with bromocriptine (discussed next). Although side effects include hepatitis with long-term use, dantrolene is generally well tolerated.

Bromocriptine

Bromocriptine, a postsynaptic D_2-receptor agonist used in Parkinson's disease, is used to counteract presumed dopamine blockage in NMS at an oral dose of 2.5–10 mg every 8 hours. Because of bromocriptine's potential to cause hypotension, it must be started at a low dose and titrated upward to a therapeutic dose.

Benzodiazepines

Lorazepam, diazepam, and clonazepam have all been used in the treatment of NMS. Benzodiazepines have the advantage of being available in oral, intramuscular, and intravenous formulations and may be effective as monotherapy.

Amantadine

Amantadine, which has anticholinergic side effects and is a weak NMDA receptor antagonist, is used as an adjunctive treatment for moderate to severe cases of NMS at a dose of 100 mg orally 2–4 times/day.

Electroconvulsive Therapy

ECT has been found useful in cases of NMS that are refractory to pharmacological treatment (Strawn et al. 2007). Most pediatric case studies have used bilateral electrode placement, as recommended by the American Academy of Child and Adolescent Psychiatry practice parameter for the use of ECT in minors (Ghaziuddin et al. 2004, 2017).

Neuroleptics

There is a reported 30% risk of NMS recurrence if the offending antipsychotic agent is restarted (Caroff and Mann 1999). Because of this high risk, patients with severe psychiatric disorders requiring ongoing antipsychotic treatment can be given a trial of low doses of a medication with low D_2 affinity after a washout period of at least 5–14 days.

Serotonin Syndrome

Serotonin syndrome, a potentially life-threatening condition precipitated by the use of serotonergic agents, can be a consequence of prescribed medications, accidental drug interactions, and/or intentional overdose (Simon and Keenaghan 2019). Although this syndrome is frequently overlooked, consultants should always consider the diagnosis in the pediatric setting, particularly in patients being prescribed combinations of serotonergic medications, or in cases with the potential for drug-drug interactions (see Chapter 17, "Psychopharmacological Approaches and Considerations"). Cases are frequently underdiagnosed and self-limiting, though there can be significant mortality in severe cases.

Epidemiology

The incidence of serotonin syndrome is unknown, although the increased use of serotonergic agents has increased its occurrence in the pediatric setting. It is important for consultants to keep this syndrome on the list of potential differential diagnoses in patients with acute mental status changes.

Clinical Presentation

Serotonin syndrome comprises a clinical triad of mental status change, autonomic hyperactivity, and neuromuscular excitation, although not all of these findings are present in all patients with this syndrome (Boyer and Shannon 2005; Brown et al. 2000). Of the various criteria for serotonin syndrome, the most widely accepted are the Hunter criteria (Table 6–7) (Dunkley et al. 2003). Signs and symptoms may include agitation, anxiety, restlessness, disorientation, diaphoresis, hyperthermia, tachycardia, nausea, vomiting, tremor, muscle rigidity, hyperreflexia, myoclonus, dilated pupils, ocular clonus, dry mucous membranes, flushed skin, increased bowel sounds, and bilateral Babinski signs (Simon and Keenaghan 2019). Altered mental status and autonomic dysfunction are present in approximately 40% of cases, while neuromuscular excitation is present in 50% (Iqbal et al. 2012). Symptoms of toxicity usually start within 1 hour of medication administration in 30% of patients and within 6 hours in 60% of patients (Mason et al. 2000). Clonus and hyperreflexia are generally more pronounced in the lower limbs (Uddin et al. 2017). Serotonin syndrome is usually self-limited and may resolve spontaneously after discontinuation of the serotonergic agents.

Etiology

The etiology of serotonin syndrome includes a wide range of commonly used drugs (Table 6–8) (Simon and Keenaghan 2019). Selective serotonin reuptake inhibitors (SSRIs), meperidine, tramadol, pentazocine, metoclopramide, valproate, carbamazepine, dextromethorphan, and cyclobenzaprine act by impairing the reuptake of serotonin from the synaptic cleft in the presynaptic neuron. Trazodone, bupropion, tricyclic antidepressants, and St. John's wort similarly impair serotonin reuptake. Monoamine oxidase inhibitors (MAOIs) (phenelzine, tranylcypromine, isocarboxazid, and selegiline), buspirone, ergot derivatives, fentanyl, and lysergic acid diethylamide (LSD) act as direct serotonin agonists. Tryptophan acts by increasing serotonin formation, whereas amphetamines, cocaine, 3,4-methylenedioxymethamphetamine (MDMA, or ecstasy), and levodopa increase serotonin release. Drug-drug interactions that can cause serotonin syndrome include linezolid (an antibiotic that has MAOI properties) and SSRIs, as well as combinations of SSRIs, trazodone, buspirone, venlafaxine, ondansetron, metoclopramide, and sumatriptan (Boyer and Shannon 2005).

Pathophysiology

Serotonin syndrome is hypothesized to be caused by excess serotonergic agonism of the central and peripheral nervous system serotonergic receptors. Stimulation of the postsynaptic 5-HT_{1A} and 5-HT_{2A} receptors from a single drug or combination of drugs produces serotonin syndrome (Simon and Keenaghan 2019). However, serum serotonin levels often do not correlate closely with clinical symptoms. Other neurotransmitters, including norepinephrine, GABA, and dopamine, and NMDA receptor antagonists may also be involved (Katus and Frucht 2016).

Table 6–7.   Hunter criteria for the diagnosis of serotonin syndrome

1.   History of exposure to a serotonergic drug

2.   Plus one or more of the following:

- Spontaneous clonus

- Inducible clonus with agitation and diaphoresis

- Ocular clonus with agitation and diaphoresis

- Tremor and hyperreflexia

- Hypertonia

- Temperature over 38°C with ocular or inducible clonus

Source.   Dunkley et al. 2003.

Assessment

Serotonin syndrome can be difficult to clinically separate from NMS and anticholinergic toxicity (see Table 6–6). However, clonus, bradyreflexia, and nausea and vomiting are not commonly seen in NMS. The diagnostic workup should include a complete blood count, electrolytes, blood urea nitrogen and creatinine, creatine phosphokinases, hepatic transaminases, coagulation studies, urinalysis, urine toxicology screen, neuroimaging, and lumbar puncture (Simon and Keenaghan 2019).

Treatment

The main treatment principles for serotonin syndrome include 1) discontinuing all serotonergic agents, 2) supportive care and normalization of vital signs, 3) sedation with benzodiazepines, and 4) administration of serotonin antagonists (Uddin et al. 2017). Antipyretics tend not to be effective. Severe cases require the control of agitation and autonomic instability (including hyperthermia, tachycardia, muscle rigidity, and dizziness). In rare cases, neuromuscular paralysis and intubation, as well as administration of 5-HT$_{2A}$ antagonists, including cyproheptadine given orally or via nasogastric tube, may be indicated. Caution needs to be exercised with the use of cyproheptadine because of side effects of sedation and hypotension.

Table 6–8.   Medications that can precipitate serotonin
                  syndrome

Class	Drugs
Antidepressants	Monoamine oxidase inhibitors:
	Phenelzine, tranylcypromine, selegiline, isocarboxazid, clorgiline
	Selective serotonin reuptake inhibitors:
	Citalopram, escitalopram, fluoxetine, fluvoxamine, sertraline
	Serotonin-norepinephrine reuptake inhibitors:
	Venlafaxine, desvenlafaxine, duloxetine
	Dopamine-norepinephrine reuptake inhibitors:
	Bupropion
	Tricyclic antidepressants:
	Amitriptyline, imipramine, desipramine, clomipramine
	Trazodone, vilazodone, nefazodone
Antiepileptics and mood stabilizers	Valproate
	Carbamazepine
	Lithium
Antimicrobials	Linezolid
	Ritonavir
Antiemetics	Metoclopramide
	Serotonin 5-HT$_3$ receptor antagonists:
	Ondansetron, dolasetron, granisetron, palonosetron
Migraine medications	Triptans:
	Sumatriptan, rizatriptan
	Ergot derivatives:
	Ergotamine, methylergonovine

Table 6–8. Medications that can precipitate serotonin syndrome *(continued)*

Class	Drugs
Pain medications	Opioids:
	Meperidine, tramadol, fentanyl, pentazocine
Illicit drugs	Amphetamines
	Cocaine
	3,4-Methylenedioxymethamphetamine (MDMA, or ecstasy)
	Lysergic acid diethylamide (LSD)
	Procarbazine
	Dextromethorphan
Other	Cyclobenzaprine
	Sibutramine
	Levodopa
	Amphetamine/amphetamine derivatives:
	Dextroamphetamine, fenfluramine, phentermine
Over-the-counter supplements	St. John's wort
	Ginseng
	Tryptophan

Source. Reprinted from Katus LE, Frucht SJ: "Management of Serotonin Syndrome and Neuroleptic Malignant Syndrome." *Current Treatment Options in Neurology* 18(9):39, 2016. Copyright © 2016, Springer. Used with permission.

Autoimmune Encephalitis

Autoimmune encephalitis (AIE) describes a group of inflammatory brain diseases which have subacute onset (within a 3-month time period) of neurocognitive symptoms affecting multiple domains and whose etiology is thought to be related to circulating autoantibodies that target areas of the central nervous system (CNS) (Mooneyham et al. 2018). Antibodies may target intracellular antigens, synaptic receptors, ion channels, and other cell-surface antigens

(Graus et al. 2016). For diagnostic criteria for one of the dozen or so identified subtypes of AIE to be met, patients must have changes in psychiatric symptoms, mental status, or short-term memory, along with new onset of seizures, focal CNS changes, pleocytosis in the cerebrospinal fluid (CSF), or magnetic resonance imaging (MRI) findings consistent with brain inflammation (Tran et al. 2018). An association with paraneoplastic processes, including ovarian or testicular teratoma, has been described (Brenton and Goodkin 2016).

Clinical Presentation

Symptoms routinely seen during the active phase of AIE include agitation, catatonia, delirium, seizures, psychotic symptoms including hallucinations, and changes in speech including mutism. As the disease progresses, it may lead to involuntary motor movements, respiratory compromise, autonomic instability, and, in severe cases, coma. Symptoms have an abrupt onset and may progress rapidly over time and include changes in cognition and memory, sleep disturbances, enuresis, encopresis developmental regression, and symptoms of anxiety, including those resembling obsessive-compulsive disorder (OCD). Disturbances in gait and balance and treatment-refractory seizures are also seen.

Assessment

Although there is no consensus regarding the battery of diagnostic tests for AIE, it is important to consider an extensive list of tests including tests of blood and cerebrospinal fluid as well as radiological and other tests (Table 6–9).

Differential Diagnosis

The differential diagnosis in AIE is extensive, including entities such as acute encephalitis and postinfectious encephalitis (Graus et al. 2016). In this section, we selectively review the following disorders that consultants may encounter: anti–NMDA receptor encephalitis, limbic encephalitis, Hashimoto's encephalopathy, and seronegative AIE.

Anti–NMDA Receptor Encephalitis

Anti–NMDA receptor encephalitis is a leading cause of seropositive AIE in children, with immunoglobulin G (IgG) antibodies directed against the GluN1

Table 6–9.   Laboratory evaluation considerations in suspected autoimmune encephalitis

Basic hematological and chemistry tests

Complete blood cell count

Electrolyte levels

Glucose level

Liver function tests

Thyroid function tests

Glucose level

Serum urea nitrogen

Creatinine level

Urinary analysis

Other laboratory test considerations based on clinical presentation

Angiotensin-converting enzyme level

Anti-Sm, anti-Ro, anti-La antibodies

Anti-DNAse B

Antistreptolysin O (ASO) titer

Antinuclear antibody

Antiphospholid antibodies

Antithyroid antibody panel

C-reactive protein test

Complement C3, C4

Creatine kinase

Erythrocyte sedimentation rate

Mycoplasma immunoglobulins G and M (IgG and IgM)

Serum autoimmune encephalitis antibody panel (NMDA, GAD 65, GABA, AMPA, VGKC)

Serum immunoglobulins

Serum ceruloplasmin 24-hour urine copper

Von Willebrand factor antigen

Table 6–9.   Laboratory evaluation considerations in suspected autoimmune encephalitis *(continued)*

Cerebrospinal fluid tests

Opening pressure

Cell count

Glucose

Protein

Gram stain

Culture and sensitivity

Angiotensin-converting enzyme level

CSF autoimmune encephalitis antibody panel (NMDA, GAD 65, GABA, AMPA, VGKC)

Oligoclonal bands/IgG index

CSF polymerase chain reaction for intro virus, herpes simplex virus, and zoster virus

Radiological and other tests

Electroencephalography

Magnetic resonance imaging (brain)

Positron emission tomography

Magnetic resonance angiography

Testicular/ovarian ultrasound

Note.   AMPA = α-amino-3-hydroxy-5-methyl-4-isoxazalepropionic acid; CSF = cerebrospinal fluid; GABA = γ=aminobutyric acid; GAD 65 = glutamic acid decarboxylase; NMDA = *N*-methyl-D-aspartate; VGKC = voltage-gated potassium channel.
Source.   Adapted from Mooneyham et al. 2018, p. 40; Tran et al. 2018, p. 172.

subunits of the NMDA receptor that are located in the forebrain and the hypothalamic-pituitary and limbic systems. This subtype of AIE accounts for 4% of all cases of AIE. Approximately 40% of these cases present in patients under age 18 years. It is more common in girls, but boys are more likely to be affected among patients under age 12 years. Up to 50% of the females are found to have ovarian teratoma (Armangue et al. 2012). It is hypothesized that inactivation of the GABA-ergic neurons, which have higher concentrations of NMDA receptors, may account for the symptoms. It is also possible that disinhibition of the basal ganglia can contribute to psychomotor agitation. Patients with this subtype of AIE frequently present first with psychiatric symptoms, including agitation.

Clinical presentation. Anti–NMDA receptor encephalitis commonly starts with the prodrome of fever and headaches lasting days to weeks, often without other symptoms, followed by the onset of behavioral and psychiatric symptoms (Figure 6–1). These include anxiety and sleep disturbance, psychotic symptoms, combative and disinhibited behavior, and catatonia (Mooneyham et al. 2018). Later, patients may develop seizures, movement disorders (including choreoathetosis, dystonia, and muscle rigidity), impaired level of consciousness, autonomic instability, and respiratory difficulties. Children under age 12 years may present with behavioral changes, including aggression and agitation, mutism, and dyskinesias, and seizures (Armangue et al. 2012). Either generalized or focal seizures occur in up to 80% of patients at onset (Brenton and Goodkin 2016). About 25% of patients have residual brain impairment, and the same percentage of patients experience a relapse.

Diagnosis. The presence of the NMDA-receptor antibody in the blood or CSF is the confirmatory test for this AIE subtype. The CSF may show elevated protein, oligoclonal bands, and lymphocytic pleocytosis. MRI may show increased signal T_2-weighted FLAIR (fluid-attenuated inversion recovery) in the medial aspect of the temporal lobes as well as leptomeningeal enhancement, whereas the electroencephalogram may show diffuse slowing. Seizures may be seen in up to 60% of cases (Wright and Vincent 2017). It is important to rule out infectious, metabolic, and other autoimmune etiologies for all patients and to request MRI of the abdomen and pelvis for female patients to screen for ovarian teratoma, which is present in approximately 30% of girls age 18 or younger with this AIE subtype (Brenton and Goodkin 2016).

Limbic Encephalitis

Limbic encephalitis (LE) affects the amygdala, hypothalamus, and other parts of the limbic system (Tran et al. 2018). Classic symptoms include the rapid development of confusion, working memory deficits, mood changes, and sei-

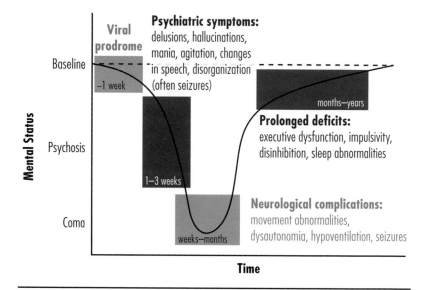

Figure 6–1.   Typical course of anti–NMDA receptor encephalitis.

Source.   Reprinted from Kayser MS, Dalmau J: "Anti-NMDA Receptor Encephalitis, Autoimmunity, and Psychosis." *Schizophrenia Research* 176(1):36–40, 2014, p. 37. Copyright © 2014, Schizophrenia International Research Society. Used with permission from Elsevier.

zures. The subacute development of short-term memory loss is considered the hallmark of this disorder, but it may not be identified because of the presence of other symptoms (Graus et al. 2016). LE has two commonly identified subtypes: voltage-gated potassium channel (VGKC) antibody encephalitis and anti-glutamic acid decarboxylase (GAD)–associated encephalitis.

Clinical presentation.   Adult patients with VGKC antibody encephalitis present with psychiatric symptoms, seizures, and subacute short-term memory loss (Tran et al. 2018). This subtype has not been defined as clearly in the pediatric population, although case series have shown that it does occur in pediatric patients. Symptoms generally include subacute cognitive and memory decline, medically refractory seizures or status epilepticus, and psychiatric symptoms. Presenting symptoms may include developmental regression.

Patients with GAD carboxylase encephalitis are predominantly young women (median age of 23 years) who have predominant focal seizures, cognitive and memory decline, progressive developmental delay, and psychiatric symptoms. There is no evidence of cancer as in anti–NMDA receptor encephalitis (Graus et al. 2016).

Diagnosis. This subtype of LE involves antibody activity targeted directly against neuronal proteins that couple with the transmembrane-selective potassium pore. Abnormalities evident on MRI include T_2-weighted FLAIR in the medial temporal lobes and hippocampal atrophy; electroencephalographic changes and pleocytosis in the CSF may support the diagnosis (Mooneyham et al. 2018).

Hashimoto's Encephalopathy

Hashimoto's encephalopathy (HE) has neurological and psychiatric symptoms associated with increased levels of antithyroid antibodies evident in both euthyroid and hypothyroid individuals. It is most commonly diagnosed in females, with a median age at diagnosis of 14 years. It is believed that the antithyroid antibodies may be markers of an autoimmune response rather than directly targeting thyroid or brain tissue. Given that some patients with HE respond well to corticosteroids, the term "steroid-responsive encephalopathy associated with autoimmune thyroiditis" is sometimes used.

Clinical presentation. HE has a diverse range of presentations, although in children the sudden onset of seizures is common (Mooneyham et al. 2018). Patients generally present, however, with the more insidious onset of altered consciousness and behavior changes such as aggression or labile mood, confusion, and hallucinations. Patients can also have cognitive decline and movement disorders.

Diagnosis. A diagnosis of HE is generally made following the identification of elevated antithyroid antibodies, including antithyroglobulin and antithyroid peroxidase serum antibodies. Many children have normal thyroid function. The CSF may show elevated protein levels, and the electroencephalogram may show slowing consistent with encephalopathy. MRI findings are generally normal in the majority of pediatric patients.

Seronegative Autoimmune Encephalitis

A subset of patients with suspected AIE have negative antibody testing. Data from the California Encephalitis Project indicate that 62% of encephalopathies are seronegative (Glaser et al. 2003). The diagnosis of seronegative autoimmune encephalitis is made on the basis of changes in mental status or short-term memory losses, rule-out of other AIE syndromes, and the absence of serum or CSF autoantibodies but the presence of specific MRI, CSF, or brain biopsy findings (Graus et al. 2016). Patients with this AEI subtype require particular vigilance because rapid treatment of the inflammatory response is required even in the absence of autoantibodies.

Treatment

Immunomodulatory Treatments

First-line treatment in suspected cases of AIE includes immunomodulatory treatment with intravenous steroids, intravenous immunoglobulin (IVIG), and plasmapheresis (Mooneyham et al. 2018). Systemic side effects of steroids are more frequently seen with oral steroids than with intermittent intravenous steroid pulses. Treatment should be initiated early in any cases of suspected AIE, given the risks of complications arising from delays in treatment. However, diagnostic tests should be obtained prior to initiating treatment. Plasmapheresis, which results in short-term depletion of peripheral antibodies, is thought to be less likely to be effective for children with ongoing autoimmune disease. Evidence regarding the preferred order of treatments has not yet been established. For patients who do not respond to first-line therapies, agents may include rituximab and cyclophosphamide. Mycophenolate, azathioprine, and mofetil may be used for maintenance treatment. HE tends to be highly responsive to steroids.

Psychiatric Treatment

Treatment of the co-occurring psychiatric symptoms in AIE is complicated given that the use of antipsychotics prior to immunomodulatory treatment may result in an exacerbation of symptoms. In general, it is better to use antipsychotics in conjunction with or after the administration of immunomodulatory treatments (Mooneyham et al. 2018). Treatment should target the symptoms that are compromising safety, such as impulsivity, aggression, the refusal to eat or drink, and suicidality (Tran et al. 2018). Of note, patients with

AIE are at higher risk of NMS and catatonia. The treatment of patients with co-occurring delirium and catatonia is also complicated by the fact that antipsychotics may worsen symptoms of catatonia. In addition, it may be difficult to differentiate between the symptoms of NMS and the symptoms of AIE. As a result, agitation, particularly in the presence of catatonia, is best managed with benzodiazepines. Only anecdotal data are available on the use of antipsychotics, including haloperidol, olanzapine, risperidone, and quetiapine, for psychotic symptoms.

Patients with AIE may be left with residual symptoms of anxiety, inattention, impulsivity, depression, psychosis, and OCD (Mooneyham et al. 2018). Psychiatric treatment should target each of these specific symptoms and should continue as long as necessary. Patients should be carefully observed for potential flares or relapse. Close collaboration with the medical team is absolutely essential.

Pediatric Acute-Onset Neuropsychiatric Syndrome

Pediatric acute-onset neuropsychiatric syndrome (PANS) is characterized by the unusually abrupt onset (<72 hours) of obsessive-compulsive symptoms or severe eating restrictions and at least two of the following seven categories of symptoms: anxiety (in particular, separation anxiety); emotional liability or depression; irritability, aggression, and/or severe oppositional behavior; behavioral/developmental regression; deterioration in school performance (related to attention deficit–like behaviors, memory deficits, and cognitive changes); sensory or motor abnormalities; and somatic signs and symptoms, including sleep disturbances, enuresis, or urinary frequency (Swedo et al. 2012, 2017). PANS is also often found to have a relapsing and remitting course of symptom severity. The syndrome is thought to have a variety of potential etiologies, including psychological trauma; underlying neurological, endocrine, and metabolic disorders; and postinfectious autoimmune and neuroinflammatory disorders, such as pediatric autoimmune neuropsychiatric disorder associated with streptococcal infections (PANDAS), cerebral vasculitis, neuropsychiatric lupus, and others (Chang et al. 2015; Swedo et al. 2017).

Along with an association with Group A β-hemolytic streptococcal (GABHS) infections, PANDAS is characterized by the very sudden onset of OCD and/ or tic disorders along with associated neurological difficulties, such as involuntary motor hyperactivity or choreiform movements, generally in patients ages 3 years to puberty (Gilbert et al. 2018). Unlike PANDAS, PANS does not require that neurological difficulties be present (Gilbert et al. 2018).

Epidemiology

There has been controversy in the pediatric community about the validity of the PANS diagnosis, in particular with respect to the lack of adequate evidence-based treatment studies (Gilbert et al. 2018). This debate likely has contributed to the unavailability of incidence data for PANS (as well as PANDAS). Dr. Susan Swedo, chief of the Section of Behavioral Pediatrics at the National Institute of Mental Health (NIMH) and the first to identify these disorders, has estimated that they affect about 1% of elementary school children (Pupillo 2017). Some data suggest a preponderance of males with prepubertal onset of symptoms, as well as a high rate of autoimmune disorders in first-degree relatives (Calaprice et al. 2017).

Clinical Features

In addition to the acute onset of OCD symptoms or food refusal in patients with PANS, the syndrome is characterized by the complexity and variety of disabling symptoms, including separation anxiety, emotional lability, personality changes, behavioral regression, irritability, aggression, and oppositional behavior, as well as deterioration in school performance (Murphy et al. 2014). PANS patients may present with sleep disturbances, enuresis, or urinary frequency (Chang et al. 2015). Some patients have been reported to develop sensitivity to light and other sensory issues, such as a refusal to wear shoes or clothing (Chang et al. 2015). OCD symptoms are often extreme (e.g., licking shoes or barking). PANS may represent a subset of avoidant/restrictive food intake disorder.

Pathophysiology

PANS has been described as a clinically heterogeneous disorder with a number of etiologies and disease mechanisms related to inflammatory and postinfectious autoimmune responses, with some clinical series documenting immune abnormalities in 75%–80% of patients (Frankovich et al. 2017). For instance, proposed biomarkers for PANS include autoantibodies to dopamine D_1 and D_2 receptors, β-tubulin, and lysoganglioside-GM1 as well as calcium calmodulin dependent protein kinase II activity previously linked to Sydenham's chorea (Hesselmark and Bejerot 2017). Although most instances of PANS are suspected to be postinfectious in origin, only GABHS infection has been consistently associated with PANDAS (Chang et al. 2015). Antibodies for GABHS are postulated to target brain proteins and stimulate or block receptors in the basal ganglia. Anti–basal ganglia antibodies have also been detected in some but not all youth diagnosed with PANDAS (Murphy et al. 2014). Infectious agents other than GABHS that may be associated with the onset of PANS include *Mycoplasma pneumoniae*, *Borrelia burgdorferi* (Lyme disease), and influenza (Chang et al. 2015).

Differential Diagnosis

A number of pediatric conditions should be considered in the differential diagnosis (Table 6–10). Unlike obsessive-compulsive symptoms in PANS/PANDAS, OCD is characterized by more insidious onset, is not episodic in nature, has no infectious trigger, and tends to have a later age at onset (10 years vs. <7 years for PANS) (Murphy et al. 2014).

Assessment

PANS is a clinical diagnosis that requires the completion of a comprehensive multidisciplinary diagnostic assessment (Chang et al. 2015). It is considered a diagnosis of exclusion that should only be made when a patient's symptoms are not better explained by a known neurological or medical disorder (Swedo et al. 2017). The evaluation should include a complete medical and psychiatric history, physical examination, laboratory testing of blood (and possibly CSF), and selected paraclinical evaluations, such as magnetic resonance imaging, electrocardiogram/echocardiography, electroencephalography, and polysomnography (Chang et al. 2015; Swedo et al. 2017).

Laboratory tests should include complete blood cell count, erythrocyte sedimentation rate, C-reactive protein, and throat culture for GABHS titers (antistreptolysin O and antideoxyribonuclease B). Additional tests to consider

Table 6–10.   Differential diagnosis of pediatric acute-onset neuropsychiatric syndrome (PANS)

Autoimmune encephalitis	Metabolic/mitochondrial
Postinfectious	Mitochondrial encephalomyopathy
Acute disseminated encephalomyelitis	Cerebral folate deficiency
Sydenham chorea	Wilson's disease
Paraneoplastic	**Psychiatric disorder**
NMDAR antibody encephalitis	Obsessive-compulsive disorder
Voltage-gated antibody disorders	Anorexia nervosa
Movement disorder	Avoidance/restrictive food intake disorder
Tourette syndrome	Bipolar disorder
Transient tic disorder	
Autoimmune disease	
Neuropsychiatric lupus	
Antiphospholipid antibody syndrome	

Note.   NMDAR = *N*-methyl-D-aspartate receptor.
Source.   Chang et al. 2015; Murphy et al. 2014.

include antinuclear antibody (with elevated inflammatory markers such as fatigue, rash, or joint pain), antiphospholipid antibody (with chorea, petechiae, migraines, stroke, thrombosis, or thrombocytopenia), and antibody tests for mycoplasma/influenza and *N*-methyl-D-aspartate receptor (Chang et al. 2015). Reviews have not supported the use of the Cunningham Panel, a commercially available set of immunological assays, in the diagnosis of PANS (Hesselmark and Bejerot 2017).

Treatment

Members of the PANS/PANDAS Research Consortium have proposed three modes of intervention: 1) removing the source of inflammation with antimicrobial interventions, 2) treating disturbances of the immune system with immunomodulatory and/or anti-inflammatory therapies, and 3) treating the symptoms with psychotherapy and psychopharmacology (Swedo et al. 2017). It is important for consultants to note that currently there is no strong evidence in support of treatment with cognitive-behavioral therapy, SSRIs, neuroleptics, antibiotics, tonsillectomy, or immunomodulation (Gilbert et al. 2018; Sigra et al. 2018; Williams et al. 2016). Until more valid and well-designed research has been done, treatment needs to be approached on a case-by-case basis, allowing for treatment if a response can be expected (i.e., antibiotics to prevent recurring infections or intravenous immunoglobulin [IVIG] with clinical evidence of neuroinflammation) (Sigra et al. 2018).

Antimicrobial Treatment

An initial course of antibiotics is recommended when there is objective evidence of infection. Treatment of GABHS infection with penicillin, cephalosporin, or amoxicillin may lead to symptom relief in patients with PANS, whereas azithromycin should be used to treat mycoplasma pneumoniae or Lyme disease. Risks of long-term treatment with antibiotics include gastrointestinal side effects and the growth of antibiotic-resistant organisms.

Immunomodulatory Treatments

Immune therapies that have been proposed to treat neuroinflammatory processes or postinfectious autoimmune reactions include corticosteroids, therapeutic plasma exchange, IVIG, anti-CD20 monoclonal antibodies (rituximab), and mycophenolate (Sigra et al. 2018). The use of nonsteroidal anti-inflammatory drugs (NSAIDs) has also been suggested.

Psychotherapeutic Treatment

Management of symptoms of OCD, anxiety, depression, mood lability, attention-deficit/hyperactivity disorder, and aggression follows principles of treatment used in psychiatric disorders not attributed to PANS (Thienemann et al. 2017). Both pharmacological treatments (in particular SSRIs) and nonpharmacological treatments (including cognitive-behavioral therapy) should be offered with the expectation that full benefits may take weeks to months to occur. NIMH has made available an overview of PANDAS (available at: https://www.nimh.nih.gov/health/publications/pandas/index.shtml) that can be used with patients and their families to help facilitate communication and understanding of this often perplexing and difficult to diagnose illness.

References

American Psychiatric Association: Diagnostic and Statistical Manual of Mental Disorders, 5th Edition. Arlington, VA, American Psychiatric Association, 2013

American Psychiatric Association, Task Force on Electroconvulsive Therapy: The practice of ECT: recommendations for treatment, training and privileging. Convuls Ther 6(2):85–120, 1990 11659302

Armangue T, Petit-Pedrol M, Dalmau J: Autoimmune encephalitis in children. J Child Neurol 27(11):1460–1469, 2012 22935553

Benarous X, Consoli A, Raffin M, et al: Validation of the Pediatric Catatonia Rating Scale (PCRS). Schizophr Res 176(2–3):378–386, 2016 27377978

Boyer EW, Shannon M: The serotonin syndrome. N Engl J Med 352(11):1112–1120, 2005 15784664

Brenton JN, Goodkin HP: Antibody-mediated autoimmune encephalitis in childhood. Pediatr Neurol 60:13–23, 2016 27343023

Brown TM, Stoudemire A, Fogel BS, et al: Psychopharmacology in the medical patient, in Psychiatric Care of the Medical Patient, 2nd Edition. Edited by Stoudemire A, Fogel BS, Greenberg DB. Oxford, Oxford University Press, 2000, pp 329–372

Bush G, Fink M, Petrides G, et al: Catatonia. I. Rating scale and standardized examination. Acta Psychiatr Scand 93(2):129–136, 1996 8686483

Calaprice D, Tona J, Parker-Athill EC, et al: A survey of pediatric acute-onset neuropsychiatric syndrome characteristics and course. J Child Adolesc Psychopharmacol 27(7):607–618, 2017 28140619

Caroff SC, Mann S: Neuroleptic malignant syndrome. Med Clin North Am 33:650–659, 1999

Chang K, Frankovich J, Cooperstock M, et al; PANS Collaborative Consortium: Clinical evaluation of youth with pediatric acute-onset neuropsychiatric syndrome (PANS): recommendations from the 2013 PANS Consensus Conference. J Child Adolesc Psychopharmacol 25(1):3–13, 2015 25325534

Cohen D, Flament M, Dubos PF, et al: Case series: catatonic syndrome in young people. J Am Acad Child Adolesc Psychiatry 38(8):1040–1046, 1999 10434497

Consoli A, Raffin M, Laurent C, et al: Medical and developmental risk factors of catatonia in children and adolescents: a prospective case-control study. Schizophr Res 137(1–3):151–158, 2012 22401837

Dhossche DM, Wachtel LE: Catatonia is hidden in plain sight among different pediatric disorders: a review article. Pediatr Neurol 43(5):307–315, 2010 20933172

Dunkley EJS, Isbister GK, Sibbritt D, et al: The Hunter Serotonin Toxicity Criteria: simple and accurate diagnostic decision rules for serotonin toxicity. QJM 96(9):635–642, 2003 12925718

Fink M: Is catatonia a primary indication for ECT? Convuls Ther 6(1):1–4, 1990 11941041

Florance NR, Davis RL, Lam C, et al: Anti-N-methyl-D-aspartate receptor (NMDAR) encephalitis in children and adolescents. Ann Neurol 66(1):11–18, 2009 19670433

Frankovich J, Swedo S, Murphy T, et al: Clinical management of pediatric acute-onset neuropsychiatric syndrome: part II—use of immunomodulatory therapies. J Child Adolesc Psychopharmacol 27:574–593, 2017

Freudenreich O, Francis A, Fricchione GL: Psychosis, mania, and catatonia, in The American Psychiatric Association Publishing Textbook of Psychosomatic Medicine and Consultation-Liaison Psychiatry, 3rd ed. Edited by Levenson JL. Washington, DC, American Psychiatric Publishing, 2019, pp 249–279

Ghaziuddin N, Kutcher SP, Knapp P, et al; Work Group on Quality Issues; AACAP: Practice parameter for use of electroconvulsive therapy with adolescents. J Am Acad Child Adolesc Psychiatry 43(12):1521–1539, 2004 15564821

Ghaziuddin N, Hendriks M, Patel P, et al: Neuroleptic malignant syndrome/malignant catatonia in child psychiatry: literature review and a case series. J Child Adolesc Psychopharmacol 27(4):359–365, 2017 28398818

Gilbert DL, Mink JW, Singer HS: A pediatric neurology perspective on pediatric autoimmune neuropsychiatric disorder associated with streptococcal infection and pediatric acute-onset neuropsychiatric syndrome. J Pediatr 199:243–251, 2018 29793872

Glaser CA, Gilliam S, Schnurr D, et al; California Encephalitis Project, 1998–2000: In search of encephalitis etiologies: diagnostic challenges in the California Encephalitis Project, 1998–2000. Clin Infect Dis 36(6):731–742, 2003 12627357

Graus F, Titulaer MJ, Balu R, et al: A clinical approach to diagnosis of autoimmune encephalitis. Lancet Neurol 15(4):391–404, 2016 26906964

Gurrera RJ, Mortillaro G, Velamoor V, et al: A validation study of the international consensus diagnostic criteria for neuroleptic malignant syndrome. J Clin Psychopharmacol 37(1):67–71, 2017 28027111

Hauptman AJ, Benjamin S: The differential diagnosis and treatment of catatonia in children and adolescents. Harv Rev Psychiatry 24(6):379–395, 2016 27824634

Hesselmark E, Bejerot S: Biomarkers for diagnosis of pediatric acute neuropsychiatric syndrome (PANS)—sensitivity and specificity of the Cunningham Panel. J Neuroimmunol 312:31–37, 2017 28919236

Iqbal MM, Basil MJ, Kaplan J, et al: Overview of serotonin syndrome. Ann Clin Psychiatry 24(4):310–318, 2012 23145389

Katus LE, Frucht SJ: Management of serotonin syndrome and neuroleptic malignant syndrome. Curr Treat Options Neurol 18(9):39, 2016 27469512

Lang FU, Lang S, Becker T, et al: Neuroleptic malignant syndrome or catatonia? Trying to solve the catatonic dilemma. Psychopharmacology (Berl) 232(1):1–5, 2015 25407348

Lima NN, Nascimento VB, Peixoto JA, et al: Electroconvulsive therapy use in adolescents: a systematic review. Ann Gen Psychiatry 12(1):17, 2013 23718899

Mann SC, Caroff SN, Fricchione G, et al: Central dopamine hypoactivity and the pathogenesis of neuroleptic malignant syndrome. Psychiatr Ann 30(5):363–374, 2000

Mason PJ, Morris VA, Balcezak TJ: Serotonin syndrome: presentation of 2 cases and review of the literature. Medicine (Baltimore) 79(4):201–209, 2000 10941349

Modi S, Dharaiya D, Schultz L, et al: Neuroleptic malignant syndrome: complications, outcomes, and mortality. Neurocrit Care 24(1):97–103, 2016 26223336

Mooneyham GC, Gallentine W, Van Mater H: Evaluation and management of autoimmune encephalitis: a clinical overview for the practicing child psychiatrist. Child Adolesc Psychiatr Clin N Am 27(1):37–52, 2018 29157501

Murphy TK, Gerardi DM, Leckman JF: Pediatric acute-onset neuropsychiatric syndrome. Psychiatr Clin North Am 37(3):353–374, 2014 25150567

Peglow S, Prem V, McDaniel W: Treatment of catatonia with zolpidem. J Neuropsychiatry Clin Neurosci 25(3):E13, 2013 24026726

Pileggi DJ, Cook AM: Neuroleptic malignant syndrome. Ann Pharmacother 50(11):973–981, 2016 27423483

Pupillo J: PANDAS/PANS treatments, awareness evolve, but some experts skeptical. AAP News, 2017

Sahlholm K, Zeberg H, Nilsson J, et al: The fast-off hypothesis revisited: a functional kinetic study of antipsychotic antagonism of the dopamine D2 receptor. Eur Neuropsychopharmacol 26(3):467–476, 2016 26811292

Sani G, Serra G, Kotzalidis GD, et al: The role of memantine in the treatment of psychiatric disorders other than the dementias: a review of current preclinical and clinical evidence. CNS Drugs 26(8):663–690, 2012 22784018

Sigra S, Hesselmark E, Bejerot S: Treatment of PANDAS and PANS: a systematic review. Neurosci Biobehav Rev 86:51–65, 2018 29309797

Simon LV, Keenaghan M: Serotonin Syndrome. Treasure Island, FL, StatPearls Publishing, 2019

Strawn JR, Keck PE Jr, Caroff SN: Neuroleptic malignant syndrome. Am J Psychiatry 164(6):870–876, 2007 17541044

Swedo S, Leckman J, Rose N: From research subgroup to clinical syndrome: modifying the PANDAS criteria to describe PANS. Pediatrics and Therapeutics 2:1–8, 2012

Swedo SE, Frankovich J, Murphy TK: Overview of treatment of pediatric acute-onset neuropsychiatric syndrome. J Child Adolesc Psychopharmacol 27(7):562–565, 2017 28722464

Thienemann M, Murphy T, Leckman J, et al: Clinical management of pediatric acute-onset neuropsychiatric syndrome: part I—psychiatric and behavioral interventions. J Child Adolesc Psychopharmacol 27(7):566–573, 2017 28722481

Tran P, Frankovich J, Van Mater H, et al: Pediatric inflammatory brain disease, in Complex Disorders in Pediatric Psychiatry. Edited by Driver D, Thomas SS. St Louis, MO, Elsevier, 2018 pp 169–188

Tse L, Barr AM, Scarapicchia V, et al: Neuroleptic malignant syndrome: a review from a clinically oriented perspective. Curr Neuropharmacol 13(3):395–406, 2015 26411967

Uddin MF, Alweis R, Shah SR, et al: Controversies in serotonin syndrome diagnosis and management: a review. J Clin Diagn Res 11(9):OE05–OE07, 2017 29207768

Velamoor R: Neuroleptic malignant syndrome: a neuro-psychiatric emergency: recognition, prevention, and management. Asian J Psychiatr 29:106–109, 2017 29061403

Weiss M, Allan B, Greenaway M: Treatment of catatonia with electroconvulsive therapy in adolescents. J Child Adolesc Psychopharmacol 22(1):96–100, 2012 22339614

Williams KA, Swedo SE, Farmer CA, et al: Randomized, controlled trial of intravenous immunoglobulin for pediatric autoimmune neuropsychiatric disorders associated with streptococcal infections. J Am Acad Child Adolesc Psychiatry 55(10):860–867.e2, 2016 27663941

Wing L, Shah A: Catatonia in autistic spectrum disorders. Br J Psychiatry 176:357–362, 2000 10827884

Wright S, Vincent A: Pediatric autoimmune epileptic encephalopathies. J Child Neurol 32(4):418–428, 2017 28056633

7

Depressive Symptoms and Disorders

Depressive disorders are a critical public health problem that affects individuals across the life span. Meta-analyses of epidemiological studies suggest that the point prevalence of depression is 2.8% for children under age 13 years and 5.6% for youth ages 13–18 years (Jane Costello et al. 2006). Studies have shown that the average age at onset of major depression is 11–14 years, with a steady increase in incidence across adolescence, as is evident in the doubling of the rate from ages 13–14 years (8.4%) to ages 17–18 years (15.4%) (Merikangas et al. 2010). Besides placing youth at risk for suicide, untreated or inadequately treated depression can become intractable to treatment, and affected individuals incur progressively greater social, educational, and economic consequences over time (Walter et al. 2018).

Estimates of major depression prevalence in physically ill youth range from 11% to 29% depending on the population sample and the methodology used (Allgaier et al. 2012a). Some prevalence variation depends on the specific illness, with some studies showing, for example, elevated rates of depression in youth with chronic fatigue syndrome, chronic pain, cleft lip and palate deformities, and epilepsy, and others demonstrating inconsistent findings for arthritis, cancer, cystic fibrosis, diabetes, HIV infection, and sickle cell disease (Pinquart and Shen 2011).

Pediatric primary care providers have been found to detect only 12.5% of youth with diagnoses of depression (Allgaier et al. 2012b). When depression co-occurs with a physical illness, the possibility for missed diagnosis of depression may be even greater. For example, healthy children and adolescents not infrequently present with irritability or somatic complaints rather than classic complaints of sadness. In the pediatric setting, it is common for physically ill pediatric patients and their families to emphasize somatic complaints rather than mood or cognitive symptoms. Pediatric providers themselves naturally tend to focus more on physical signs and symptoms and may even be reluctant to stigmatize patients by suggesting a psychiatric diagnosis. One commonly held belief is that depression is an understandable reaction to the stress of a physical illness and therefore does not warrant treatment. Furthermore, many of the neurovegetative symptoms used to diagnose depression, such as fatigue, sleep, or decreased appetite, can be the direct physiological effects of an illness and/or its treatment (Table 7–1). Nevertheless, concern about depression in the physically ill child or adolescent is one of the most frequent reasons for psychiatric consultation.

Clinical Considerations in the Physically Ill Child

Depression as a Continuum

In the pediatric setting, the term *depression* is used with different meanings. It may refer to an array of clinical conditions ranging from a transient mood change requiring no treatment to a severe depressive disorder associated with thoughts of death that requires psychiatric hospitalization (Beasley and Beardslee 1998). By remembering this continuum, consultants will be prepared to implement a stepped care approach whereby the intensity of recommended treatment ascends based on the severity of the patient's presentation (see Chapter 1, "Pediatric Consultation-Liaison Psychiatry").

Table 7–1. Overlap between DSM-5 symptoms of depression and physical illness symptoms and treatment

DSM-5 diagnostic item	Physical illness confound
Weight loss	Cancer chemotherapy agents
Decreased appetite	Chronic disease
	Cancer
	Cystic fibrosis
	Diabetes mellitus
	Inflammatory bowel disease
	Renal failure
	Infection (e.g., HIV, tuberculosis)
	Malabsorption
	Vitamin deficiency
Weight gain	Anticonvulsant medications
Increased appetite	Antihistaminergic medications
	Corticosteroids
	Cushing's disease
	Hypogonadism
	Hypothalamic lesions
	Hypothyroidism
	Insulinoma
	Polycystic ovary disease
Insomnia	Alcohol
	Asthma
	Caffeine
	Corticosteroids
	Duodenal ulcers

Table 7–1.   Overlap between DSM-5 symptoms of depression and physical illness symptoms and treatment *(continued)*

DSM-5 diagnostic item	Physical illness confound
Insomnia *(continued)*	Hyperthyroidism
	Nocturia
	Pain
	Psychostimulant medications
	Restless legs syndrome
	Sleep apnea
	Sympathomimetic amines
Hypersomnia	Brain tumors
	Diabetic ketoacidosis
	Encephalitis
	Hypercapnia
	Hypothyroidism
	Liver failure
	Opiates
	Sleep apnea (daytime hypersomnia)
	Uremia
Fatigue/loss of energy	Addison's disease
	Anemia
	Anticonvulsant medications
	Chronic disease
	Endocarditis
	Guillain-Barré syndrome
	Heart failure
	Hepatitis
	Mononucleosis

Table 7–1.   Overlap between DSM-5 symptoms of depression and physical illness symptoms and treatment *(continued)*

DSM-5 diagnostic item	Physical illness confound
Fatigue/loss of energy *(continued)*	Chronic disease *(continued)*
	Motor neuron disease
	Multiple sclerosis
	Muscular dystrophy
	Narcolepsy
	Poliomyelitis
	Rheumatoid arthritis
	Tumors
	Uremia
	Vitamin B_{12} deficiency
Difficulty with thinking/concentration	Cirrhosis
	Dementia
	Huntington's disease
	Lead poisoning
	Marijuana
	Metachromatic leukodystrophy
	Opiates
Loss of interest in sex	Cirrhosis
	Hemochromatosis
	Hormonal disorder
	Substance abuse
Psychomotor agitation	Hypercalcemia
	Psychostimulant medications
	Reye's syndrome
	Substance withdrawal or abuse
	Wernicke-Korsakoff syndrome

Depression and Physical Symptom Perception

Patients with symptoms of depression have more medically unexplained symptoms even when the severity of their medical illness is taken into account (Katon et al. 2001). Patients with comorbid depressive and physical illnesses can have a heightened awareness of, and a tendency to focus on, the physical symptoms of their illness, including their perception of pain (Margetić et al. 2005). Common physical complaints that can accompany depression include joint pain, limb pain, back pain, gastrointestinal problems, fatigue, weakness, and appetite changes. Chronic abdominal pain and headaches are particularly associated with depression in children, although diarrhea, insomnia, and nervousness also occur.

There is preliminary evidence from patients with comorbid depression and inflammatory bowel disease (IBD) of the following depression subtypes: 1) mild—diverse low-grade depressive symptoms; 2) somatic—severe fatigue, appetite change, anhedonia, decreased motor activity, and depressed mood with concurrent high-dose steroid therapy and the highest IBD activity; and 3) cognitive despair—highest rates of self-reported depressive symptoms, and anxiety with IBD symptoms in the relative absence of inflammation (Szigethy et al. 2014b). These findings, together with those from other studies (Hood et al. 2012; Miller and Cole 2012), suggest a link between depression and inflammation that consultants can consider in their assessments.

As noted above, clinical depression may go undiagnosed in patients because the physical symptoms associated with depression may be interpreted as symptoms of a physical illness. These patients frequently deny having any emotional disturbance and may resist referrals to psychiatric treatment. The term *alexithymia* describes a personality construct that is characterized by difficulties identifying, differentiating, and articulating emotions and that is associated with physical health impairment and somatization (Cameron et al. 2014). The relationship between alexithymia and pediatric somatic complaints requires further study (Natalucci et al. 2018).

Patients with a high number of physical symptoms are more likely to have a depressive illness. Kişlal et al. (2005) reported elevated rates of depression in adolescents admitted for evaluation of pediatric issues. Similarly, Knook et al. (2011) found that 28% of the children referred for an evaluation of unexplained pain had clinically relevant psychiatric disorders consisting of anxiety, depressive, and disruptive disorders. Finally, it is important to consider that physical symptoms, in particular pain complaints, tend to increase the duration of the patient's depressed mood. Treatment that does not address pain and other physical symptoms is likely to be associated with incomplete response to the treatment of depression. By contrast, improvement in physical symptoms is correlated with improvement in symptoms of depression.

Depression as a Co-occurring Symptom

Sad or irritable mood can accompany nearly all DSM-5 disorders (American Psychiatric Association 2013) but can also be a normative response to a physical illness. Consultants will find that the co-occurrence of anxiety and depressive symptoms is particularly common in patients with physical illness. The symptom pattern that predominates in a clinical presentation can depend on several factors, including the time course of the physical illness and its treatment as well as whether the anxiety and depressive symptoms meet DSM-5 diagnostic criteria for a mental disorder.

Depression and Functional Impairment

Studies of physically ill adult patients have suggested a strong relationship between depression and functional impairment. Depressed patients tend to have a poor perception of their physical health and more impairment in their social and academic functioning. In a cross-sectional study of more than 130,000 individuals with chronic physical illness, a strong association was found between major depression, health care use, and role impairment (Stein et al. 2006). In fact, the presence of depression may be better than the severity of physical illness at predicting functional impairment over time. By contrast, as symptoms of depression improve, so do ratings on measures of functional impairment (Ormel et al. 1993).

Depression and Health Care Behaviors

The presence of a depressive disorder may have economic implications. Children with internalizing symptoms, such as depression and anxiety, have been shown to have higher rates of health care utilization and higher health care costs (Bernal et al. 2000; Haarasilta et al. 2003). Depression is associated with an approximately 50% increase in medical costs for chronic medical illness, even after adjustment for severity of physical illness (Katon 2003). Major depression has been associated with higher rates of adverse health-risk behaviors, including overeating, smoking, and a sedentary lifestyle (Goodman and Whitaker 2002). Depression and anxiety are risk factors for adolescent smoking and obesity in early adulthood. Depressive disorders may affect the patient's motivation as well as adherence to the pediatric treatment. For example, patients with co-occurring diabetes mellitus and depression have decreased adherence to the prescribed diet as well as poorer diabetic control (Ciechanowski et al. 2000).

Morbidity and Mortality

Depression and physical illness occurring together have a worse prognosis than when they occur in isolation. The presence of depression is associated with higher morbidity and mortality rates in adults with medical illnesses such as cancer, renal failure, and coronary artery disease. Adolescents with sickle cell disease have been reported to have twice the rate of attempted suicide compared with their healthy peers (Bhatt-Poulose et al. 2016). Death rates are increased in patients with diagnoses of stroke and those on renal dialysis. Patients with physical illnesses are at greater risk of relapse of depression symptoms, as is evident in the 5-year depression recurrence rate of 92% in adults with comorbid depression and diabetes mellitus (Lustman et al. 1997). The risk of suicide is increased in physically ill patients, particularly adults with diagnoses of cancer or HIV, those on renal dialysis, or those with chronic pain (Bhatt-Poulose et al. 2016).

Differential Diagnosis of Depressive Illness in the Physically Ill Child or Adolescent

When faced with the assessment and management of depression symptoms in the pediatric setting, consultants will likely find that patients 1) have a primary depressive or bipolar disorder; 2) have a psychological reaction to the stress of a physical illness; 3) exhibit the direct physiological effects of a medical or substance-induced condition and/or its treatment; or 4) a combination of these (Figure 7–1).

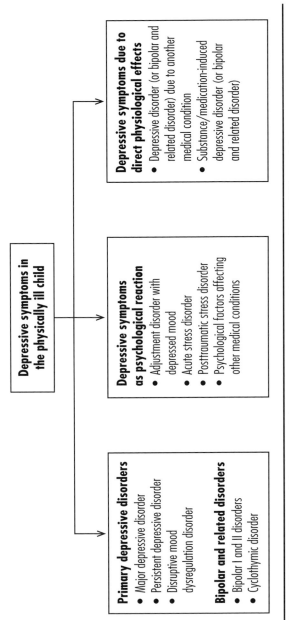

Figure 7–1.   Differential diagnosis of depressive symptoms in the physically ill child or adolescent.

Primary Depressive Disorder

DSM-5 diagnostic criteria for major depressive disorder and persistent depressive disorder (dysthymia) are given in Boxes 7–1 and 7–2, respectively. Major depressive disorder is characterized by the presence of five (or more) of the following symptoms that occur most of the day, nearly every day, in the same 2-week period: depressed mood or pervasive anhedonia (at least one of these must be present); significant weight or appetite change; insomnia or hypersomnia; psychomotor agitation or retardation; fatigue or loss of energy; worthlessness or guilt; indecisiveness or reduced concentration; and recurrent thoughts of death, recurrent suicidal ideation without a plan, or a suicide attempt or plan (American Psychiatric Association 2013). In persistent depressive disorder or dysthymia in children, the depressed mood (including irritability) is chronic and occurs most of the day, for more days than not, for at least 1 year (American Psychiatric Association 2013).

Box 7–1.   DSM-5 Diagnostic Criteria for
            Major Depressive Disorder

A. Five (or more) of the following symptoms have been present during the same 2-week period and represent a change from previous functioning; at least one of the symptoms is either (1) depressed mood or (2) loss of interest or pleasure.

Note: Do not include symptoms that are clearly attributable to another medical condition.

   1. Depressed mood most of the day, nearly every day, as indicated by either subjective report (e.g., feels sad, empty, hopeless) or observation made by others (e.g., appears tearful). (**Note:** In children and adolescents, can be irritable mood.)
   2. Markedly diminished interest or pleasure in all, or almost all, activities most of the day, nearly every day (as indicated by either subjective account or observation).
   3. Significant weight loss when not dieting or weight gain (e.g., a change of more than 5% of body weight in a month), or decrease or increase in appetite nearly every day. (**Note:** In children, consider failure to make expected weight gain.)
   4. Insomnia or hypersomnia nearly every day.

5. Psychomotor agitation or retardation nearly every day (observable by others, not merely subjective feelings of restlessness or being slowed down).
6. Fatigue or loss of energy nearly every day.
7. Feelings of worthlessness or excessive or inappropriate guilt (which may be delusional) nearly every day (not merely self-reproach or guilt about being sick).
8. Diminished ability to think or concentrate, or indecisiveness, nearly every day (either by subjective account or as observed by others).
9. Recurrent thoughts of death (not just fear of dying), recurrent suicidal ideation without a specific plan, or a suicide attempt or a specific plan for committing suicide.

B. The symptoms cause clinically significant distress or impairment in social, occupational, or other important areas of functioning.
C. The episode is not attributable to the physiological effects of a substance or another medical condition.

Note: Criteria A–C represent a major depressive episode.

Note[1]**:** Responses to a significant loss (e.g., bereavement, financial ruin, losses from a natural disaster, a serious medical illness or disability) may

---

[1]In distinguishing grief from a major depressive episode (MDE), it is useful to consider that in grief the predominant affect is feelings of emptiness and loss, while in an MDE it is persistent depressed mood and the inability to anticipate happiness or pleasure. The dysphoria in grief is likely to decrease in intensity over days to weeks and occurs in waves, the so-called pangs of grief. These waves tend to be associated with thoughts or reminders of the deceased. The depressed mood of an MDE is more persistent and not tied to specific thoughts or preoccupations. The pain of grief may be accompanied by positive emotions and humor that are uncharacteristic of the pervasive unhappiness and misery characteristic of an MDE. The thought content associated with grief generally features a preoccupation with thoughts and memories of the deceased, rather than the self-critical or pessimistic ruminations seen in an MDE. In grief, self-esteem is generally preserved, whereas in an MDE feelings of worthlessness and self-loathing are common. If self-derogatory ideation is present in grief, it typically involves perceived failings vis-à-vis the deceased (e.g., not visiting frequently enough, not telling the deceased how much he or she was loved). If a bereaved individual thinks about death and dying, such thoughts are generally focused on the deceased and possibly about "joining" the deceased, whereas in an MDE such thoughts are focused on ending one's own life because of feeling worthless, undeserving of life, or unable to cope with the pain of depression.

include the feelings of intense sadness, rumination about the loss, insomnia, poor appetite, and weight loss noted in Criterion A, which may resemble a depressive episode. Although such symptoms may be understandable or considered appropriate to the loss, the presence of a major depressive episode in addition to the normal response to a significant loss should also be carefully considered. This decision inevitably requires the exercise of clinical judgment based on the individual's history and the cultural norms for the expression of distress in the context of loss.

D. The occurrence of the major depressive episode is not better explained by schizoaffective disorder, schizophrenia, schizophreniform disorder, delusional disorder, or other specified and unspecified schizophrenia spectrum and other psychotic disorders.

E. There has never been a manic episode or a hypomanic episode.
    Note: This exclusion does not apply if all of the manic-like or hypomanic-like episodes are substance-induced or are attributable to the physiological effects of another medical condition.

Specify:
   With anxious distress
   With mixed features
   With melancholic features
   With atypical features
   With mood-congruent psychotic features
   With mood-incongruent psychotic features
   With catatonia
   With peripartum onset
   With seasonal pattern

Source.   Reprinted from American Psychiatric Association: *Diagnostic and Statistical Manual of Mental Disorders*, 5th Edition. Arlington, VA, American Psychiatric Association, 2013. Copyright © 2013 American Psychiatric Association. Used with permission.

Box 7–2.   DSM-5 Diagnostic Criteria for
            Persistent Depressive Disorder (Dysthymia)

This disorder represents a consolidation of DSM-IV-defined chronic major depressive disorder and dysthymic disorder.

A. Depressed mood for most of the day, for more days than not, as indicated by either subjective account or observation by others, for at least 2 years.

Note: In children and adolescents, mood can be irritable and duration must be at least 1 year.

B. Presence, while depressed, of two (or more) of the following:

1. Poor appetite or overeating.
2. Insomnia or hypersomnia.
3. Low energy or fatigue.
4. Low self-esteem.
5. Poor concentration or difficulty making decisions.
6. Feelings of hopelessness.

C. During the 2-year period (1 year for children or adolescents) of the disturbance, the individual has never been without the symptoms in Criteria A and B for more than 2 months at a time.

D. Criteria for a major depressive disorder may be continuously present for 2 years.

E. There has never been a manic episode or a hypomanic episode, and criteria have never been met for cyclothymic disorder.

F. The disturbance is not better explained by a persistent schizoaffective disorder, schizophrenia, delusional disorder, or other specified or unspecified schizophrenia spectrum and other psychotic disorder.

G. The symptoms are not attributable to the physiological effects of a substance (e.g., a drug of abuse, a medication) or another medical condition (e.g., hypothyroidism).

H. The symptoms cause clinically significant distress or impairment in social, occupational, or other important areas of functioning.

Note: Because the criteria for a major depressive episode include four symptoms that are absent from the symptom list for persistent depressive disorder (dysthymia), a very limited number of individuals will have depressive symptoms that have persisted longer than 2 years but will not meet criteria for persistent depressive disorder. If full criteria for a major depressive episode have been met at some point during the current episode of illness, they should be given a diagnosis of major depressive disorder. Otherwise, a diagnosis of other specified depressive disorder or unspecified depressive disorder is warranted.

Specify if:
With anxious distress
With mixed features
With melancholic features
With atypical features

With mood-congruent psychotic features
With mood-incongruent psychotic features
With peripartum onset

Specify if:

In partial remission
In full remission

Specify if:

Early onset: If onset is before age 21 years.
Late onset: If onset is at age 21 years or older.

Specify if (for most recent 2 years of persistent depressive disorder):

With pure dysthymic syndrome: Full criteria for a major depressive episode have not been met in at least the preceding 2 years.

With persistent major depressive episode: Full criteria for a major depressive episode have been met throughout the preceding 2-year period.

With intermittent major depressive episodes, with current episode: Full criteria for a major depressive episode are currently met, but there have been periods of at least 8 weeks in at least the preceding 2 years with symptoms below the threshold for a full major depressive episode.

With intermittent major depressive episodes, without current episode: Full criteria for a major depressive episode are not currently met, but there has been one or more major depressive episodes in at least the preceding 2 years.

Specify current severity:

Mild
Moderate
Severe

Source.   Reprinted from American Psychiatric Association: *Diagnostic and Statistical Manual of Mental Disorders*, 5th Edition. Arlington, VA, American Psychiatric Association, 2013. Copyright © 2013 American Psychiatric Association. Used with permission.

In the pediatric setting, patients with primary depression are much more likely to have more intense suicidal thoughts, feelings of helplessness, dysphoria, guilt, distractibility, and discouragement than are those patients experiencing depressive symptoms as a psychological reaction or due to the direct effects of their illness. As mentioned in the introduction to this chapter, the neurovegetative or somatic symptoms of depression may complicate the diagnosis because many pediatric conditions and their treatments are accompanied by similar symptoms. Past individual and family histories of depressive episodes and their responses to treatment can be helpful to consultants in determining the presence of a primary disorder.

Bipolar and Related Disorders

In DSM-5, the essential feature of a bipolar I disorder is a distinct period in which abnormally, persistently elevated, expansive, or irritable mood and persistently increased activity or energy occur most of the day, nearly every day, in the same 1-week period (Box 7–3). Nearly all individuals with these symptoms have or will experience a significant depressive episode. A bipolar II diagnosis requires the lifetime experience of at least one episode of major depression and a hypomanic episode (American Psychiatric Association 2013). In cyclothymic disorder in children or adolescents, hypomanic and depressive periods are experienced over at least 1 year but do not reach full criteria for an episode of mania, hypomania, or major depression (American Psychiatric Association 2013).

Box 7–3.   DSM-5 Diagnostic Criteria for Bipolar I Disorder

For a diagnosis of bipolar I disorder, it is necessary to meet the following criteria for a manic episode. The manic episode may have been preceded by and may be followed by hypomanic or major depressive episodes.

Manic Episode

A. A distinct period of abnormally and persistently elevated, expansive, or irritable mood and abnormally and persistently increased activity or energy, lasting at least 1 week and present most of the day, nearly every day (or any duration if hospitalization is necessary).

B. During the period of mood disturbance and increased energy or activity, three (or more) of the following symptoms (four if the mood is only irritable) are present to a significant degree and represent a noticeable change from usual behavior:

   1. Inflated self-esteem or grandiosity.
   2. Decreased need for sleep (e.g., feels rested after only 3 hours of sleep).

3. More talkative than usual or pressure to keep talking.
4. Flight of ideas or subjective experience that thoughts are racing.
5. Distractibility (i.e., attention too easily drawn to unimportant or irrelevant external stimuli), as reported or observed.
6. Increase in goal-directed activity (either socially, at work or school, or sexually) or psychomotor agitation (i.e., purposeless non-goal-directed activity).
7. Excessive involvement in activities that have a high potential for painful consequences (e.g., engaging in unrestrained buying sprees, sexual indiscretions, or foolish business investments).

C. The mood disturbance is sufficiently severe to cause marked impairment in social or occupational functioning or to necessitate hospitalization to prevent harm to self or others, or there are psychotic features.

D. The episode is not attributable to the physiological effects of a substance (e.g., a drug of abuse, a medication, other treatment) or another medical condition.

Note: A full manic episode that emerges during antidepressant treatment (e.g., medication, electroconvulsive therapy) but persists at a fully syndromal level beyond the physiological effect of that treatment is sufficient evidence for a manic episode and, therefore, a bipolar I diagnosis.

Note: Criteria A–D constitute a manic episode. At least one lifetime manic episode is required for the diagnosis of bipolar I disorder.

Hypomanic Episode

A. A distinct period of abnormally and persistently elevated, expansive, or irritable mood and abnormally and persistently increased activity or energy, lasting at least 4 consecutive days and present most of the day, nearly every day.

B. During the period of mood disturbance and increased energy and activity, three (or more) of the following symptoms (four if the mood is only irritable) have persisted, represent a noticeable change from usual behavior, and have been present to a significant degree:

1. Inflated self-esteem or grandiosity.
2. Decreased need for sleep (e.g., feels rested after only 3 hours of sleep).
3. More talkative than usual or pressure to keep talking.
4. Flight of ideas or subjective experience that thoughts are racing.

5. Distractibility (i.e., attention too easily drawn to unimportant or irrelevant external stimuli), as reported or observed.
6. Increase in goal-directed activity (either socially, at work or school, or sexually) or psychomotor agitation.
7. Excessive involvement in activities that have a high potential for painful consequences (e.g., engaging in unrestrained buying sprees, sexual indiscretions, or foolish business investments).

C. The episode is associated with an unequivocal change in functioning that is uncharacteristic of the individual when not symptomatic.
D. The disturbance in mood and the change in functioning are observable by others.
E. The episode is not severe enough to cause marked impairment in social or occupational functioning or to necessitate hospitalization. If there are psychotic features, the episode is, by definition, manic.
F. The episode is not attributable to the physiological effects of a substance (e.g., a drug of abuse, a medication, other treatment) or another medical condition.

Note: A full hypomanic episode that emerges during antidepressant treatment (e.g., medication, electroconvulsive therapy) but persists at a fully syndromal level beyond the physiological effect of that treatment is sufficient evidence for a hypomanic episode diagnosis. However, caution is indicated so that one or two symptoms (particularly increased irritability, edginess, or agitation following antidepressant use) are not taken as sufficient for diagnosis of a hypomanic episode, nor necessarily indicative of a bipolar diathesis.

Note: Criteria A–F constitute a hypomanic episode. Hypomanic episodes are common in bipolar I disorder but are not required for the diagnosis of bipolar I disorder.

Major Depressive Episode

A. Five (or more) of the following symptoms have been present during the same 2-week period and represent a change from previous functioning; at least one of the symptoms is either (1) depressed mood or (2) loss of interest or pleasure.

Note: Do not include symptoms that are clearly attributable to another medical condition.

1. Depressed mood most of the day, nearly every day, as indicated by either subjective report (e.g., feels sad, empty, or hopeless) or observation made by others (e.g., appears tearful). (**Note:** In children and adolescents, can be irritable mood.)

2. Markedly diminished interest or pleasure in all, or almost all, activities most of the day, nearly every day (as indicated by either subjective account or observation).

3. Significant weight loss when not dieting or weight gain (e.g., a change of more than 5% of body weight in a month), or decrease or increase in appetite nearly every day. (**Note:** In children, consider failure to make expected weight gain.)

4. Insomnia or hypersomnia nearly every day.

5. Psychomotor agitation or retardation nearly every day (observable by others; not merely subjective feelings of restlessness or being slowed down).

6. Fatigue or loss of energy nearly every day.

7. Feelings of worthlessness or excessive or inappropriate guilt (which may be delusional) nearly every day (not merely self-reproach or guilt about being sick).

8. Diminished ability to think or concentrate, or indecisiveness, nearly every day (either by subjective account or as observed by others).

9. Recurrent thoughts of death (not just fear of dying), recurrent suicidal ideation without a specific plan, or a suicide attempt or a specific plan for committing suicide.

B. The symptoms cause clinically significant distress or impairment in social, occupational, or other important areas of functioning.

C. The episode is not attributable to the physiological effects of a substance or another medical condition.

Note: Criteria A–C constitute a major depressive episode. Major depressive episodes are common in bipolar I disorder but are not required for the diagnosis of bipolar I disorder.

Note: Responses to a significant loss (e.g., bereavement, financial ruin, losses from a natural disaster, a serious medical illness or disability) may include the feelings of intense sadness, rumination about the loss, insomnia, poor appetite, and weight loss noted in Criterion A, which may resemble a depressive episode. Although such symptoms may be understandable or considered appropriate to the loss, the presence of a major depressive episode in addition to the normal response to a significant loss should also be carefully considered. This decision inevitably requires the exercise of clinical judgment based on the individual's history and the cultural norms for the expression of distress in the context of loss (see footnote 1 earlier in this chapter).

Bipolar I Disorder

A. Criteria have been met for at least one manic episode (Criteria A–D under "Manic Episode" above).

B. The occurrence of the manic and major depressive episode(s) is not better explained by schizoaffective disorder, schizophrenia, schizophreniform disorder, delusional disorder, or other specified or unspecified schizophrenia spectrum and other psychotic disorder.

Specify:
With anxious distress
With mixed features
With rapid cycling
With melancholic features
With atypical features
With mood-congruent psychotic features
With mood-incongruent psychotic features
With catatonia
With peripartum onset
With seasonal pattern

Source. Reprinted from American Psychiatric Association: *Diagnostic and Statistical Manual of Mental Disorders*, 5th Edition. Arlington, VA, American Psychiatric Association, 2013. Copyright © 2013 American Psychiatric Association. Used with permission.

Presentation of a primary bipolar illness is rare in the pediatric setting, especially in children younger than 12 years. In this setting, manic symptoms and agitation accompanied by depressive symptoms are more likely related to the direct physiological effects causing a neurocognitive disorder, such as delirium, than to bipolar illness. *Secondary mania* is the term sometimes given to manic or hypomanic episodes that are secondary to a pediatric condition or are induced by exposure to medications or toxic factors. Consultants should also be alert to the presentation of disruptive, impulse-control, or conduct disorders, as well as disruptive mood dysregulation disorder. The latter disorder is a depressive disorder diagnosis introduced in DSM-5 that describes the presentation of children with persistent irritability and frequent episodes of extreme behavior dyscontrol (three or more temper tantrums per week with persistent irritability or anger between episodes), who typically develop depressive and anxiety disorders over time rather than bipolar disorders (American Psychiatric Association 2013).

Depressive Symptoms as Psychological Reaction

The stress of having a physical illness and receiving treatment may trigger feelings of helplessness and result in depressive symptoms, particularly in the early phases after the diagnosis. This dysphoric mood is a normal reactive or situational response to an aversive event. It tends to be milder in form and more responsive to distraction and support without the disabling personal distress or impaired functioning of a primary depressive disorder.

Depressive symptoms often accompany behavioral regression, which is a common psychological response to physical illness and its treatment. For example, behavioral regression in the hospital is well known and can range from a normative response of a patient to cooperatively allow others to take care of him or her to more troubling emotional or behavioral responses. Besides the association with depressive symptoms, regressed behavior is manifested in several ways, including clinginess, fearfulness, social withdrawal, oppositionality, and tearfulness. In situations of acute medical stress, it is common for older children and adolescents to display behaviors that are more characteristic of younger children. Regressed behavior in the hospital generally resolves spontaneously when the stress of the illness or hospitalization is over.

During the evaluation of a child referred with symptoms of depression, consultants should consider a number of possible conditions that occur in the context of psychological reactions to illness and/or hospitalization.

Adjustment Disorder With Depressed Mood

The essential feature of adjustment disorder with depressed mood is the presence of depressive symptoms that do not meet criteria for major depression yet are associated with significant personal distress and/or impairment in social or occupational functioning (American Psychiatric Association 2013). Adjustment disorder with depressed mood is frequently seen at some point during the treatment of a patient with serious pediatric illness. For example, estimates of adjustment problems range from 36% to 60% in children with diabetes mellitus (LeBlanc et al. 2003). Consultants can have difficulty differentiating between the depressive symptoms of an adjustment disorder in the context of a pediatric illness versus that of a major depressive disorder.

Bereavement

It is important to differentiate grief that occurs as part of normal bereavement in children who have a life-threatening illness from adjustment disorder with depressed mood and from primary depressive disorders (Table 7–2). Children in the terminal stages of an illness frequently cycle in and out of symptoms of depression, anger, anxiety, and fear (Brown and Sourkes 2010). Feelings of sadness tend to be intermittent and often do not meet criteria for a major depression. Fleeting thoughts of suicide are not uncommon in terminally ill patients; however, these thoughts often reflect patients' wish not to suffer rather than a true wish to die. It is important for both the parents and the medical team to be able to tolerate the child's sadness and accept these feelings as part of a normal mourning process.

It is common for the medical team to call in consultants in the terminal stages of the child's illness with a request for antidepressant medication, motivated by feelings of helplessness on the part of the staff. In these cases, it is important to help the child, the family, and the pediatric team to manage their feelings of loss and to interpret the depressive symptoms as an important part of a normal grieving process. Consultants should consider involving a palliative care specialist if available (see Chapter 13, "Pediatric Cancer, Stem Cell Transplantation, and Palliative Care").

Acute Stress Disorder and Posttraumatic Stress Disorder

Acute stress disorder (ASD) and posttraumatic stress disorder (PTSD) are discussed in more detail in Chapter 8, "Anxiety Symptoms and Trauma/Stress Reactions." With their concomitant anhedonia and dysphoria, these disorders have symptom overlap with adjustment disorders with depressive mood and primary depressive disorders. Consultants need to be aware that life-threatening illness is not automatically considered to be as stressful as the traumatic events associated with more typical examples of ASD and PTSD (American Psychiatric Association 2013).

Psychological Factors Affecting Other Medical Conditions

In patients diagnosed with psychological factors affecting other medical conditions, depressive symptoms are among many psychological factors (e.g., anxiety) that may adversely impact the medical management of a physical condition (American Psychiatric Association 2013; see also Chapter 8 "Anxiety Symptoms and Trauma/Stress Reactions"). Consultants should keep in mind the well-known and frequent comorbidity of anxiety and depressive symptoms.

Table 7–2. Comparison of primary depressive disorder versus normal bereavement in terminally ill patients

Primary depressive disorder characteristics	Grief characteristics
Patient's symptoms meet DSM-5 criteria for primary depressive disorder.	Symptoms of depression are specifically connected to thoughts and memories of the patient's loss and tend to come in waves.
Primary depressive disorder occurs in up to 50% of terminally ill patients with increased prevalence associated with pain or advanced disease.	Grief is a common experience in all terminally ill patients and varies along with the patient's illness progression.
Psychotherapy and/or psychiatric medications are often indicated for treatment.	Many patients may work through their feelings of grief without psychiatric treatment, although psychotherapy may be helpful.
Suicidality may be seen in cases of severe primary depressive disorder.	Patients may have thoughts of wanting their life to end but in the absence of severe pain and/or disability are rarely suicidal.
Patients with severe primary depressive disorder lose the capacity for pleasure.	Patients are able to experience pleasure in between episodes of grief.
Patients have feelings of hopelessness about the future.	Patients are able to take pleasure in anticipating future events.

Depressive Symptoms Due to Direct Physiological Effects of a Medical Condition or Its Treatment

Depressive Disorder Due to Another Medical Condition

Box 7–4 shows the DSM-5 diagnostic criteria used when the depressive disorder is due to another medical condition. In a study of 775 consecutive psychiatric consultations, 3.5% met criteria for an organic mood disorder, representing one-third of all patients diagnosed with depression (Rundell and Wise 1989). Depressive symptoms can precede physical symptoms of a medical illness, such as occurs in the classic presentation of pancreatic carcinoma (Boyd and Riba 2007). As shown in Table 7–3, a large number of other physical illnesses are etiologically related to episodes of depression as well as mania.

Box 7–4. DSM-5 Diagnostic Criteria for Depressive
Disorder Due to Another Medical Condition

A. A prominent and persistent period of depressed mood or markedly diminished interest or pleasure in all, or almost all, activities that predominates in the clinical picture.
B. There is evidence from the history, physical examination, or laboratory findings that the disturbance is the direct pathophysiological consequence of another medical condition.
C. The disturbance is not better explained by another mental disorder (e.g., adjustment disorder with depressed mood, in which the stressor is a serious medical condition).
D. The disturbance does not occur exclusively during the course of a delirium.
E. The disturbance causes clinically significant distress or impairment in social, occupational, or other important areas of functioning.

Specify if:
With depressive features: Full criteria are not met for a major depressive episode.
With major depressive–like episode: Full criteria are met (except Criterion C) for a major depressive episode.
With mixed features: Symptoms of mania or hypomania are also present but do not predominate in the clinical picture.

Source. Reprinted from American Psychiatric Association: *Diagnostic and Statistical Manual of Mental Disorders*, 5th Edition. Arlington, VA, American Psychiatric Association, 2013. Copyright © 2013 American Psychiatric Association. Used with permission.

Clinical findings suggestive of an underlying physiological etiology include an atypical clinical picture, resistance to conventional treatment modalities, and unexplained personality changes. The patient often has a flat or malaiselike mood that has a temporal relationship to the physical condition,

Table 7–3.   Physical illnesses etiologically related to episodes of
depression and mania

Illness	Depressive episode	Manic episode
Neurological disorders		
Epilepsy	+	+
Huntington's disease	+	+
Multiple sclerosis	+	+
Postconcussion	+	+
Stroke	+	+
Parkinson's disease	+	+
Wilson's disease	+	+
Sleep apnea	+	−
Subarachnoid hemorrhage	+	−
Posttraumatic encephalopathy	−	+
Idiopathic calcification of basal ganglia	−	+
Endocrine disorders		
Cushing's syndrome	+	+
Hyperthyroidism	+	+
Hypothyroidism	+	+
Addison's disease	+	−
Hyperparathyroidism	+	−
Hypoparathyroidism	+	−

Table 7–3. Physical illnesses etiologically related to episodes of depression and mania *(continued)*

Illness	Depressive episode	Manic episode
Infectious diseases		
AIDS	+	+
Encephalitis	+	+
Infectious mononucleosis	+	+
Influenza	+	+
Syphilis	+	+
Hepatitis	+	−
Pneumonia	+	−
Subacute bacterial endocarditis	+	−
Tuberculosis	+	−
Post-St. Louis type A encephalitis	−	+
Viral meningoencephalitis	−	+
Cryptococcal meningoencephalitis	−	+
Tumors		
Central nervous system	+	−
Lung	+	−
Pancreas	+	−
Gliomas	−	+
Meningiomas	−	+
Thalamic	−	+

Table 7–3. Physical illnesses etiologically related to episodes of depression and mania *(continued)*

Illness	Depressive episode	Manic episode
Miscellaneous		
Anemia	+	+
Uremia	+	+
Hemodialysis	+	+
Hypokalemia	+	−
Hyperkalemia	+	−
Failure to thrive	+	−
Porphyria	+	−
Carcinoid	−	+
Klinefelter's syndrome	−	+
Kleine-Levin syndrome	−	+
Niacin deficiency	−	+
Postoperative excitement	−	+
Vitamin B_{12} deficiency	−	+

Source. Adapted from Wise and Rundell 1988.

as well as significant physical examination (e.g., weight loss) or laboratory (e.g., increased creatinine) findings. Central nervous system lesions involving the frontal, limbic, and temporal lobes are more frequently associated with depressive disorders. Left-sided lesions are reported to be correlated with an increased risk for depression, whereas right-sided lesions are more likely to be associated with mania (Cummings 1986).

Bipolar and Related Disorder Due to Another Medical Condition

Box 7–5 lists the DSM-5 criteria for bipolar and related disorder due to another medical condition. Patients with a genetic predisposition to bipolar disorder are more likely to develop manic episodes in response to medical illness or medications. Neurological causes of mania include focal strokes in the right basotemporal or inferofrontal region, strokes or tumors in the perihypothalamic region, Huntington's disease, multiple sclerosis, head trauma, infections such as neurosyphilis and Creutzfeldt-Jakob disease, and frontotemporal dementia (Mendez 2000). Sleep deprivation may play a role in predisposing patients to manic episodes. It is not uncommon to find precipitants to manic episodes in patients with a primary bipolar disorder; however, in cases of secondary mania, the precipitation of symptoms is more directly related to the underlying medical condition and/or its treatment. Secondary manic episodes usually respond quickly to treatment of the underlying precipitating factor.

Box 7–5.   DSM-5 Diagnostic Criteria for Bipolar and Related Disorder Due to Another Medical Condition

A. A prominent and persistent period of abnormally elevated, expansive, or irritable mood and abnormally increased activity or energy that predominates in the clinical picture.
B. There is evidence from the history, physical examination, or laboratory findings that the disturbance is the direct pathophysiological consequence of another medical condition.
C. The disturbance is not better explained by another mental disorder.
D. The disturbance does not occur exclusively during the course of a delirium.
E. The disturbance causes clinically significant distress or impairment in social, occupational, or other important areas of functioning, or necessitates hospitalization to prevent harm to self or others, or there are psychotic features.

Specify if:
With manic features: Full criteria are not met for a manic or hypomanic episode.
With manic- or hypomanic-like episode: Full criteria are met except Criterion D for a manic episode or except Criterion F for a hypomanic episode.

With mixed features: Symptoms of depression are also present but do not predominate in the clinical picture.

Source. Reprinted from American Psychiatric Association: *Diagnostic and Statistical Manual of Mental Disorders*, 5th Edition. Arlington, VA, American Psychiatric Association, 2013. Copyright © 2013 American Psychiatric Association. Used with permission.

Substance/Medication-Induced Depressive and Bipolar Disorders

Substance/medication-induced depressive and bipolar disorders (Boxes 7–6 and 7–7) are more common in adults than in children and adolescents. Depression is well known to be more common in patients with substance-related disorders. Patients with severe alcohol use disorders may have symptoms of depression that can be indistinguishable from a primary depressive disorder. Most alcohol-induced depressions resolve within 2 days to 2 weeks with abstinence. Patients who are going through withdrawal from cocaine may have symptoms of depression, irritability, and anxiety that begin shortly after abstinence and may last up to 3 days.

Box 7–6.   DSM-5 Diagnostic Criteria for Substance/ Medication-Induced Depressive Disorder

---

A. A prominent and persistent disturbance in mood that predominates in the clinical picture and is characterized by depressed mood or markedly diminished interest or pleasure in all, or almost all, activities.

B. There is evidence from the history, physical examination, or laboratory findings of both (1) and (2):

　1. The symptoms in Criterion A developed during or soon after substance intoxication or withdrawal or after exposure to a medication.

　2. The involved substance/medication is capable of producing the symptoms in Criterion A.

C. The disturbance is not better explained by a depressive disorder that is not substance/medication-induced. Such evidence of an independent depressive disorder could include the following:

The symptoms preceded the onset of the substance/medication use; the symptoms persist for a substantial period of time (e.g., about 1 month) after the cessation of acute withdrawal or severe intoxication; or there is other evidence suggesting the existence of an independent non-substance/medication-induced depressive disorder (e.g., a history of recurrent non-substance/medication-related episodes).

D. The disturbance does not occur exclusively during the course of a delirium.

E. The disturbance causes clinically significant distress or impairment in social, occupational, or other important areas of functioning.

Note: This diagnosis should be made instead of a diagnosis of substance intoxication or substance withdrawal only when the symptoms in Criterion A predominate in the clinical picture and when they are sufficiently severe to warrant clinical attention.

Specify if (see Table 1 in the DSM-5 chapter "Substance-Related and Addictive Disorders" for diagnoses associated with substance class):

With onset during intoxication: If criteria are met for intoxication with the substance and the symptoms develop during intoxication.

With onset during withdrawal: If criteria are met for withdrawal from the substance and the symptoms develop during, or shortly after, withdrawal.

Source. Reprinted from American Psychiatric Association: *Diagnostic and Statistical Manual of Mental Disorders*, 5th Edition. Arlington, VA, American Psychiatric Association, 2013. Copyright © 2013 American Psychiatric Association. Used with permission.

Box 7–7.   DSM-5 Diagnostic Criteria for Substance/ Medication-Induced Bipolar and Related Disorder

A. A prominent and persistent disturbance in mood that predominates in the clinical picture and is characterized by elevated, expansive, or irritable mood, with or without depressed mood, or markedly diminished interest or pleasure in all, or almost all, activities.

B. There is evidence from the history, physical examination, or laboratory findings of both (1) and (2):

1. The symptoms in Criterion A developed during or soon after substance intoxication or withdrawal or after exposure to a medication.
2. The involved substance/medication is capable of producing the symptoms in Criterion A.

C. The disturbance is not better explained by a bipolar or related disorder that is not substance/medication-induced. Such evidence of an independent bipolar or related disorder could include the following:

> The symptoms precede the onset of the substance/medication use; the symptoms persist for a substantial period of time (e.g., about 1 month) after the cessation of acute withdrawal or severe intoxication; or there is other evidence suggesting the existence of an independent non-substance/medication-induced bipolar and related disorder (e.g., a history of recurrent non-substance/medication-related episodes).

D. The disturbance does not occur exclusively during the course of a delirium.
E. The disturbance causes clinically significant distress or impairment in social, occupational, or other important areas of functioning.

Specify if (see Table 1 in the DSM-5 chapter "Substance-Related and Addictive Disorders" for diagnoses associated with substance class):

> **With onset during intoxication:** If the criteria are met for intoxication with the substance and the symptoms develop during intoxication.
> **With onset during withdrawal:** If criteria are met for withdrawal from the substance and the symptoms develop during, or shortly after, withdrawal.

Source.   Reprinted from American Psychiatric Association: *Diagnostic and Statistical Manual of Mental Disorders*, 5th Edition. Arlington, VA, American Psychiatric Association, 2013. Copyright © 2013 American Psychiatric Association. Used with permission.

Many medications are listed as potential causes of depressive symptoms (Table 7–4). It is important for consultants to note whether there is a temporal relationship between the onset of depression and the medication in question or with changes in medication dosage. Diagnosis may also be supported by the finding that reintroduction of the suspected medication leads to a recurrence of the depression. There are no known controlled prospective studies that show an association of any medication with a primary depressive illness, and in practice it is less common that a medication alone is the most significant factor in causing disabling depressive symptomatology.

Assessment

The goal of assessment is to differentiate clinically significant depressive symptoms from everyday sadness and irritability, which are common and developmentally normative. The SIG E CAPS mnemonic (Wise and Rundell 1988) is a well-known memory aid that can ensure that all the diagnostic criteria for a major depressive episode are considered (Table 7–5). Table 7–6 outlines a useful working model that consultants can use as a guide in considering the differential diagnosis of depressive symptoms in the pediatric setting. Evaluative components in assessing depressive and manic symptoms in a pediatric setting are outlined in Table 7–7. Consultants need to carefully review available laboratory, radiographic, and other tests; on the basis of the clinical presentation, they may want to recommend additional tests.

Because depressive symptoms can go unrecognized or underestimated in youth with physical illnesses, consultants may consider using a standardized symptom rating scale to help recognize and characterize the nature and breadth of these symptoms. Although the well-known Children's Depression Inventory, 2nd Edition (CDI-2: Kovacs 2011) is too lengthy for routine use, the short version (CDI-2: Self-Report, Short Form; Kovacs 2011) has been shown to be a valid instrument for assessing medically ill children (Allgaier et al. 2012a). In addition, some scales with acceptable psychometric properties are freely available, such as the following:

- Patient Health Questionnaire-9 (PHQ-9; Richardson et al. 2010) is a 9-item self-report questionnaire assessing adolescent depression symptoms and severity (available at https://afsp.org/wp-content/uploads/2016/03/13252_AFSP_PHQ_HealthQestionnaire_m2.pdf).
- Mood and Feeling Questionnaire (MFQ; Messer et al. 1995) has a 34-item parent questionnaire and a 33-item patient questionnaire used to assess depressive symptoms in youth ages 8–18 years (available at http://devepi.duhs.duke.edu/mfq.html).

Table 7–4.   Selected medications associated with depression and mania

Associated with depression	Associated with mania
Analgesics (narcotics)	Androgens (anabolic steroids)
Methadone	Bronchodilators
Oxycodone	Albuterol
Cancer chemotherapy agents	Terbutaline
Amphotericin B	Cardiovascular
L-Asparaginase	Captopril
Interferon	Clonidine withdrawal
Procarbazine	Methyldopa
Vincristine	Corticosteroids
Vinblastine	Cancer chemotherapy agents
Cardiovascular	Procarbazine
Atenolol	Decongestants
Methyldopa	Histamine-2 receptor antagonists
Nadolol	Cimetidine
Procainamide	Psychiatric medications
Propafenone	Alprazolam
Propranolol	Antidepressants
Corticosteroids	Buspirone
Prednisone	Lorazepam
Histamine-2 receptor antagonists	Methylphenidate
Cimetidine	Triazolam

Table 7–4. Selected medications associated with depression and mania *(continued)*

Associated with depression	Associated with mania
Immunosuppressants	Miscellaneous
Cyclosporine	Amantadine
Tacrolimus	Baclofen
Interferon	Carbamazepine
Oral contraceptives	Cyclobenzaprine
	Cyproheptadine
	Metoclopramide
	Thyroid preparations
	Tolmetin
	Zidovudine

- Ask Suicide-Screening Questions (ASQ; Horowitz et al. 2012) is a screening instrument, consisting of four items, that has high sensitivity and negative predictive value and has been shown to be helpful in the assessment of suicide risk in patients presenting to pediatric emergency departments (available at https://www.nimh.nih.gov/labs-at-nimh/asq-toolkit-materials/index.shtml).

Treatment

Management of depressive symptoms in physically ill children begins with ensuring that their illness is being fully treated medically because this alone may alleviate the symptoms. Actions include aggressively managing pain and exploring possible pediatric and psychiatric diagnostic entities that may be contributing directly to a patient's dysphoria.

A number of nonpharmacological interventions can be instituted. The first step is to mobilize the patient within the constraints of his or her physical

Table 7–5.   Mnemonic for diagnostic criteria for major depressive
syndrome

SIG E CAPS ("Prescribe energy capsules")

Sleep—insomnia or hypersomnia

Interests—loss of interests or pleasure

Guilt—excessive guilt, worthlessness, hopelessness

Energy—loss of energy, or fatigue

Concentration—diminished concentration ability, indecisiveness

Appetite—decreased appetite; more than 5% weight loss or gain

Psychomotor—psychomotor retardation or agitation

Suicidality—suicidal thoughts or ideation, suicide plan, suicide attempt; includes
thoughts of death or preoccupation with death

Source.   Reprinted from Wise MG, Rundell JR: "Depression and Mania," in *Concise Guide to
Consultation Psychiatry.* Washington, DC, American Psychiatric Press, 1988, pp. 55–73. Copyright © 1988, American Psychiatric Press. Used with permission.

illness. These may include changing the hospital environment (e.g., making
the room more familiar with pictures, making sure drapes are open) or having
the patient take part in the hospital's child life or activity program. Supportive
psychotherapy and/or cognitive-behavioral therapy techniques can prove
helpful to patients (Szigethy et al. 2014a), and parents can be educated about
the impact of hospitalization on their children and the parents' importance in
this process. Principles of individual and family intervention are outlined in
Chapter 15 ("Psychotherapy in the Pediatric Setting") and Chapter 16 ("Family Interventions").

Pharmacotherapy becomes a consideration when a child has insufficient
response to the psychosocial interventions, the child's daily functioning is significantly impaired, the child's depression is sufficiently severe to interfere
with medical treatment, and/or the child has a history of previous depressive episodes, manic episodes, or psychosis. Although literature pertaining to pharmacological treatment of comorbid depression and physical illness is limited,

Table 7–6. Differential diagnosis between primary depressive illness, depressive disorder due to another medical condition, and depressive symptoms as psychological reaction

	Primary depressive illness	Depressive disorder due to another medical condition	Depressive symptoms as psychological reaction
Meets diagnostic criteria for primary depressive illness	++	+	+/−
Presence of suicidality	++	+/−	+/−
Family history of depressive disorder	++	−	+/−
Past history of depression	+	+/−	+/−
Neurovegetative symptoms of depression	++	++	−
Abnormal findings on physical examination or workup	−	++	−
Treatment with medications that cause depression	−	+	−
Presence of psychosocial stressors	+	−	++
Mood brightens when distracted	+/−	−	++
Positive response to antidepressants	++	−	−
Positive response to psychotherapy	++	−	++

Source. Adapted from Waller and Rush 1983.

Table 7–7.   Evaluative components in assessing depressive and manic symptoms in the pediatric setting

Medical-psychiatric history

Current subjective symptoms

Sources of depression/mania

Academic and social impact	Isolation
Death	Loss of control
Diagnosis of illness	Loss of privacy
Financial burden of illness	Pain
Hospital depression	Physical effects of illness
Impact on family members	Uncertainty about prognosis

Use of prescribed medications and/or drugs of abuse

History of psychiatric disorders, especially depressive and manic disorders

Family history of psychiatric disorders, especially depressive disorders

Mental status examination with emphasis on mood, cognition, and psychotic symptoms

Physical examination, with attention to focal neurological deficits

Nondominant hemisphere

Anosognosia	Hemiparesis
Constructional dyspraxia	Hyperactive tendon reflexes
Babinski sign	Left-sided neglect

Frontal lobe

Basal ganglia	Chorea
Athetosis	Parkinsonism

Table 7–7.   Evaluative components in assessing depressive and manic symptoms in the pediatric setting *(continued)*

Hematological and chemistry test considerations based on clinical presentation

Complete blood cell count	Glucose level
Electrolyte levels	Liver function tests
Calcium level	Magnesium level
Serum cortisol	Phosphorus level
Serum urea nitrogen	Urinary toxicology screen
Creatinine level	Arterial blood gas analysis

Radiographic and other test considerations based on clinical presentation

Chest radiography	Computed tomography
Magnetic resonance imaging	Lumbar puncture
Electroencephalography	Electrocardiography/24-hour monitor

clinical experience suggests that the target symptoms of depression in physical illnesses may respond to pharmacotherapy. Consultants will generally target depression with one of the selective serotonin reuptake inhibitor antidepressants. The use of a stimulant medication is another consideration for treating the physically ill child with symptoms of fatigue and malaise due to a pediatric condition. Psychopharmacological management is addressed in Chapter 17 ("Psychopharmacological Approaches and Considerations").

References

Allgaier AK, Frühe B, Pietsch K, et al: Is the Children's Depression Inventory Short version a valid screening tool in pediatric care? A comparison to its full-length version. J Psychosom Res 73(5):369–374, 2012a 23062811

Allgaier AK, Pietsch K, Frühe B, et al: Screening for depression in adolescents: validity of the Patient Health Questionnaire in pediatric care. Depress Anxiety 29(10):906–913, 2012b 22753313

American Psychiatric Association: Diagnostic and Statistical Manual of Mental Disorders, 5th Edition. Arlington, VA, American Psychiatric Association, 2013

Beasley PJ, Beardslee WR: Depression in the adolescent patient. Adolesc Med 9(2):351–362, vii, 1998 10961241

Bernal P, Estroff DB, Aboudarham JF, et al: Psychosocial morbidity: the economic burden in a pediatric health maintenance organization sample. Arch Pediatr Adolesc Med 154(3):261–266, 2000 10710024

Bhatt-Poulose K, James K, Reid M, et al: Increased rates of body dissatisfaction, depressive symptoms, and suicide attempts in Jamaican teens with sickle cell disease. Pediatr Blood Cancer 63(12):2159–2166, 2016 27393908

Boyd AD, Riba M: Depression and pancreatic cancer. J Natl Compr Canc Netw 5(1):113–116, 2007 17239331

Brown MR, Sourkes B: Pediatric palliative care, in Textbook of Pediatric Psychosomatic Medicine. Edited by Shaw RJ, DeMaso DR. Washington, DC, American Psychiatric Publishing, 2010, pp 245–257

Cameron K, Ogrodniczuk J, Hadjipavlou G: Changes in alexithymia following psychological intervention: a review. Harv Rev Psychiatry 22(3):162–178, 2014 24736520

Ciechanowski PS, Katon WJ, Russo JE: Depression and diabetes: impact of depressive symptoms on adherence, function, and costs. Arch Intern Med 160(21):3278–3285, 2000 11088090

Cummings JL: Organic psychoses: delusional disorders and secondary mania. Psychiatr Clin North Am 9(2):293–311, 1986 2873560

Goodman E, Whitaker RC: A prospective study of the role of depression in the development and persistence of adolescent obesity. Pediatrics 110(3):497–504, 2002 12205250

Haarasilta L, Marttunen M, Kaprio J, et al: Major depressive episode and health care use among adolescents and young adults. Soc Psychiatry Psychiatr Epidemiol 38(7):366–372, 2003 12861442

Hood KK, Lawrence JM, Anderson A, et al; SEARCH for Diabetes in Youth Study Group: Metabolic and inflammatory links to depression in youth with diabetes. Diabetes Care 35(12):2443–2446, 2012 23033243

Horowitz LM, Bridge JA, Teach SJ, et al: Ask Suicide-Screening Questions (ASQ): a brief instrument for the pediatric emergency department. Arch Pediatr Adolesc Med 166(12):1170–1176, 2012 23027429

Jane Costello E, Erkanli A, Angold A: Is there an epidemic of child or adolescent depression? J Child Psychol Psychiatry 47(12):1263–1271, 2006 17176381

Katon WJ: Clinical and health services relationships between major depression, depressive symptoms, and general medical illness. Biol Psychiatry 54(3):216–226, 2003 12893098

Katon WJ, Sullivan M, Walker E: Medical symptoms without identified pathology: relationship to psychiatric disorders, childhood and adult trauma, and personality traits. Ann Intern Med 134(9 Pt 2):917–925, 2001 11346329

Kişlal FM, Kutluk T, Cetin FC, et al: Psychiatric symptoms of adolescents with physical complaints admitted to an adolescence unit. Clin Pediatr (Phila) 44(2):121–130, 2005 15735829

Knook LM, Konijnenberg AY, van der Hoeven J, et al: Psychiatric disorders in children and adolescents presenting with unexplained chronic pain: what is the prevalence and clinical relevancy? Eur Child Adolesc Psychiatry 20(1):39–48, 2011 21174221

Kovacs M: The Children's Depression Inventory, 2nd Edition (CDI-2). Technical Manual. North Tonawanda, NY, Multi-Health Systems, 2011

LeBlanc LA, Goldsmith T, Patel DR: Behavioral aspects of chronic illness in children and adolescents. Pediatr Clin North Am 50(4):859–878, 2003 12964698

Lustman PJ, Griffith LS, Freedland KE, et al: The course of major depression in diabetes. Gen Hosp Psychiatry 19(2):138–143, 1997 9097068

Margetić B, Aukst-Margetić B, Bilić E, et al: Depression, anxiety and pain in children with juvenile idiopathic arthritis (JIA). Eur Psychiatry 20(3):274–276, 2005 15935428

Mendez MF: Mania in neurologic disorders. Curr Psychiatry Rep 2(5):440–445, 2000 11122994

Merikangas KR, He JP, Burstein M, et al: Lifetime prevalence of mental disorders in U.S. adolescents: results from the National Comorbidity Survey Replication—Adolescent Supplement (NCS-A). J Am Acad Child Adolesc Psychiatry 49(10):980–989, 2010 20855043

Messer SC, Angold A, Costello J, et al: Development of a short questionnaire for use in epidemiological studies of depression in children and adolescents: factor composition and structure across development. Int J Methods Psychiatr Res 5:251–262, 1995

Miller GE, Cole SW: Clustering of depression and inflammation in adolescents previously exposed to childhood adversity. Biol Psychiatry 72(1):34–40, 2012 22494534

Natalucci G, Faedda N, Calderoni D, et al: Headache and alexithymia in children and adolescents: what is the connection? Front Psychol 9:48, 2018 29449820

Ormel J, Von Korff M, Van den Brink W, et al: Depression, anxiety, and social disability show synchrony of change in primary care patients. Am J Public Health 83(3):385–390, 1993 8438977

Pinquart M, Shen Y: Depressive symptoms in children and adolescents with chronic physical illness: an updated meta-analysis. J Pediatr Psychol 36(4):375–384, 2011 21088072

Richardson LP, McCauley E, Grossman DC, et al: Evaluation of the Patient Health Questionnaire-9 Item for detecting major depression among adolescents. Pediatrics 126(6):1117–1123, 2010 21041282

Rundell JR, Wise MG: Causes of organic mood disorder. J Neuropsychiatry Clin Neurosci 1(4):398–400, 1989 2521090

Stein MB, Cox BJ, Afifi TO, et al: Does co-morbid depressive illness magnify the impact of chronic physical illness? A population-based perspective. Psychol Med 36(5):587–596, 2006 16608557

Szigethy EM, Bujoreanu SI, Youk AO, et al: Randomized efficacy trial of two psychotherapies for depression in youth with inflammatory bowel disease. J Am Acad Child Adolesc Psychiatry 53(7):726–735, 2014a 24954822

Szigethy EM, Youk AO, Benhayon D, et al: Depression subtypes in pediatric inflammatory bowel disease. J Pediatr Gastroenterol Nutr 58(5):574–581, 2014b 24345836

Waller DA, Rush AJ: Differentiating primary affective disease, organic affective syndromes, and situational depression on a pediatric service. J Am Acad Child Psychiatry 22(1):52–58, 1983 6826998

Walter HJ, Kackloudis G, Trudell EK, et al: Enhancing pediatricians' behavioral health competencies through child psychiatry consultation and education. Clin Pediatr (Phila) 57(8):958–969, 2018 29082768

Wise MG, Rundell JR: Depression and mania, in Concise Guide to Consultation Psychiatry. Washington, DC, American Psychiatric Press, 1988, pp 55–73

8

Anxiety Symptoms and Trauma/Stress Reactions

Anxiety is the anticipation of future threat, whereas fear is the emotional response to a real or perceived imminent threat (American Psychiatric Association 2013). Both are ubiquitous for children and adolescents in the pediatric setting and may significantly interfere with functioning and cause psychological distress. Anxiety and fear may be directly manifested by the physiological mechanism of a medical condition or medication and/or affect the course of a medical condition and its treatment. Symptoms of anxiety and fear may adversely impact the course of a medical condition, including through interference with treatment adherence. Although these symptoms are essential features of anxiety disorders, they also commonly occur in a large number of psychiatric disorders (e.g., depressive, substance-related, psychotic, and trauma- and stressor-related disorders) and/or may accompany another psychiatric disorder as a comorbid anxiety (Costello et al. 2011; Verduin and Kendall 2003).

In work with physically ill children and adolescents, consultants are commonly faced with untangling these diagnostic dilemmas. In general, symptoms of anxiety and fear may be 1) secondary to the presence of a comorbid primary anxiety disorder; 2) a psychological reaction to the stress of a physical illness; 3) the direct physiological effects of a medical or substance-induced condition and/or its treatment; or 4) combinations of all three (Figure 8–1).

Primary Anxiety Disorders

Anxiety disorders are among the most common childhood psychiatric disorders, with a 7.1% current prevalence for ages 3–17 years (Ghandour et al. 2019). There is a 30% estimated lifetime prevalence for any childhood anxiety disorder and a median age at onset of 11 years. Specific anxiety disorders in descending order of lifetime prevalence are specific phobia (20%), social anxiety (9%), separation anxiety (8%), panic (2%), and generalized anxiety (2%) (Kessler et al. 2005, 2012). Each type of anxiety disorder generally manifests during specific developmental phases: separation anxiety during preschool years; specific phobias during early school-age years; social anxiety during later school-age/ early adolescent years; and generalized anxiety and panic during later adolescence/young adulthood (Beesdo-Baum and Knappe 2012; Costello et al. 2003). Table 8–1 outlines the essential features of the anxiety disorders that are more commonly seen by consultants in the pediatric setting.

Factors that may play important etiological roles in anxiety disorders include insecure attachment, behavioral inhibition, parenting factors, and stressful/traumatic exposures (Clauss and Blackford 2012; Colonnesi et al. 2011; Green et al. 2010). Estimates of anxiety disorder inheritability have ranged from 20% to 50% in twin studies (Taylor et al. 2018). Accounting for the remaining variability in risk, nonshared environment factors (i.e., early life stress) can adversely impact neurochemical messaging between the prefrontal cortex and the amygdala, which are partners in the fear circuit. Learning (classical and operant conditioning) continues to be viewed as playing an important etiological and maintenance role in these disorders (Taylor et al. 2018).

Patients with chronic physical illnesses are at risk for elevated symptoms of anxiety (Ferro and Boyle 2015; Pinquart and Shen 2011). Some evidence indicates that the symptoms may be mediated by symptoms of maternal depression, family dysfunction, and/or child self-esteem (Ferro and Boyle 2015). That said, it has been noted that differences in anxiety levels between children with and without chronic illnesses but with anxiety are generally small. Anxiety symptoms appear to be most prevalent when the course of illness and emer-

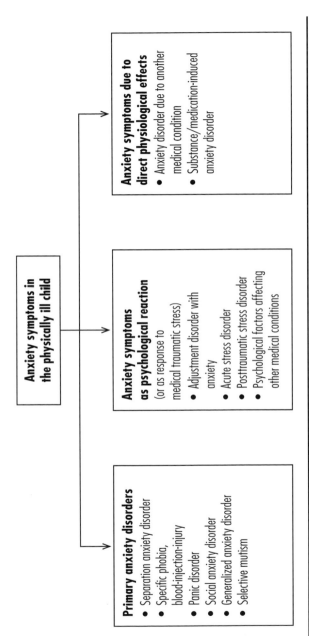

Figure 8–1. Differential diagnosis of anxiety symptoms in the physically ill child or adolescent.

Table 8–1.   Selected primary anxiety disorders to consider in the physically ill child

DSM-5 anxiety disorder	Essential features
Separation anxiety disorder	Excessive fear or anxiety concerning separation from home or attachment figures that is developmentally inappropriate
Specific phobia; blood-injection-injury	Marked fear or anxiety circumscribed to blood, injections, transfusions, other medical care, and/or injury
Panic disorder	Recurrent unexpected panic attacks with an abrupt surge of intense fear or intense discomfort from physical and cognitive symptoms that reaches peak in minutes
Social anxiety disorder	Marked or intense fear or anxiety of social situations in which the individual is scrutinized by others
Generalized anxiety disorder	Excessive anxiety and worry (apprehensive expectations) about a number of events or activities
Selective mutism	Consistent failure to speak in specific social situations in which there is an expectation for speaking

Source.   American Psychiatric Association 2013.

gence of illness symptoms are very difficult to control and/or when the child's control over his or her environment is restricted because of chronic illness (Pinquart and Shen 2011). There is increased risk for anxiety disorders in adulthood and increased suicide risk, especially for children with panic disorders and comorbid anxiety with depression.

The psychological symptoms of anxiety are routinely associated with physical signs of autonomic activity, such as palpitations, shortness of breath, tremulousness, flushing, faintness, dizziness, chest pain, dry mouth, and/or muscle tension. These physical symptoms can present consultants with particularly complex diagnostic issues in a child with a co-occurring pediatric condition.

Panic attacks are characterized by an abrupt surge of intense fear or intense discomfort that reaches its peak within minutes and during which time at least four physical or cognitive symptoms occur (Table 8–2). Consultants also need to be aware that a panic attack is not a mental disorder, because panic attacks can occur in the context of any anxiety disorder as well as in other mental disorders, including depressive disorders, posttraumatic stress disorder (PTSD), substance use disorders, and certain pediatric conditions, such as those affecting the cardiac, respiratory, vestibular, and gastrointestinal systems (American Psychiatric Association 2013).

Anxiety Symptoms as Psychological Reaction: Trauma/Stress Reactions

Anxiety and fear are common psychological reactions to the stress of a major pediatric illness and its treatment. Patients with genetic and biological vulnerabilities to anxiety symptoms are vulnerable to having intense reactions to the diagnosis and treatment of their physical illnesses, but these same pediatric conditions can induce disabling anxiety in patients with no prior history of anxiety. In their assessment, consultants should consider the following psychological sources of anxiety: illness diagnosis, physical integrity, hospital anxiety, impact of illness, and prognosis and death (Table 8–3).

Pediatric medical traumatic stress (PMTS) is a term used to characterize the psychological responses of children and their families to pain, injury, serious illness, medical procedures, and invasive or frightening treatment experiences (Kazak et al. 2006; Price et al. 2016). PMTS responses, which include anxiety and fear, are described in the following symptom triad: intrusiveness (reexperiencing), numbness (or avoidance), and hyperarousal. This PMTS triad parallels the DSM-5 acute stress disorder (ASD) and PTSD diagnostic criteria of intrusive symptoms, persistence of stimuli, and negative alterations in cognition and mood associated with a traumatic event as well as marked alterations in arousal and reactivity (American Psychiatric Association 2013). These symptoms may occur across a spectrum of severity ranging from normative/mild to moderate to severe. At the severe end of this spectrum, the diagnostic criteria for a trauma- and stressor-related disorder will be met in the context of exposure to actual or threatened death and/or serious injury (American Psychiatric Association 2013).

Table 8–2.   Physical and cognitive symptoms of a panic attack

Panic attack is defined as an abrupt surge of intense fear or intense discomfort that reaches a peak within minutes, and during which time four (or more) of the following symptoms occur:

  Palpitations, pounding heart, or accelerated heart rate

  Sweating

  Trembling or shaking

  Sensations of shortness of breath or smothering

  Feelings of choking

  Chest pain or discomfort

  Nausea or abdominal distress

  Feeling dizzy, unsteady, light-headed, or faint

  Chills or heat sensations

  Paresthesias (numbness or tingling sensations)

  Derealization (feeling of unreality) or depersonalization (being detached from
    oneself)

  Fear of losing control or "going crazy"

  Fear of dying

Note.   Culture-specific symptoms (e.g., tinnitus, neck soreness, headache, uncontrollable screaming or crying) may be seen. Such symptoms should not count as one of the four required symptoms.
Source.   Adapted from American Psychiatric Association: *Diagnostic and Statistical Manual of Mental Disorders,* 5th Edition. Arlington, VA, American Psychiatric Association, 2013. Copyright © 2013 American Psychiatric Association. Used with permission.

An integrative model has been used to understand family adjustment to experiencing PMTS whereby three consecutive time periods are considered: 1) peritrauma (during or immediately following the medical event); 2) acute medical care (early, ongoing, and evolving responses); and 3) longer-term PMTS (Kazak et al. 2006). This model assumes a range of normal reactions, preexisting psychological functioning that influence risk, the use of a developmental

Table 8–3. Psychological sources of anxiety associated with pediatric physical illness

Source of anxiety	Factors to consider
Illness diagnosis	Patients often experience symptoms of anxiety around the time of diagnosis of a physical illness. Individuals with a family history of a specific medical condition may experience anxiety symptoms due to the excessive fear that they will be similarly affected. This fear can cause elevated symptoms of anxiety related to routine pediatric appointments during the period between the initial evaluation of a symptom and its diagnosis. Anxiety may also occur when a patient has an abnormal laboratory test that does not lead to a diagnosis but does require follow-up or monitoring.
Physical integrity	Beginning around age 4 or 5, children become more concerned about bodily injury and are more cognitively aware of the physical effects of illness. As a result, they frequently experience anxiety. There may be fears about amputation, loss of vision, or pain. Adolescents in particular may worry about the cosmetic effects of an illness or treatment due to excessive concerns about social stigma.
Hospital anxiety	Hospitalized children have to adjust to the presence of pediatric staff and to disruptions to their daily routine. These children may experience anxiety about the presence of hospital staff, particularly when the staff becomes associated with stressful medical procedures or the delivery of disturbing medical information. Children younger than 4 or 5 years are particularly prone to anxiety when separated from their caretakers. Patients who have not adhered to their medical treatment or who have engaged in risk-taking behaviors may conceal important medical information because of anticipatory anxiety about the potential disapproval of their physicians.

Table 8–3.   Psychological sources of anxiety associated with pediatric physical illness *(continued)*

Source of anxiety	Factors to consider
Impact of illness	Children frequently report symptoms of anxiety related to the impact of the illness on their own lives and on family members. They may be concerned about missing school or falling behind academically. Adolescents may be particularly troubled by their separation from peers as well as by feeling "different" from others. Children may feel guilty about their need for increased parental attention and assistance. Some children report worries about the financial impact of their illness on the family because their parents have to take time off work or because of the costs of treatment.
Prognosis and death	Children may experience anxieties about their prognosis and death that can be based on both realistic and unrealistic appraisals of their illness. Children can develop symptoms of anxiety related to fears about the recurrence of an illness such as cancer. Such fears are not necessarily assuaged by a favorable statistical prognosis. A family history of medical illness or knowledge of the death of a family member or peer can influence these fears. Children may also report concerns about the emotional impact of their death on parents or siblings.

Source.   Reprinted from Guite JW, Kazak AE: "Anxiety Symptoms and Disorders," in *Textbook of Pediatric Psychosomatic Medicine.* Edited by Shaw RJ, DeMaso DR. Washington, DC, American Psychiatric Publishing, 2010, p. 104. Used with permission.

lens, and a social ecological approach that informs optimal mental health intervention, including screening, prevention, and treatment, in response to the medical trauma experienced by patients and their families (Price et al. 2016).

Funded by the U.S. Substance Abuse and Mental Health Services Administration (SAMHSA) and Health and Human Services (HHS), the National Child Traumatic Stress Network (NCTSN) has developed PMTS resources for both parents and health care providers (available at: https://www.nctsn.org/what-is-child-trauma/trauma-types/medical-trauma). The NCTSN recommends that all health care providers practice "trauma-informed care" by incorporating an understanding of traumatic stress and related responses into their patient encounters. As a means of ensuring the identification, prevention, and treatment of PMTS responses, the NCTSN has proposed that all health care providers follow the D-E-F Protocol: 1) reduce Distress (assess and manage pain, ask about fears and worries, consider grief and loss); 2) promote Emotional support (consider who and what the patient needs now, address barriers to mobilizing existing supports); and 3) remember the Family (assess parents' or siblings' distress, gauge family stressors and resources, address other needs beyond medical) (available at: https://www.nctsn.org/resources/pediatric-medical-traumatic-stress-toolkit-health-care-providers).

Trauma- and Stressor-Related Disorders

Although no longer classified as anxiety disorders in DSM-5, trauma- and stressor-related disorders have symptoms in the pediatric setting that can often be understood within an anxiety- or fear-based framework.

Adjustment Disorder

Adjustment disorder with anxiety (nervousness, worry, jitteriness, or separation anxiety) or with mixed anxiety and depressed mood occurs in response to an identifiable stressor of any severity (American Psychiatric Association 2013). The stressor may be a single event, such as an acute hospitalization, or there may be multiple stressors (e.g., multiple hospitalizations and family problems). The stressor may be recurrent or continuous and may affect the patient, the family, and/or the pediatric team. Associated with marked distress and/or significant impairment in functioning, the adjustment disorders are common accompaniments and often are the major psychological response to pediatric illness (American Psychiatric Association 2013).

Acute Stress Disorder and Posttraumatic Stress Disorder

ASD and PTSD are characterized by exposure to actual or threatened death, serious injury, or sexual violence (Boxes 8–1 and 8–2). When the full criteria for these disorders are met, features of anhedonia and dysphoria, anger or aggression, or dissociative symptoms are generally more predominant than anxiety- or fear-based symptoms.

Box 8–1.   DSM-5 Diagnostic Criteria for
            Acute Stress Disorder

A. Exposure to actual or threatened death, serious injury, or sexual violence in one (or more) of the following ways:

   1. Directly experiencing the traumatic event(s).
   2. Witnessing, in person, the event(s) as it occurred to others.
   3. Learning that the event(s) occurred to a close family member or
      close friend. **Note:** In cases of actual or threatened death of a
      family member or friend, the event(s) must have been violent or
      accidental.
   4. Experiencing repeated or extreme exposure to aversive details
      of the traumatic event(s) (e.g., first responders collecting human
      remains, police officers repeatedly exposed to details of child
      abuse).

      Note: This does not apply to exposure through electronic media,
      television, movies, or pictures, unless this exposure is work
      related.

B. Presence of nine (or more) of the following symptoms from any of
   the five categories of intrusion, negative mood, dissociation, avoidance, and arousal, beginning or worsening after the traumatic
   event(s) occurred:

   Intrusion Symptoms

   1. Recurrent, involuntary, and intrusive distressing memories of
      the traumatic event(s). **Note:** In children, repetitive play may
      occur in which themes or aspects of the traumatic event(s) are
      expressed.
   2. Recurrent distressing dreams in which the content and/or af-
      fect of the dream are related to the event(s). **Note:** In children,
      there may be frightening dreams without recognizable content.
   3. Dissociative reactions (e.g., flashbacks) in which the individual
      feels or acts as if the traumatic event(s) were recurring. (Such
      reactions may occur on a continuum, with the most extreme
      expression being a complete loss of awareness of present sur-
      roundings.) **Note:** In children, trauma-specific reenactment
      may occur in play.

4. Intense or prolonged psychological distress or marked physiological reactions in response to internal or external cues that symbolize or resemble an aspect of the traumatic event(s).

Negative Mood

5. Persistent inability to experience positive emotions (e.g., inability to experience happiness, satisfaction, or loving feelings).

Dissociative Symptoms

6. An altered sense of the reality of one's surroundings or oneself (e.g., seeing oneself from another's perspective, being in a daze, time slowing).
7. Inability to remember an important aspect of the traumatic event(s) (typically due to dissociative amnesia and not to other factors such as head injury, alcohol, or drugs).

Avoidance Symptoms

8. Efforts to avoid distressing memories, thoughts, or feelings about or closely associated with the traumatic event(s).
9. Efforts to avoid external reminders (people, places, conversations, activities, objects, situations) that arouse distressing memories, thoughts, or feelings about or closely associated with the traumatic event(s).

Arousal Symptoms

10. Sleep disturbance (e.g., difficulty falling or staying asleep, restless sleep).
11. Irritable behavior and angry outbursts (with little or no provocation), typically expressed as verbal or physical aggression toward people or objects.
12. Hypervigilance.
13. Problems with concentration.
14. Exaggerated startle response.

C. Duration of the disturbance (symptoms in Criterion B) is 3 days to 1 month after trauma exposure.

Note: Symptoms typically begin immediately after the trauma, but persistence for at least 3 days and up to a month is needed to meet disorder criteria.

D. The disturbance causes clinically significant distress or impairment in social, occupational, or other important areas of functioning.

E. The disturbance is not attributable to the physiological effects of a substance (e.g., medication or alcohol) or another medical condition (e.g., mild traumatic brain injury) and is not better explained by brief psychotic disorder.

Source. Reprinted from American Psychiatric Association: *Diagnostic and Statistical Manual of Mental Disorders*, 5th Edition. Arlington, VA, American Psychiatric Association, 2013. Copyright © 2013 American Psychiatric Association. Used with permission.

Box 8–2.   DSM-5 Diagnostic Criteria for Posttraumatic Stress Disorder

---

Posttraumatic Stress Disorder

Note: The following criteria apply to adults, adolescents, and children older than 6 years. For children 6 years and younger, see corresponding criteria below.

A. Exposure to actual or threatened death, serious injury, or sexual violence in one (or more) of the following ways:

   1. Directly experiencing the traumatic event(s).
   2. Witnessing, in person, the event(s) as it occurred to others.
   3. Learning that the traumatic event(s) occurred to a close family member or close friend. In cases of actual or threatened death of a family member or friend, the event(s) must have been violent or accidental.
   4. Experiencing repeated or extreme exposure to aversive details of the traumatic event(s) (e.g., first responders collecting human remains; police officers repeatedly exposed to details of child abuse).

      Note: Criterion A4 does not apply to exposure through electronic media, television, movies, or pictures, unless this exposure is work related.

B. Presence of one (or more) of the following intrusion symptoms associated with the traumatic event(s), beginning after the traumatic event(s) occurred:

   1. Recurrent, involuntary, and intrusive distressing memories of the traumatic event(s).

> **Note:** In children older than 6 years, repetitive play may occur in which themes or aspects of the traumatic event(s) are expressed.

2. Recurrent distressing dreams in which the content and/or affect of the dream are related to the traumatic event(s).

> **Note:** In children, there may be frightening dreams without recognizable content.

3. Dissociative reactions (e.g., flashbacks) in which the individual feels or acts as if the traumatic event(s) were recurring. (Such reactions may occur on a continuum, with the most extreme expression being a complete loss of awareness of present surroundings.)

> **Note:** In children, trauma-specific reenactment may occur in play.

4. Intense or prolonged psychological distress at exposure to internal or external cues that symbolize or resemble an aspect of the traumatic event(s).
5. Marked physiological reactions to internal or external cues that symbolize or resemble an aspect of the traumatic event(s).

C. Persistent avoidance of stimuli associated with the traumatic event(s), beginning after the traumatic event(s) occurred, as evidenced by one or both of the following:

1. Avoidance of or efforts to avoid distressing memories, thoughts, or feelings about or closely associated with the traumatic event(s).
2. Avoidance of or efforts to avoid external reminders (people, places, conversations, activities, objects, situations) that arouse distressing memories, thoughts, or feelings about or closely associated with the traumatic event(s).

D. Negative alterations in cognitions and mood associated with the traumatic event(s), beginning or worsening after the traumatic event(s) occurred, as evidenced by two (or more) of the following:

1. Inability to remember an important aspect of the traumatic event(s) (typically due to dissociative amnesia and not to other factors such as head injury, alcohol, or drugs).
2. Persistent and exaggerated negative beliefs or expectations about oneself, others, or the world (e.g., "I am bad," "No one can

be trusted," "The world is completely dangerous," "My whole nervous system is permanently ruined").

3. Persistent, distorted cognitions about the cause or consequences of the traumatic event(s) that lead the individual to blame himself/herself or others.

4. Persistent negative emotional state (e.g., fear, horror, anger, guilt, or shame).

5. Markedly diminished interest or participation in significant activities.

6. Feelings of detachment or estrangement from others.

7. Persistent inability to experience positive emotions (e.g., inability to experience happiness, satisfaction, or loving feelings).

E. Marked alterations in arousal and reactivity associated with the traumatic event(s), beginning or worsening after the traumatic event(s) occurred, as evidenced by two (or more) of the following:

1. Irritable behavior and angry outbursts (with little or no provocation) typically expressed as verbal or physical aggression toward people or objects.

2. Reckless or self-destructive behavior.

3. Hypervigilance.

4. Exaggerated startle response.

5. Problems with concentration.

6. Sleep disturbance (e.g., difficulty falling or staying asleep or restless sleep).

F. Duration of the disturbance (Criteria B, C, D, and E) is more than 1 month.

G. The disturbance causes clinically significant distress or impairment in social, occupational, or other important areas of functioning.

H. The disturbance is not attributable to the physiological effects of a substance (e.g., medication, alcohol) or another medical condition.

Specify whether:

With dissociative symptoms: The individual's symptoms meet the criteria for posttraumatic stress disorder, and in addition, in response to the stressor, the individual experiences persistent or recurrent symptoms of either of the following:

1. **Depersonalization:** Persistent or recurrent experiences of feeling detached from, and as if one were an outside observer of, one's mental processes or body (e.g., feeling as though one

were in a dream; feeling a sense of unreality of self or body or of time moving slowly).

2. **Derealization:** Persistent or recurrent experiences of unreality of surroundings (e.g., the world around the individual is experienced as unreal, dreamlike, distant, or distorted).

Note: To use this subtype, the dissociative symptoms must not be attributable to the physiological effects of a substance (e.g., blackouts, behavior during alcohol intoxication) or another medical condition (e.g., complex partial seizures).

Specify if:

With delayed expression: If the full diagnostic criteria are not met until at least 6 months after the event (although the onset and expression of some symptoms may be immediate).

Source. Reprinted from American Psychiatric Association: *Diagnostic and Statistical Manual of Mental Disorders*, 5th Edition. Arlington, VA, American Psychiatric Association, 2013. Copyright © 2013 American Psychiatric Association. Used with permission.

Consultants should be aware that a life-threatening illness or debilitating pediatric condition is not necessarily considered a traumatic event. Medical incidents that qualify as traumatic events consistent with ASD or PTSD are characterized by being sudden and catastrophic (American Psychiatric Association 2013). As mentioned above, less stressful events should lead consultants to use adjustment disorder as a more applicable diagnosis. That said, life-threatening illness has been thought to differ from the traumatic events generally associated with more typical examples of ASD and PTSD. In a physical illness, the threat to the individual arises internally and cannot be separated from the patient (Green et al. 1997). There is a qualitative difference between threats to the individual that are externally located (e.g., the threat following an assault or motor vehicle accident) and the threat of a disease that is located within the patient. Intrusive thoughts about physical illnesses tend to be ruminative and future oriented rather than focused on the recollection of a past trauma. This is particularly the case in chronic physical illnesses such as cancer or cystic fibrosis. Similarly, hyperarousal is commonly experienced as increased sensitivity to physical symptoms and may resemble hypochondriasis.

Nonetheless, there are numerous reports of an increased prevalence of posttraumatic stress symptoms in both physically ill patients and family members across a variety of illnesses, including cancer (Hobbie et al. 2000; Ljung-man et al. 2014; Stuber et al. 1996, 1997, 2010), diabetes (Rechenberg et al. 2017), epilepsy (Carmassi et al. 2017), infant death (Christiansen 2017), pulmonary hypertension (Mullen et al. 2014), neonatal intensive care (Shaw et al. 2006), and solid organ transplantation (Farley et al. 2007; Shemesh et al. 2000; Supelana et al. 2016; Young et al. 2003).

Psychological Factors Affecting Other Medical Conditions

The essential feature of the somatic symptom disorder diagnosis of psychological factors affecting other medical conditions is the presence of one or more clinically significant psychological or behavioral factors that adversely affect a pediatric condition by increasing the risk for suffering, death, or disability (American Psychiatric Association 2013). Anxiety is but one of many psychological factors that may adversely influence a physical condition. Anxiety symptoms that aggravate asthma or ulcerative colitis are two clinical examples. In contrast, when the anxiety symptoms are in response to a pediatric condition, consultants would more properly code the presence of an adjustment disorder with anxiety.

Anxiety Symptoms Due to Direct Physiological Effects

Anxiety Disorder Due to Another Medical Condition

The essential feature in anxiety disorder due to another medical condition is the presence of clinically significant anxiety that is judged to be best explained as a physiological effect of another medical condition (Box 8–3) (American Psychiatric Association 2013). Many pediatric conditions may result in symptoms of anxiety, and it is important to consider this diagnosis as a possibility if the history is not typical for a primary anxiety disorder, if the disturbance is inconsistent with a psychological reaction, and/or if anxiety symptoms are resistant to treatment. Pediatric etiologies are more likely when physical symptoms of anxiety, such as shortness of breath, tachycardia, or tremor, are marked. Table 8–4 lists some of the common medical conditions that are associated with symptoms of anxiety.

Box 8–3.   DSM-5 Diagnostic Criteria for Anxiety Disorder
Due to Another Medical Condition

A. Panic attacks or anxiety is predominant in the clinical picture.
B. There is evidence from the history, physical examination, or laboratory findings that the disturbance is the direct pathophysiological consequence of another medical condition.
C. The disturbance is not better explained by another mental disorder.
D. The disturbance does not occur exclusively during the course of a delirium.
E. The disturbance causes clinically significant distress or impairment in social, occupational, or other important areas of functioning.

Source.   Reprinted from American Psychiatric Association: *Diagnostic and Statistical Manual of Mental Disorders,* 5th Edition. Arlington, VA, American Psychiatric Association, 2013. Copyright © 2013 American Psychiatric Association. Used with permission.

Anxiety Symptoms in Specific Physical Conditions

Consultants will observe anxiety symptoms in a wide variety of pediatric conditions. There will be the noncategorical effects of anxiety that are experienced by all patients facing a physical illness and its treatment. From this perspective, children and their families are seen as experiencing stress in the context of being ill and not as a result of specific factors associated with a particular disease. For example, invasive pediatric procedures (e.g., venipuncture, intravenous lines) are common across illness types and can cause anxiety. In this context, anxiety symptoms are more dependent on the correlates of adjustment in childhood physical illness (see Chapter 2, "Coping and Adaptation in Physically Ill Children"). That said, this section provides brief highlights regarding a number of commonly encountered pediatric conditions associated with anxiety symptoms.

Cancer

Anxiety is common at various points throughout the diagnosis and treatment of pediatric cancer (Pao and Kazak 2015). Patients often experience increased anxiety during initial diagnosis, relapse, and even routine follow-up visits. Reference has been made to the increased rates of problematic PMTS experi-

Table 8–4.   Selected medical conditions etiologically related to anxiety symptoms

Neurological disorders	**Cardiac**
Delirium/dementia	Arrhythmias
Mass lesions	Congestive heart failure
Postconcussive syndrome	Hypovolemia
Poststroke	Valvular disease
Seizure	**Miscellaneous**
Vertigo	Anaphylaxis
Endocrine disorders	Asthma
Carcinoid syndrome	Diabetes mellitus
Hyperadrenalism	Hyperkalemia
Hypercalcemia	Hyperthermia
Hyperthyroid	Hypoxia
Hypocalcemia	Inflammatory bowel disease
Hypoglycemia	Pancreatic tumor
Hypomagnesemia	Pneumothorax
Hypothyroid	Porphyria
Pheochromocytoma	Pulmonary edema
	Pulmonary embolism
	Systemic lupus erythematosus

enced by patients and family members (Kazak et al. 2006; Price et al. 2016). Anxiety symptoms can interfere with a patient's ability to tolerate important components of medical treatment, including bone marrow aspirates, central line access, repeated venipunctures, and preparations for radiation therapy. Anticipatory nausea and vomiting are common and frequently have an anxiety component (Guite and Kazak 2010). Several of the medications used in the treatment of cancer include symptoms of anxiety as possible side effects. Antiemetic medications, such as prochlorperazine or metoclopramide, can cause symptoms of akathisia that may be misdiagnosed as anxiety. Anxiety symptoms are also elevated in patients experiencing disease-related pain.

Gastrointestinal Disorders

Studies suggest that patients with pediatric inflammatory bowel disease (IBD) are vulnerable to developing psychiatric disorders, including symptoms of anxiety and depression (Guite and Kazak 2010; Szigethy et al. 2014a). There is preliminary evidence for IBD depression profiles, including one subgroup with a predominately somatic presentation (depressed mood with high-dose steroid therapy) and another with a more cognitive presentation (highest rates of depression and anxiety) (Szigethy et al. 2014b). Pediatric patients with organic or functional gastrointestinal disorders have been found to have significantly elevated levels of anxiety compared to healthy comparators (Guite and Kazak 2010). There is significant comorbidity between recurrent abdominal pain and anxiety disorders. Pediatric patients with functional gastrointestinal disorders are at increased risk for psychological distress, disability, and health service use over time (Guite and Kazak 2010).

Heart Disease

A meta-analysis reviewing the psychological functioning of patients with congenital heart disease found that older children and adolescents displayed an increased risk of internalizing and, to a lesser extent, externalizing behavior problems (Karsdorp et al. 2007). Anxiety symptoms can appear as a direct result of cardiac failure caused by worsening congenital heart disease or an acute myocarditis. Anxiety states can occur early in the course of an unrecognized subacute bacterial endocarditis. Although the emotional functioning of patients with pediatric heart disease is generally not in the psychopathology range, those children who are at higher risk for anxiety often have other risk factors (e.g., cognitive deficits or family functioning problems) that need to be considered in the presentation (DeMaso 2004). Patients with single ventricle congenital heart disease display a high risk for psychiatric morbidity, particularly anxiety disorders and attention-deficit/hyperactivity disorder (DeMaso et al. 2017).

Hormone-Secreting Tumors

Pheochromocytoma is a rare disorder associated with catecholamine secretion from a tumor in the renal medulla. This secretion can result in acute, episodic, or chronic symptoms of anxiety often associated with hypertension. Clinical symptoms include increased heart rate, increased blood pressure, myocardial contractility, and vasoconstriction. Patients may present with headache, sweating, palpitations, apprehension, and a sense of impending doom (Goebel-Fabbri et al. 2005). Other patients may present with classic symptoms of a panic attack. Thyroid adenoma or carcinoma, parathyroid gland, adrenocorticotropic hormone–producing tumors, and insulinomas are other hormone-secreting tumors associated with anxiety symptoms.

Pulmonary Disease

Hypoxia, a condition in which a patient experiences symptoms of air hunger, may provoke anxiety in any individual. Consultants should be alert to this etiology, particularly in high-risk situations such as occur in the intensive care unit. After experiencing a lack of oxygen, some patients may develop secondary anxiety symptoms that interfere with efforts to wean them from the ventilator. Posttraumatic stress symptoms have also been reported in patients who experience episodes of acute respiratory distress syndrome (Shaw et al. 2001). Patients may develop posttraumatic stress symptoms without any conscious recollection of the specific traumatic events that occurred during their intensive care unit treatments. Posttraumatic stress symptoms have been reported in pediatric patients with asthma who present with symptoms of acute respiratory distress (Shaw et al. 2002).

Youth with asthma have more anxiety and other internalizing problems than do healthy peers (Guite and Kazak 2010; Katon et al. 2004). The strong overlap of symptoms of asthma and anxiety can make the differential diagnosis confusing. Asthma and anxiety disorders, particularly panic disorder, can manifest together in the same individual (Guite and Kazak 2010). The anxiety may be secondary to the stress of asthma, or hypercapnia and hyperventilation may predispose the individual to panic attacks. Episodes of respiratory distress and the side effects of asthma medications may increase anxiety. In addition, anxiety and psychological distress are thought to provoke and increase the severity of asthma attacks.

High rates of anxiety and depression have been found in patients with cystic fibrosis, with anxiety symptoms being more prevalent than depressive ones (Cruz et al. 2009). Although uncommon in children, pulmonary edema also has been associated with symptoms of anxiety.

Seizure Disorders

Anxiety disorders frequently co-occur with seizure disorders, with prevalence rates of depression and anxiety disorders reported to be 16%–31% among children with epilepsy assessed through epidemiological samples (Caplan et al. 2005; Plioplys et al. 2007). Complex partial seizures and panic attacks may have overlapping symptoms, including fear, depersonalization, dizziness, and paresthesias; this overlap can make it difficult to differentiate panic attacks from complex seizures based purely on clinical symptoms.

Traumatic Brain Injury and Postconcussive Syndrome

Patients who have sustained traumatic brain injury have an increased prevalence of anxiety disorders, including generalized anxiety disorder and PTSD (Whelan-Goodinson et al. 2009). Although these symptoms are in general transient, some patients develop more sustained symptoms. Even when cerebral concussion does not result in any irreversible anatomic lesions, it may be followed with periods of retrograde amnesia. A small proportion of individuals, after receiving a concussion, may develop a constellation of symptoms that include anxiety, impairment of sleep and appetite, irritability, lightheadedness, headaches, and poor concentration (Goldberg and Posner 2000).

Thyroid Disease

Patients with thyroid disorders often experience anxiety symptoms. Hyperthyroidism is associated with symptoms of anxiety and may be difficult to differentiate from a primary anxiety disorder. Signs indicating thyrotoxicosis include persistent acute anxiety, warm and dry hands, and fatigue accompanied by the desire to be active (Colón and Popkin 1996). Anxiety symptoms usually resolve when the underlying thyroid condition is treated, but anxiety can be treated with β-blockers during the acute treatment phase. Consultants may consider routine thyroid function tests in patients presenting with new-onset anxiety, with anxiety disorders that are resistant to treatment, or with anxiety that is accompanied by prominent physical symptoms. Although less common, anxiety also has been reported in patients with hypothyroidism.

Substance/Medication-Induced Anxiety Disorder

The essential features of substance/medication-induced anxiety disorder are the prominent symptoms of anxiety or panic that are judged to be due to the effects of a substance (American Psychiatric Association 2013). Anxiety may be induced by a variety of substances or medications, due to either the direct effect of a substance or a withdrawal reaction (Table 8–5). Corticosteroids, anticholinergic medications, β-adrenergic agonists, and asthma medications are all potential causes of anxiety, particularly if the medication has recently been started or the dosage has been changed.

Assessment

Once anxiety symptoms are identified as a concern, consultants must differentiate clinically significant anxiety from everyday worries and fears, which are common and developmentally normative (Table 8–6). In the pediatric setting, consultants should carefully review available laboratory, radiographic, and other tests; on the basis of the clinical presentation, they may want to recommend additional tests.

Although standardized symptom rating scales are not diagnostic, consultants may consider using them to support an anxiety diagnosis, characterize the nature and breadth of specific symptoms, and quantify pretreatment severity. Two of the various freely available scales that have acceptable psychometric properties are the Screen for Child Anxiety Related Emotional Disorders (SCARED; available at: https://www.pediatricbipolar.pitt.edu/resources/instruments) and the Generalized Anxiety Disorder–7 (GAD-7; available at: https://www.phqscreeners.com/sites/g/files/g10049256/f/201412/GAD-7_English.pdf).

Treatment

Treatment of anxiety symptoms and trauma/stress reactions in physically ill children and adolescents follows the same principles as in healthy children. Cognitive-behavioral therapy (CBT), selective reuptake inhibitors, or combinations of these are the first-line treatments for anxiety disorders (Thabrew et al. 2018; Wang et al. 2017). There is less support for the use of serotonin-norepinephrine reuptake inhibitors and insufficient evidence to support the use of benzodiazepines in the treatment of anxiety disorders (Wang et al. 2017). The latter can be helpful for acute-situation anxiety, but their use should be time limited and closely monitored to ensure there is no adverse impact, such as worsening of

Table 8–5.   Selected medications and substances associated with anxiety symptoms

Direct effect of medication/substance

β-Adrenergic agonists	Corticosteroids
Amphetamines	Dopaminergics
Androgens	Estrogens
Anticholinergics	Insulin
Antidepressants (including SSRIs)	Metronidazole
Antiemetics	Progestins
Antipsychotics	Sumatriptans
Baclofen	Sympathomimetics
Caffeine	Theophylline
Cocaine	Thyroid preparations

Withdrawal of medication/substance

Alcohol	Caffeine
Barbiturates	Opiates
Benzodiazepines	SSRIs

Note.   SSRI = selective serotonin reuptake inhibitor.

delirium. Additional information is provided in Chapter 17 ("Psychopharmacological Approaches and Considerations").

Psychotherapy in the hospital setting is generally brief, in large part due to the short lengths of stay. In this setting, supportive psychotherapy and reassurance can play an important role in correcting patients' misconceptions about the significance of physical symptoms. CBT techniques that have proven useful and effective include the Coping Cat program (Crawley et al. 2013; Kendall and Bertzos 2006) and trauma-focused CBT (Cohen et al. 2012; Ramirez de Arellano et al. 2014). Behavioral interventions, such as systematic desensitization, help to treat phobias that interfere with medical treatment. Guided imagery, progressive muscle relaxation, and hypnosis are

Table 8–6. Evaluative components in assessing anxiety symptoms in the pediatric setting

Medical-psychiatric history

Current subjective symptoms

Sources of anxiety

Academic and social impact	Isolation
Death	Loss of control
Diagnosis of illness	Loss of privacy
Financial burden of illness	Pain
Hospital anxiety	Physical effects of illness
Impact on family members	Uncertainty about prognosis

Use of prescribed medications and/or drugs of abuse

History of psychiatric disorders, especially anxiety disorders

Family history of psychiatric disorders, especially anxiety disorders

Mental status examination

Hematological and chemistry test considerations based on clinical presentation

Complete blood cell count	Glucose level
Electrolyte levels	Liver function tests
Calcium level	Magnesium level
Serum cortisol	Phosphorus level
Serum urea nitrogen	Urinary toxicology screen
Creatinine level	Arterial blood gas analysis

Radiographic and other test considerations based on clinical presentation

Chest radiography	Lumbar puncture
Computed tomography	Electroencephalography
Magnetic resonance imaging	Electrocardiography/24-hour monitor

potentially helpful in the inpatient setting. Effective treatment of pain, when pain is present, is a critical part of managing any disabling anxiety symptoms. More information about treatment is discussed in Chapter 15, "Individual Psychotherapy"; Chapter 16, "Family Interventions"; and Chapter 18, "Preparation for Procedures."

References

American Psychiatric Association: Diagnostic and Statistical Manual for Mental Disorders, 5th Edition. Arlington, VA, American Psychiatric Association, 2013

Beesdo-Baum K, Knappe S: Developmental epidemiology of anxiety disorders. Child Adolesc Psychiatr Clin N Am 21(3):457–478, 2012 22800989

Caplan R, Siddarth P, Gurbani S, et al: Depression and anxiety disorders in pediatric epilepsy. Epilepsia 46(5):720–730, 2005 15857439

Carmassi C, Corsi M, Gesi C, et al: DSM-5 criteria for PTSD in parents of pediatric patients with epilepsy: What are the changes with respect to DSM-IV TR? Epilepsy Behav 70(Pt A):97–103, 2017 28412608

Christiansen DM: Posttraumatic stress disorder in parents following infant death: a systematic review. Clin Psychol Rev 51:60–74, 2017 27838460

Clauss JA, Blackford JU: Behavioral inhibition and risk for developing social anxiety disorder: a meta-analytic study. J Am Acad Child Adolesc Psychiatry 51(10):1066–1075.e1, 2012 23021481

Cohen JA, Mannarino AP, Kliethermes M, et al: Trauma-focused CBT for youth with complex trauma. Child Abuse Negl 36(6):528–541, 2012 22749612

Colón EA, Popkin MK: Anxiety and panic, in Textbook of Consultation-Liaison Psychiatry. Edited by Rundell JR, Wise MG. Washington DC, American Psychiatric Press, 1996, pp 403–425

Colonnesi C, Draijer EM, Jan J M Stams G, et al: The relation between insecure attachment and child anxiety: a meta-analytic review. J Clin Child Adolesc Psychol 40(4):630–645, 2011 21722034

Costello EJ, Mustillo S, Erkanli A, et al: Prevalence and development of psychiatric disorders in childhood and adolescence. Arch Gen Psychiatry 60(8):837–844, 2003 12912767

Costello EJ, Egger HL, Copeland W, et al: The developmental epidemiology of anxiety disorders: phenomenology, prevalence, and comorbidity. Anxiety Disord Child Adolesc Res Assess Intervent 2:56–75, 2011

Crawley SA, Kendall PC, Benjamin CL, et al: Brief cognitive-behavioral therapy for anxious youth: feasibility and initial outcomes. Cognit Behav Pract 20(2):134–146, 2013 24244089

Cruz I, Marciel KK, Quittner AL, et al: Anxiety and depression in cystic fibrosis. Semin Respir Crit Care Med 30(5):569–578, 2009 19760544

DeMaso DR: Pediatric heart disease, in Handbook of Pediatric Psychology in School Settings. Edited by Brown RT. Hillsdale, NJ, Lawrence Erlbaum, 2004, pp 283–297

DeMaso DR, Calderon J, Taylor GA, et al: Psychiatric disorders in adolescents with single ventricle congenital heart disease. Pediatrics 139:e20162241, 2017 28148729

Farley LM, DeMaso DR, D'Angelo E, et al: Parenting stress and parental post-traumatic stress disorder in families after pediatric heart transplantation. J Heart Lung Transplant 26(2):120–126, 2007 17258144

Ferro MA, Boyle MH: The impact of chronic physical illness, maternal depressive symptoms, family functioning, and self-esteem on symptoms of anxiety and depression in children. J Abnorm Child Psychol 43(1):177–187, 2015 24938212

Ghandour RM, Sherman LJ, Vladutiu CJ, et al: Prevalence and treatment of depression, anxiety, and conduct problems in US children. J Pediatr 206:256–267.e3, 2019 30322701

Goebel-Fabbri A, Musen G, Sparks CR, et al: Endocrine and metabolic disorders, in The American Psychiatric Publishing Textbook of Psychosomatic Medicine. Edited by Levenson JL. Washington, DC, American Psychiatric Publishing, 2005, pp 495–515

Goldberg RJ, Posner DA: Anxiety in the medically ill, in Psychiatric Care of the Medical Patient, 2nd Edition. Edited by Stoudemire A, Fogel BS, Greenberg DB. New York, Oxford University Press, 2000, pp 165–180

Green BL, Epstein SA, Krupnick JL, et al: Trauma and medical illness: assessing trauma-related disorders in medical settings, in Assessing Psychological Trauma and PTSD. Edited by Wilson JP, Keane TM. New York, Guilford, 1997, pp 160–191

Green JG, McLaughlin KA, Berglund PA, et al: Childhood adversities and adult psychiatric disorders in the national comorbidity survey replication I: associations with first onset of DSM-IV disorders. Arch Gen Psychiatry 67(2):113–123, 2010 20124111

Guite JW, Kazak AE: Anxiety symptoms and disorders, in Textbook of Pediatric Psychosomatic Medicine. Edited by Shaw RJ, DeMaso DR. Washington, DC, American Psychiatric Publishing, 2010, pp 101–119

Hobbie WL, Stuber M, Meeske K, et al: Symptoms of posttraumatic stress in young adult survivors of childhood cancer. J Clin Oncol 18(24):4060–4066, 2000 11118467

Karsdorp PA, Everaerd W, Kindt M, et al: Psychological and cognitive functioning in children and adolescents with congenital heart disease: a meta-analysis. J Pediatr Psychol 32(5):527–541, 2007 17182669

Katon WJ, Richardson L, Lozano P, et al: The relationship of asthma and anxiety disorders. Psychosom Med 66(3):349–355, 2004 15184694

Kazak AE, Kassam-Adams N, Schneider S, et al: An integrative model of pediatric medical traumatic stress. J Pediatr Psychol 31(4):343–355, 2006 16093522

Kendall PC, Bertzos KA: Cognitive-Behavioral Therapy for Anxious Children: Therapist Manual. Ardmore, PA, Workbook Publishing, 2006

Kessler RC, Berglund P, Demler O, et al: Lifetime prevalence and age-of-onset distributions of DSM-IV disorders in the National Comorbidity Survey Replication. Arch Gen Psychiatry 62(6):593–602, 2005 15939837

Kessler RC, Avenevoli S, Costello EJ, et al: Prevalence, persistence, and sociodemographic correlates of DSM-IV disorders in the National Comorbidity Survey Replication Adolescent Supplement. Arch Gen Psychiatry 69(4):372–380, 2012 22147808

Ljungman L, Cernvall M, Grönqvist H, et al: Long-term positive and negative psychological late effects for parents of childhood cancer survivors: a systematic review. PLoS One 9(7):e103340, 2014 25058607

Mullen MP, Andrus J, Labella MH, et al: Quality of life and parental adjustment in pediatric pulmonary hypertension. Chest 145(2):237–244, 2014 24030476

Pao M, Kazak AE: Anxiety and depression, in Pediatric Psycho-Oncology, 2nd Edition. Edited by Wiener LS, Pao M, Kazak AE, et al. New York, Oxford University Press, 2015, pp 105–118

Pinquart M, Shen Y: Anxiety in children and adolescents with chronic physical illnesses: a meta-analysis. Acta Paediatr 100(8):1069–1076, 2011 21332786

Plioplys S, Dunn DW, Caplan R: 10-year research update review: psychiatric problems in children with epilepsy. J Am Acad Child Adolesc Psychiatry 46(11):1389–1402, 2007 18049289

Price J, Kassam-Adams N, Alderfer MA, et al: Systematic review: a reevaluation and update of the integrative (trajectory) model of pediatric medical traumatic stress. J Pediatr Psychol 41(1):86–97, 2016 26319585

Ramirez de Arellano MA, Lyman DR, Jobe-Shields L, et al: Trauma-focused cognitive behavioral therapy: assessing the evidence. Psychiatr Serv 65:591–602, 2014 24638076

Rechenberg K, Grey M, Sadler L: Stress and posttraumatic stress in mothers of children with Type 1 diabetes. J Fam Nurs 23(2):201–225, 2017 28795899

Shaw RJ, Harvey JE, Nelson KL, et al: Linguistic analysis to assess medically related posttraumatic stress symptoms. Psychosomatics 42(1):35–40, 2001 11161119

Shaw RJ, Robinson TE, Steiner H: Acute stress disorder following ventilation. Psychosomatics 43(1):74–76, 2002 11927764

Shaw RJ, Deblois T, Ikuta L, et al: Acute stress disorder among parents of infants in the neonatal intensive care nursery. Psychosomatics 47(3):206–212, 2006 16684937

Shemesh E, Lurie S, Stuber ML, et al: A pilot study of posttraumatic stress and non-adherence in pediatric liver transplant recipients. Pediatrics 105(2):E29, 2000 10654989

Stuber ML, Christakis DA, Houskamp B, et al: Posttrauma symptoms in childhood leukemia survivors and their parents. Psychosomatics 37(3):254–261, 1996 8849502

Stuber ML, Kazak AE, Meeske K, et al: Predictors of posttraumatic stress symptoms in childhood cancer survivors. Pediatrics 100(6):958–964, 1997 9374564

Stuber ML, Meeske KA, Krull KR, et al: Prevalence and predictors of posttraumatic stress disorder in adult survivors of childhood cancer. Pediatrics 125(5):e1124–e1134, 2010 20435702

Supelana C, Annunziato RA, Kaplan D, et al: PTSD in solid organ transplant recipients: Current understanding and future implications. Pediatr Transplant 20(1):23–33, 2016 26648058

Szigethy EM, Bujoreanu SI, Youk AO, et al: Randomized efficacy trial of two psychotherapies for depression in youth with inflammatory bowel disease. J Am Acad Child Adolesc Psychiatry 53(7):726–735, 2014a 24954822

Szigethy EM, Youk AO, Benhayon D, et al: Depression subtypes in pediatric inflammatory bowel disease. J Pediatr Gastroenterol Nutr 58(5):574–581, 2014b 24345836

Taylor JH, Lebowitz ER, Silverman WK: Anxiety disorders, in Lewis's Child and Adolescent Psychiatry, 5th Edition. Edited by Martin A, Bloch MH, Volkmar FR. Philadelphia, PA, Wolters Kluwer, 2018, pp 509–518

Thabrew H, Stasiak K, Hetrick SE, et al: Psychological therapies for anxiety and depression in children and adolescents with long-term physical conditions. Cochrane Database Syst Rev 12:CD012488, 2018 30578633

Verduin TL, Kendall PC: Differential occurrence of comorbidity within childhood anxiety disorders. J Clin Child Adolesc Psychol 32(2):290–295, 2003 12679288

Wang Z, Whiteside S, Sim L, et al: Anxiety in children, in Comparative Effectiveness Review No 192. (Prepared by the Mayo Clinic Evidence-Based Practice Center under Contract No 290-2015-00013-I) (AHRQ Publ No 17-EHC023-EF). Rockville, MD, Agency for Healthcare Research and Quality, 2017

Whelan-Goodinson R, Ponsford J, Johnston L, et al: Psychiatric disorders following traumatic brain injury: their nature and frequency. J Head Trauma Rehabil 24(5):324–332, 2009 19858966

Young GS, Mintzer LL, Seacord D, et al: Symptoms of posttraumatic stress disorder in parents of transplant recipients: incidence, severity, and related factors. Pediatrics 111(6 Pt 1):e725–e731, 2003 12777592

9

Somatic Symptom and Related Disorders

Medically unexplained physical symptoms are common in children and adolescents. Although frequently chronic and disabling, these symptoms do not often result in referrals for psychiatric evaluation or treatment (Mayou et al. 2003). The DSM-5 somatic symptom and related disorders (SSRDs) are those disorders in which physical symptoms are unexplained or for which the patient's response to an underlying medical condition is disproportionate and debilitating (American Psychiatric Association 2013). The SSRDs are a source of significant health care costs, including the provision of unnecessary and potentially harmful medical interventions (Malas et al. 2017).

The principal diagnosis in this category, somatic symptom disorder (SSD), is characterized by the presence of distressing somatic symptoms associated with abnormal thoughts, feelings, and behaviors in response to the symptoms. Other SSRD diagnoses include conversion disorder, illness anxiety disorder, psychological factors affecting other medical conditions (discussed in Chapter 8, "Anxiety Symptoms and Trauma/Stress Reactions"), and factitious disorder (discussed in Chapter 11, "Fabricated or Induced Illness Symptoms"). This chapter includes a discussion of risk factors for pediatric somatization, descriptions of the SSRDs, and approaches to help guide consultants in the assessment and management of SSRDs.

Risk Factors for Pediatric Somatization

The term *somatization*, which is relevant in the context of SSRDs, is defined as a pattern of seeking medical help for physical symptoms that cannot be fully explained by pathophysiological mechanisms but are nevertheless attributed to physical disease by the sufferer. Somatization has been described as the tendency to experience and express psychological distress through somatic complaints (Abbey 2005). It has been suggested that somatization occurs universally in young children, who have not yet developed the cognitive and linguistic skills needed to comprehend and communicate their feelings (Stoudemire 1991). Somatization is common in cultures that accept physical illness but not psychological symptoms as a reason for disability.

Between 10% and 30% of children worldwide experience physical symptoms that are seemingly unexplained by a physical illness (Ibeziako and De-Maso 2015). Community surveys of youth suggest that recurrent somatic complaints generally fall into four symptom clusters: cardiovascular, gastrointestinal, pain/weakness, and pseudoneurological (Garber et al. 1991). The prevalence of somatization is roughly equal among boys and girls in early childhood, but in adolescence, girls are five times more likely than boys to have somatic complaints (Martel 2013). Youth with a history of somatization are more likely to experience emotional and behavioral difficulties, be absent from school, and perform poorly academically. Studies have demonstrated that children and adolescents with functional somatic symptoms are significantly more likely than their unaffected peers to experience anxiety and depressive symptoms (Campo 2012). Youth with conversion disorder—specifically nonepileptic seizures—have significant comorbid psychopathology, including internalizing disorders and posttraumatic stress disorders (Plioplys et al. 2014).

Genetic factors, stressful life events, personality traits and coping styles, cognitive and learning difficulties, learned complaints, family factors, childhood physical illness, and sociocultural background are risk factors that have been associated with pediatric somatization. These are discussed in the following subsections.

Genetic Factors

Somatization clusters in families. This is particularly true for SSD, which occurs in 10%–20% of first-degree relatives of patients with this disorder. Rates of somatization show a concordance of up to 29% in monozygotic twin studies (Kaplan et al. 1994). Genetic factors have been hypothesized to contribute to the development of personality traits that may predispose to somatization when combined with environmental factors (Campo and Fritsch 1994). Children are believed to be more prone to adopt somatic ways to express emotional distress if they observe their parents using similar strategies, particularly if the emotional expression of distress is considered inappropriate (Stuart and Noyes 1999). Some studies indicate that parental physical illness may be associated with childhood somatization (Kaplan et al. 1994).

Stressful Life Events

Stressful life events, including childhood trauma, physical and sexual abuse, bullying, and exposure to natural disasters, have all been associated with the development of somatization (Bedard-Thomas et al. 2018; Ibeziako et al. 2016; Malas et al. 2017). In one study, just over one-third of patients with SSRDs had a history of bullying victimization; compared with nonbullied patients, the bullied patients had higher rates of comorbid anxiety, suicidal histories, family psychiatric histories, and learning difficulties, and they reported more significant life events within the year before hospitalization (Ibeziako et al. 2016). Youth with psychogenic nonepileptic seizures tend to have higher rates of bullying and more lifetime adversity, including physical and sexual abuse, compared with their siblings (Plioplys et al. 2014).

Personality Traits and Coping Styles

Somatization has been postulated to occur in individuals who are unable to verbalize emotional distress and instead use physical symptoms as means of expression (Shapiro 1996). The term *alexithymia* has been used to describe individuals with somatic concerns who do not have a verbal vocabulary to describe their moods (Natalucci et al. 2018). Physical symptoms have been referred to as a form of body language for children who have difficulty expressing emotions verbally. Examples include individuals who have difficulties with disclosing traumatic events or expressing anger and high-achieving children who cannot admit they are under too much pressure. Personality traits of introspectiveness (the tendency to think about oneself), poor self-concept, and pessimism have been associated with somatization (Abbey 2005), as have insecurity, perfectionism, and conscientiousness (Thomson et al. 2014).

Somatic complaints in adults have also been linked to what has been referred to as *somatosensory amplification*, or the tendency to experience normal somatic sensations as intense, noxious, and disturbing (Barsky et al. 1988; Köteles and Witthöft 2017). Patients with this form of somatization tend to be hypervigilant to their own bodily sensations, overreact to these sensations, and interpret them as indicating physical illness. Neuroimaging studies have found five neuronal areas—premotor and supplementary motor cortexes, middle frontal gyrus, anterior cingulate cortex, insula, and posterior cingulate cortex—that differ between patients with SSRDs and healthy controls; this finding largely overlaps with the circuit network model of somatosensory amplification (Boeckle et al. 2016).

Cognitive and Learning Difficulties

Children with difficulties learning and using academic skills, particularly in the context of high parental expectations, tend to have increased rates of somatization (Kingma et al. 2011). Compared with unaffected siblings, youth with "functional" neurological disorders have been found to score lower on tests of Full Scale IQ, vocabulary level, and mathematics, as well as to have more learning difficulties (Plioplys et al. 2014). Between 40% and 60% of patients with psychogenic nonepileptic seizures are reported to have learning and subtle language problems despite normal IQs (Doss et al. 2017).

Learned Complaints

In operant conditioning, behaviors that are rewarded will increase in strength or frequency, whereas behaviors that are inhibited or punished will decrease. Under this learning principle, attention and sympathy from others and/or decrease in responsibilities (*secondary gain*) can reinforce somatic complaints. If somatic symptoms are reinforced, such as by increased parental attention and/ or avoidance of unpleasant school pressures, early in the course of developing an SSRD, this reinforcement appears to increase the likelihood that the somatic complaints will become more ingrained and less amenable to change. In sum, youth can gain benefits from assuming a sick role, which can increase their reluctance to give up their symptoms.

Social learning theory suggests that somatic symptoms may be a result of "modeling" or "observational learning" within the family (Jamison and Walker 1992). Family members with similar physical complaints (*symptom models*) are common in patients with SSRDs (Ibeziako and DeMaso 2015).

Family Factors

In family systems theory, somatization can serve the function of drawing attention away from other areas of tension within a family (Stuart and Noyes 1999). The concept of *enmeshment* refers to the blurring of intergenerational boundaries with overinvolved and hyperresponsive family interactions. Family enmeshment combined with overprotectiveness, rigidity, and lack of conflict resolution has been postulated to predispose family members to the development of somatization (Minuchin et al. 1978; see Chapter 16, "Family Interventions"). It has been suggested that children in such families with significant degrees of conflict may develop somatic complaints as a mechanism to avoid any emotional expression that may exacerbate familial stress. In the home setting, experiences associated with somatization include frequent family conflicts, family enmeshment, and parental divorce (Malas et al. 2017).

Childhood Physical Illness

Studies have shown a relationship between a past history of physical illness and somatization (Dell and Campo 2011). Up to 67% of men and 78% of women who reported frequent somatic symptoms in adulthood had reported frequent somatic symptoms 5 years earlier when they were in high school (Poikolainen et al. 2000).

Sociocultural Background

SSRDs have been reported to be more common in rural areas and among individuals of lower socioeconomic status (American Psychiatric Association 2013; Gureje et al. 1997). Spells or visions are common aspects of culturally sanctioned religious and healing rituals, and falling down with loss or alteration in consciousness is a feature in a variety of culture-specific syndromes.

Somatic Symptom and Related Disorders

As mentioned in the introduction to this chapter, DSM-5 recognizes five SSRDs, three of which will be summarized in this chapter: somatic symptom, conversion, and illness anxiety disorders. Table 9–1 compares clinical features of these three disorders.

Somatic Symptom Disorder

Introduced in DSM-5, SSD consolidated and replaced previous diagnoses of somatization disorder, undifferentiated somatoform disorder, and pain disorder. SSD is characterized by the presence of one or more somatic complaints accompanied by significant distress and/or impairment that may or may not be associated with a medical condition (Box 9–1) (American Psychiatric Association 2013). Some patients have only one severe symptom, most commonly pain (see Chapter 10, "Pediatric Pain"). The diagnoses of SSD and a co-occurring pediatric illness are not mutually exclusive because the SSD diagnosis is based on the presence of positive symptoms and the fact that patients have disproportionate and persistent thoughts about the seriousness of their symptoms, have persistently high levels of anxiety, and/or devote excessive time and energy to the symptoms or health concerns (American Psychiatric Association 2013). When symptoms are persistent and/or severe, SSD can result in disabling impairment, school absenteeism, and increased health care utilization and the potential for unnecessary diagnostic evaluation and treatment intervention (Malas et al. 2017).

Box 9–1.   DSM-5 Diagnostic Criteria for
           Somatic Symptom Disorder

A. One or more somatic symptoms that are distressing or result in significant disruption of daily life.
B. Excessive thoughts, feelings, or behaviors related to the somatic symptoms or associated health concerns as manifested by at least one of the following:

    1. Disproportionate and persistent thoughts about the seriousness of one's symptoms.

2. Persistently high level of anxiety about health or symptoms.
3. Excessive time and energy devoted to these symptoms or health concerns.

C. Although any one somatic symptom may not be continuously present, the state of being symptomatic is persistent (typically more than 6 months).

Specify if:
With predominant pain (previously pain disorder): This specifier is for individuals whose somatic symptoms predominantly involve pain.

Specify if:
Persistent: A persistent course is characterized by severe symptoms, marked impairment, and long duration (more than 6 months).

Specify current severity:
Mild: Only one of the symptoms specified in Criterion B is fulfilled.
Moderate: Two or more of the symptoms specified in Criterion B are fulfilled.
Severe: Two or more of the symptoms specified in Criterion B are fulfilled, plus there are multiple somatic complaints (or one very severe somatic symptom).

Source.   Reprinted from American Psychiatric Association: *Diagnostic and Statistical Manual of Mental Disorders*, 5th Edition. Arlington, VA, American Psychiatric Association, 2013. Copyright © 2013 American Psychiatric Association. Used with permission.

Epidemiology

Although the prevalence of SSD remains unclear because of its relatively recent introduction in DSM-5, prevalence may be approximated based on prevalence rates of somatization, which is estimated to occur in 5%–13% of patients on inpatient pediatric units (Malas et al. 2018). Somatization is the second leading request for pediatric consultation in the hospital setting (Shaw et al. 2016). Although the criteria used to define youth with frequent unexplained somatic complaints vary, surveys examining somatic complaints in youth have identified polysymptomatic "somatizers," with reported prevalence rates of 4.5%–10% in adolescent boys and 10.7%–15% in adolescent girls (Campo and Fritsch 1994).

Table 9–1.   A comparison of clinical features in somatic symptom, conversion, and illness anxiety disorders

	Somatic symptom disorder	Conversion disorder	Illness anxiety disorder
Clinical presentation	Polysymptomatic Recurrent Chronic "Sickly" by history	Monosymptomatic Mostly acute Simulates disease	Disease concern or preoccupation
Demographic/epidemiologic features	Female predominance Familial pattern	Female predominance in adolescence Rural and lower social class Less educated and psychologically unsophisticated	Equal male:female ratio Previous physical disease
Diagnostic features	Review of system profusely positive Multiple physician contacts Polysurgical	Simulation incompatible with known physiologic mechanisms or anatomy	Disease conviction amplifies symptoms Obsessional
Management strategy	Build therapeutic alliance Schedule regular appointments Requires crisis intervention	Build therapeutic alliance Suggestion and persuasion Multiple techniques	Build therapeutic alliance Document symptoms Psychosocial review

Table 9–1. A comparison of clinical features in somatic symptom, conversion, and illness anxiety disorders *(continued)*

	Somatic symptom disorder	Conversion disorder	Illness anxiety disorder
Prognosis	Poor to fair	Excellent unless chronic	Fair to good; waxes and wanes
Associated disturbances	Anxiety and depressive disorder Conduct disorder Substance abuse	Drug/alcohol dependence Somatization disorder Histrionic personality traits Depression	Depression Panic disorder Obsessive-compulsive disorder
Primary differential presentation	Physical disease Depression Anxiety	Neurological disease	Physical disease Personality disorder Delusional disorder
Psychological processes contributing to symptoms	Unconscious Cultural Developmental	Unconscious Psychological stress or conflict may be present Secondary gain Symptom model	Unconscious Stress-bereavement Developmental factors

Source. Adapted from Folks DG, Ford CV, Houck CA: "Somatoform Disorders, Factitious Disorders, and Malingering," in *Clinical Psychiatry for Medical Students.* Edited by Stoudemire A. Philadelphia, PA, Lippincott Williams & Wilkins, 1998, pp 343–381. Copyright © 1998, Lippincott Williams & Wilkins. Used with permission.

Clinical Features

Youth with SSD most commonly present in pediatric settings, as opposed to psychiatry specialty settings, with symptoms including headaches, fatigue, muscle aches, abdominal distress, back pain, and/or blurred vision (Garber et al. 1991). Prepubertal children are more likely to report complaints of headache and abdominal pain; complaints of limb pain, fatigue, and muscle aches appear to increase with age. Specific constellations of symptoms may result in the diagnosis of syndromes such as irritable bowel syndrome, chronic fatigue, or fibromyalgia. In severe and persistent SSD, there is often a history of concurrent treatment from several physicians, resulting in fragmented care and contradictory treatment plans along with multiple workups for the same symptoms. Comorbid anxiety and depressive symptoms are common, as are conduct or substance-related disorders.

Conversion Disorder

Conversion disorder is defined by the presence of one or more symptoms of altered voluntary motor or sensory function causing significant distress or impairment that is not better explained by another medical, neurological, or mental disorder (Box 9–2) (American Psychiatric Association 2013). The symptoms must also be viewed as abnormal within the individual's own culture. "Functional" and "psychogenic" are alternative names that have been used to describe conversion disorder symptoms. In cases where there is evidence of nonepileptic seizure activity, terms such as "pediatric psychogenic nonepileptic seizures," "nonelectrical seizures," "conversion seizures," or "nonepileptic events" have all been used to describe the problem (Doss and Plioplys 2018).

Box 9–2.   DSM-5 Diagnostic Criteria for Conversion
           Disorder (Functional Neurological Symptom
           Disorder)

A. One or more symptoms of altered voluntary motor or sensory function.
B. Clinical findings provide evidence of incompatibility between the symptom and recognized neurological or medical conditions.
C. The symptom or deficit is not better explained by another medical or mental disorder.

D. The symptom or deficit causes clinically significant distress or impairment in social, occupational, or other important areas of functioning or warrants medical evaluation.

Specify symptom type:

With weakness or paralysis
With abnormal movement (e.g., tremor, dystonic movement, myoclonus, gait disorder)
With swallowing symptoms
With speech symptom (e.g., dysphonia, slurred speech)
With attacks or seizures
With anesthesia or sensory loss
With special sensory symptom (e.g., visual, olfactory, or hearing disturbance)
With mixed symptoms

Specify if:

Acute episode: Symptoms present for less than 6 months.
Persistent: Symptoms occurring for 6 months or more.

Specify if:

With psychological stressor *(specify stressor)*
Without psychological stressor

Source. Reprinted from American Psychiatric Association: *Diagnostic and Statistical Manual of Mental Disorders*, 5th Edition. Arlington, VA, American Psychiatric Association, 2013. Copyright © 2013 American Psychiatric Association. Used with permission.

The term *conversion* derives from the psychoanalytic concept that the somatic symptom is the result of an unconscious resolution of a psychological conflict—commonly a sexual or aggressive impulse—in which the mind "converts" psychological distress into a physical symptom. The resulting reduction in anxiety was thought to explain the phenomenon of *la belle indifférence*, or the apparent lack of concern sometimes observed in patients with conversion disorder. *Primary gain* is obtained by keeping a conflict out of consciousness and minimizing anxiety. The symptom is thought to allow the partial expression of the forbidden wish but in a disguised form, so that the patient does not need to consciously confront the unacceptable impulse. *Secondary gain* in the form of increased attention from caregivers or being excused from various pressures or responsibilities is viewed as contributing to the development or continuation of conversion symptoms.

Epidemiology

In studies of pediatric patients, the incidence of conversion disorder varies between 0.5% and 10% (DeMaso and Beasley 2005). Conversion disorder is three times more common in adolescents than in preadolescents, and it rarely occurs in children younger than 5 years. Females tend to outnumber males in adolescence, but the ratio is more equal in younger children. Psychogenic nonepileptic seizures have been reported to account for up to 25% of all admissions to inpatient epilepsy monitoring units, with an estimated 300,000–400,000 individuals with this condition in the United States (Doss and Plioplys 2018; LaFrance et al. 2013). Conversion disorder is more common in rural populations, among those from lower socioeconomic status, and in adolescents who are under pressure to perform in academic or athletic settings.

Clinical Features

Conversion disorder includes motor and sensory symptoms as well as loss of consciousness. Motor symptoms include seizures, abnormal movements, disturbances in gait, weakness, paralysis, and/or tremors. Sensory symptoms include anesthesia and paresthesia, commonly in one of the extremities, as well as deafness, blindness, and/or tunnel vision. Classically the presenting symptoms do not conform to known physiological pathways and/or anatomic distribution; for example, sensory deficits may follow a "stocking-glove" distribution and end abruptly at the wrist or ankle.

The onset of conversion symptoms is generally acute, and individual symptoms are generally short-lived, remitting within 2 weeks in most hospitalized patients (American Psychiatric Association 2013). Symptoms may briefly disappear when the patient is distracted. There may be a symptom model in the family or in another important person in the patient's life. The hypothesis that patients may serve as their own symptom model is supported in the finding that one-third of patients with psychogenic nonepileptic seizures have a co-occurring diagnosis of epilepsy (Plioplys et al. 2014). Table 9–2 lists clinical features that can be used by consultants to aid in differentiating psychogenic nonepileptic seizures from epilepsy.

Good prognostic factors of conversion disorder include sudden onset, the presence of an easily identifiable stressor, good premorbid adjustment, and absence of comorbid medical or psychiatric disorders. Patients with psychogenic nonepileptic seizures appear to have a poorer prognosis than those with paral-

Table 9–2.   Differential diagnosis of pediatric psychogenic nonepileptic seizures (PNES) and epilepsy

Clinical features	PNES	Epilepsy
Electroencephalogram: ictal/interictal	Normal	Abnormal/ variable
Duration	Often prolonged	Short
Pattern	Variable	Stereotyped
Frequency	Generally higher frequency	Paroxysmal/ cluster
Occurring in the presence of others	Yes	Variable
Occurrence during sleep	Rare	Yes
Onset	Gradual	Sudden
Incontinence	Rare	Infrequent
Biting	Tongue	Cheek
Scream	During spell	At onset
Convulsion	Bizarre, thrashing, sexual movements	Tonic/clonic
Injury	Infrequent, mild	Infrequent, severe
Pupillary reaction	Normal	Slow, nonreactive
Memory of seizure	Variable but sometimes intact	Usually amnestic
Orientation after event	Clear	Confused
Effect of suggestion or hypnosis	Precipitate or terminate	No effect
Effect of antiepileptic medications	Minimal	Decreased seizure frequency

Source.   Adapted from Maldonado and Spiegel 2001.

ysis or blindness. Comorbid mood, separation, and anxiety disorders are common. Stressful family events, such as recent divorce, current marital conflict, or death of a close family member, are frequently seen with conversion symptoms (Wyllie et al. 1999). The recurrence of symptoms is not uncommon, occurring in 20%–25% of cases within 1 year (American Psychiatric Association 2013).

Illness Anxiety Disorder

Individuals with illness anxiety disorder (or hypochondriasis, as it was previously classified) are preoccupied with having or acquiring a serious illness in the absence of any significant somatic symptoms (American Psychiatric Association 2013). Patients have a high level of anxiety about their physical health and repeatedly engage in excessive health-related behaviors such as checking for signs of illness. This preoccupation is based on the misinterpretation of physical symptoms or signs and is severe enough to cause clinically significant distress or functional impairment but is not of delusional intensity (American Psychiatric Association 2013).

Epidemiology

Illness anxiety disorder is thought to be a chronic and relapsing condition with age at onset in early and middle adulthood: men and women are equally affected (American Psychiatric Association 2013). The prevalence of hypochondriasis ranges from 1% to 5% in the general population and from 4% to 6% of general medical outpatients (Hart and Björgvinsson 2010). On rare occasions, adolescents may manifest similar levels of illness concern along with impairment, but their symptoms generally do not meet diagnostic criteria; for example, unrealistic concerns about having a physical illness such as cancer may lead to an "other specified or unspecified SSRD diagnosis" (Fritz et al. 1997).

Clinical Features

The core symptoms of illness anxiety disorder include a fear of disease, the conviction of having a disease, and bodily preoccupation/absorption associated with multiple somatic complaints (Folks et al. 2000). Patients often complain of poor relationships with their physicians and report feelings of anger and "doctor shopping" behavior. These patients appear to be particularly prone to somatosensory amplification and may experience significant secondary gain as a result of their adoption of the sick role. Complications may arise as a result of exposure to unnecessary treatments and procedures. Coexisting psychiatric conditions, including depression, panic disorder, and generalized anxiety disorder, are present in approximately two-thirds of patients with illness anxiety disorder (Barsky 2001).

Assessment

The biological, psychiatric, and social dimensions need to be evaluated both separately and in relation to each other in all patients with suspected SSRDs (Ibeziako and DeMaso 2015). Patients should undergo a complete and comprehensive medical workup to rule out serious medical illness, but an effort should be made to avoid unnecessary and potentially harmful tests and procedures. Ideally, if somatization is suspected, psychiatric consultation should be included early in this workup process. Again, it is important for consultants to remember that the diagnosis of SSRD and the presence of physical illness are not mutually exclusive. When somatization is presumed, the likelihood of subsequently discovering a previously undiagnosed physical disease is less than 10% (Campo and Fritz 2001). Nevertheless, certain physical illnesses are notoriously overlooked and should be carefully considered as part of the diagnostic workup for problematic somatic symptoms (Table 9–3).

The psychiatric differential diagnosis for patients with potential SSRDs includes depressive, bipolar, anxiety, obsessive-compulsive, body dysmorphic, and delusional disorders. Because the presence of intentionally produced symptoms is not uncommon in SSRDs, consultants may need to differentiate SSRD conditions, in which most symptoms are unconsciously produced, from factitious disorder and malingering, in which the symptoms are predominately consciously produced (see Chapter 11, "Fabricated or Induced Illness Symptoms"). In malingering, the essential feature is the intentional production of false or grossly exaggerated physical or psychological symptoms motivated by external incentives, such as avoiding work, obtaining financial compensation, evading criminal prosecution, or obtaining drugs (American Psychiatric Association 2013).

Referral by the pediatric team for psychiatric consultation is difficult to accept for many families because patients with SSRDs and their families present with the belief that there is a medical cause for their problem. A common

Table 9–3.   Selected medical conditions to consider in the differential diagnosis of youth presenting with disabling somatic symptoms

AIDS	Lyme disease
Acquired myopathies	Migraine headaches
Acute intermittent porphyria	Multiple sclerosis
Angina	Myasthenia gravis
Basal ganglia disease	Narcolepsy
Brain tumors	Optic neuritis
Cardiac arrhythmias	Periodic paralysis
Chronic systemic infections	Postural orthostatic hypertension syndrome
Creutzfeldt-Jakob disease	Polymyositis
Guillain-Barré syndrome	Seizure disorders
Hyperparathyroidism	Superior mesenteric artery syndrome
Hyperthyroidism	Systemic lupus erythematosus

response to referral is for the family to react adversely and think that their child's symptoms are not being taken seriously. It is helpful for the primary physician of the pediatric team to frame the consultation as a routine part of a comprehensive medical workup as well as an opportunity to assess the level of stress connected with the current physical symptoms. The pediatric team should not "send the family away" after consultation but rather should communicate to the family that the psychiatric results will be integrated into their findings to obtain a more complete understanding of the child's symptoms. Consultants must be prepared to address the family's concerns and to reassure the family that the consultant's involvement does not mean that the medical workup has been abandoned.

There are a number of key elements for consultants to consider in their assessments for the presence of an SSRD (Table 9–4). These include the presence of psychosocial stressors, comorbid depression or anxiety disorders, a history of somatization in the child or the parents, the presence of a model of illness behavior, and evidence of secondary gain resulting from the symptoms. Symptoms may not follow known physiological principles or anatomical patterns and may respond to suggestion or placebo. Video-electroencephalographic monitoring has been increasingly used to investigate seizure disorders. The lack of electrical evidence in the face of a seizure makes conversion disorder or functional neurological disorder a likely diagnosis.

Consultants may also consider using standardized symptom rating scales, although such scales are not diagnostic, to characterize the nature and breadth of the somatic symptoms as well as quantify pretreatment severity. Several validated rating scales may be useful in screening youth for possible SSRDs (Malas et al. 2017). The Children's Somatization Inventory (Walker et al. 2009) is a 24- or 35-item self- and parent-report instrument used to identify common somatic complaints in the previous 2 weeks. The Children's Psychosomatic Symptom Checklist (Wisniewski et al. 1988) is a 12-item self-report instrument that evaluates the frequency and severity of 12 somatic symptoms. The Somatic Symptom Checklist (Williams and Hollis 1999) is a 31-item instrument used to assess the lifetime presence of somatic symptoms. The Functional Disability Inventory (Walker and Greene 1991) is a 15-item self-report instrument used to assess the presence and severity of functional disability over the past 2 weeks. Consultants may also consider screening tools for common comorbid psychiatric disorders, such as anxiety and depression (see Chapter 7, "Depressive Symptoms and Disorders," and Chapter 8, "Anxiety Symptoms and Trauma/Stress Reactions").

Treatment

Effective treatment of an SSRD begins with the development of a positive working relationship between patient, family, pediatric team, and mental health providers based on a shared understanding of the diagnosis, the formulation, and a management plan that generally incorporates a number of different treatment modalities that target the factors that are believed to be associated with the development of somatization (Figure 9–1) (Shaw et al. 2010).

Stepwise Approach for Consultants

Guidelines for a stepwise approach that consultants can use to develop and implement an integrated medical and psychiatric treatment approach to SSRDs

Table 9–4. Key elements to consider in the psychiatric assessment of somatic symptom and related disorders in children and adolescents

Medical findings suggestive of somatic symptom and related disorders

- Absence of findings despite thorough medical workup

    - Lack of electrical evidence on video-electroencephalographic monitoring

- Inconsistent findings on examination

    - Sensory changes inconsistent with anatomical distribution (e.g., splitting at the midline; loss of sensation of entire face but not scalp; discrepancy between pain and temperature sensation; absence of Romberg sign)

    - Absence of functional impairment despite claims of profound weakness (e.g., impairment of fine motor function on testing, yet able to dress and undress)

    - Face-hand test (deflecting falling arm from face)

    - Hoover's sign (patient pushes down with "paretic" leg when attempting to raise unaffected leg and fails to press down with unaffected leg when raising "paretic" leg)

    - Astasia-abasia (staggering gait, momentarily balancing, but never actually falling)

    - Dragging a "weak" leg as though it were a totally lifeless object instead of circumduction of the leg

    - Psychogenic deafness responding to unexpected words or noises

    - Tunnel vision

    - Movement disorder with normal concurrent electroencephalogram

    - Symptoms suggestive of conversion seizures.

    - Increased symptoms in the presence of family or medical staff

    - Periods of normal function when distracted

- Temporal relationship between onset of symptom and psychosocial stressor

Table 9–4.   Key elements to consider in the psychiatric assessment of somatic symptom and related disorders in children and adolescents *(continued)*

Psychiatric findings suggestive of somatic symptom and related disorders

- Excessive thoughts, feelings, or behaviors related to the somatic symptoms or associated health concerns (see Boxes 9–1 and 9–2)

- Co-occurring psychiatric disorder

- Learning difficulties and academic failure

- Stressful life events (including childhood trauma and bullying)

- Symptom model(s)

Family beliefs regarding somatic symptoms

- Belief in a single undiagnosed primary medical cause

  - Investment in further medical workup

  - Fear about serious medical illness

- Belief in the role of environmental triggers

- Belief in the role of psychological factors

- Beliefs regarding symptom management

  - Awareness of nonpharmacological approaches

  - Belief that the child should rest and be excused from usual responsibilities

Family medical history

- Family history of unexplained somatic symptoms

- Pattern of reinforcement of illness behavior in the family

Impact of somatic symptoms

- Emotional (e.g., depression/anxiety vs. *la belle indifférence*)

- Family (e.g., disruption of work schedule, impact on marital relationship, impact on distraction from family conflict)

- Social and peer relationships

- Academic (e.g., absenteeism, placement in home teaching)

Table 9–4. Key elements to consider in the psychiatric assessment of somatic symptom and related disorders in children and adolescents *(continued)*

Reinforcement of somatic symptoms

- Reinforcement by parents

    - Medical journals and diaries of symptoms kept by parents

    - Parent home from work

- Increased attention from family and/or friends

- Increased attention from medical providers

- Avoidance of school, social, or athletic stressor

are outlined in Table 9–5. The formulation of the problem is the crucial first step in treatment. As mentioned previously, patients and their families routinely present to their physicians with the belief that their symptoms are caused by a medical illness alone. This view needs to be reframed from this narrow medical model perspective to a comprehensive biopsychosocial understanding. Upon completion of the assessment, consultants should communicate their formulation to the medical team, generally in an interdisciplinary provider meeting, to ensure that a consensus has been reached regarding the diagnosis and treatment plan and to facilitate adequate and consistent communication among all providers.

In these meetings, consultants must remain alert for the countertransference reactions that are sometimes engendered in the medical team, who feel frustrated by the time consumed in caring for patients and the never-ending recurrent complaints from individuals who might be perceived as deserving of the sick role, which may cause the medical team to avoid or to spend less time communicating with these patients (Ibeziako and DeMaso 2012).

After a consensus on diagnosis and management has been reached with the medical team, the next step is to hold an informing conference or interdisciplinary informing family meeting that includes both the primary managing physician and the family (Ibeziako and DeMaso 2012; Ibeziako et al. 2019). It is important in this meeting that the managing physician present the medical and psychosocial findings to the patient and family in a supportive

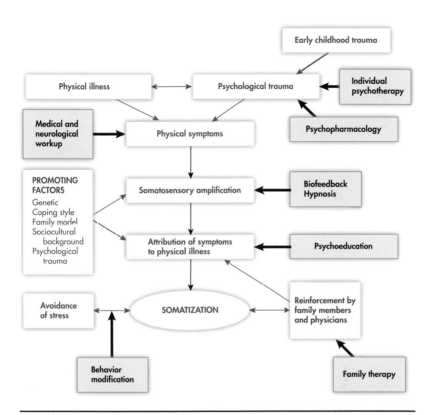

Figure 9–1. Treatment approaches to pediatric somatization.

Source. Reprinted from Shaw RJ, Spratt EG, Bernard RS, et al.: "Somatoform Disorders," in *Textbook of Pediatric Psychosomatic Medicine.* Edited by Shaw RJ, DeMaso DR. Washington, DC, American Psychiatric Publishing, 2010, pp 121–139. Copyright © 2010, American Psychiatric Publishing. Used with permission.

and nonjudgmental manner. If patients and their families believe that the managing physician understands and empathizes with the degree of distress produced by the somatic symptoms, then they are more likely to be active participants in treatment. Consultants may or may not elect to attend this meeting, depending on the comfort and expertise of the managing physician and the severity of the SSRD. Table 9–6 provides guidelines on how to present the diagnosis of a conversion disorder to the family; this approach may be modified for other types of SSRD.

Table 9–5.   Guidelines to a stepwise approach for consultants to developing an integrated medical and psychiatric treatment approach to somatic symptom and related disorders

1.   Complete a psychiatric assessment

- Review histories, examinations, and studies by pediatrician and pediatric specialists

- Perform patient and family interviews

- Elicit diagnostic criteria

- Develop a developmental biopsychosocial formulation of the patient and family

2.   Convey the biopsychosocial formulation to the pediatrician and medical team

- Remember that somatoform illness is not a diagnosis by exclusion

- Remember that symptoms can be in significant excess of what would be expected from the physical findings that are present

- Remember that physical findings may have accounted for early symptoms but may no longer be the etiology for the current symptoms

3.   Convene an informing conference between the pediatrician and the family

- Convey integrated medical and psychiatric findings to family

- Because the family has a medical model as their frame of reference, help reframe this understanding of symptoms into a developmental biopsychosocial formulation

4.   Implement treatment interventions in both medical and psychiatric domains

- Consider the following medical interventions:

    - Set up ongoing pediatric follow-up appointments

    - Physical therapy or other face-saving remedies may be added depending on symptoms

Table 9–5. Guidelines to a stepwise approach for consultants to developing an integrated medical and psychiatric treatment approach to somatic symptom and related disorders *(continued)*

5. Consider the following psychiatric interventions

    • Implement cognitive-behavioral intervention

    • Implement psychotherapy

    • Implement family therapy

    • Assess for the presence of target symptoms for psychotropic medications

Source. Reprinted from Ibeziako PI, DeMaso DR: "The Somatoform Disorders," in *Clinical Child Psychiatry,* 3rd Edition. Edited by Klykylo WM, Kay JL. Indianapolis, IN, Wiley, 2012, pp. 458–474. Copyright © 2012, John Wiley & Sons. Used with permission.

The American Academy of Child and Adolescent Psychiatry (AACAP) SSRD workgroup, consisting of expert pediatric consultation-liaison psychiatrists from multiple institutions across North America, has moved to standardize a stepwise approach across institutions (Ibeziako et al. 2019). Paralleling the stepwise approach just described, the workgroup's clinical pathway outlines five steps from admission to discharge in the recognition, assessment, and treatment of SSRDs in the pediatric hospital: 1) medical providers' early recognition of potential somatization due to the presence of inconsistent history and examination with or without psychosocial stressor; 2) early interdisciplinary assessment with a comprehensive biopsychosocial approach with consultation at the time somatization is suspected; 3) an interdisciplinary provider meeting involving all providers to review findings and achieve consensus on the problem and intervention plan; 4) an interdisciplinary meeting to communicate the diagnosis and management plan to the family; and 5) interdisciplinary management with focus on implementing a treatment plan to improve patient functioning and ultimate hospital discharge (Ibeziako et al. 2019). The SSRD workgroup has also developed short scripts and handouts to standardize and facilitate communication around the five steps (Ibeziako et al. 2019), in addition to an educational brochure, "Physical Symptoms of Emotional Distress: Somatic Symptoms and Related Disorders," which can be shared with families (American Academy of Child and Adolescent Psychiatry 2017).

Table 9–6.   An approach to conveying the diagnosis of pediatric psychogenic nonepileptic seizures to patients and their families

1. Present objective evidence of absence of seizure activity associated with episodes.

2. Explain the common reasons for seizure episodes (e.g., epilepsy, cardiac, and/or emotional).

3. Give the good news that the patient does not have epilepsy.

4. Cite common examples of physical phenomena, such as fainting or hand sweating, that may be related to emotional arousal.

5. Acknowledge the patient's suffering.

6. Acknowledge the family's concern.

7. Emphasize that the events are not under voluntary control.

8. Explain that remote and recent events may contribute to the episodes, even if the patient is not feeling stressed.

9. Emphasize the physically disabling nature of the events and the importance of prompt, intensive, and appropriate treatment.

Source.   Adapted from Chabolla et al. 1996.

Unfortunately, some families remain resistant to mental health intervention. In these situations, consultants can help by advising pediatric teams about alternative ways in which they can decrease reinforcement for a patient's sick role and lessen psychosocial stressors. Consultants can also provide advice to teams regarding the needs for social service intervention in cases of parental or medical neglect, such as when parents seek multiple unnecessary medical procedures or fail to pursue necessary mental health treatment (Ibeziako et al. 2019).

With family acceptance of a biopsychosocial formulation of the problem, an integrated medical and psychiatric treatment approach focused on the development and implementation of a treatment plan to improve the patient's functioning, and not a continued search for a cause of the presenting symptoms, can be implemented (Ibeziako and DeMaso 2012). In the treatment of these disorders, it is helpful to establish realistic goals that emphasize improvements in functioning rather than the illusion that the symptoms can be completely re-moved. This approach also includes ongoing monitoring and treatment for possible physical illness, often by the patient's primary care physician, in addition to the recommended mental health interventions.

Role of the Primary Care Physician

Primary care physicians can schedule frequent, brief, and ongoing pediatric visits while avoiding unnecessary medical investigations and procedures. This arrangement allows patients to receive attention from a primary physician without having to develop somatic symptoms. This practice has been shown to reduce overall health care utilization and to improve patient satisfaction (Burton et al. 2012). Over time, the physician may learn more about the connections between psychosocial stressors and the patient's somatic complaints. It may be helpful for attention to be paid to the anxiety the patient experiences in relation to the physical symptoms rather than to the symptoms themselves. Reassurance that a serious or life-threatening illness is not present is necessary but generally insufficient to alleviate the anxiety of the patient (Campo and Fritz 2001).

The Rehabilitation Model

Taking a rehabilitative approach is generally useful in the treatment of SSRDs. This approach acknowledges the reality of the symptoms, emphasizes the necessary involvement of mind and body in the recovery process, and shifts the focus from "cure" to "return to normal functioning" while allowing youth to "save face" through the promotion of physical recovery as the primary goal (Ibeziako and DeMaso 2012). Patients become active participants in their recovery and in doing so are more able to relinquish the sick role. Parents are encouraged to view their child as capable, strong, and competent rather than passive, helpless, and fragile. Success is measured by the ability to return to school and the resumption of normal social and recreational activities.

Rehabilitative approaches include the use of intensive physical and occupational therapies that emphasize the recovery of function and offer face-saving remedies for the patient. Physical therapy may be particularly helpful in restoring function in cases of conversion disorder (Abbey 2005). This approach can be combined with a behavioral modification program that provides incentives for improvements in functioning while removing secondary gain for illness behavior.

For severely disabled patients, it may be advisable to recommend admission to an inpatient medical-psychiatric treatment program that specializes in SSRDs. Other options to consider are day treatment or partial hospitalization programs. These approaches have the benefit of temporarily removing the child from the home environment, where the family may be playing an unwitting role in reinforcing the child's symptoms.

Psychotherapy

Meta-analyses have shown that psychological treatments improve symptom load, disability, and school attendance in children and adolescents suffering from various functional somatic symptoms, including functional abdominal symptoms, fatigue, tension-type headache, and musculoskeletal pains (Bonvanie et al. 2017).

The efficacy of cognitive-behavioral therapy (CBT) has been supported in patients with SSRDs (Allen and Woolfolk 2010; Kroenke 2007; Tsui et al. 2017). CBT approaches target distorted beliefs about the meaning of somatic symptoms and draw attention to the factors that increase worries about health, including the excessive focus on physical symptoms or misinterpretation of these symptoms. CBT appears to be more generally effective when combined with a package of multimodal treatment interventions that include relaxation training, self-hypnosis, and biofeedback (Dell and Campo 2011). Hypnosis, which may be used as a diagnostic technique in conversion disorder, may be used as a treatment technique by providing the patient with a face-saving method of obtaining control over symptoms (Maldonado and Spiegel 2000; Tsui et al. 2017). Caplan et al. (2017) have developed a comprehensive treatment guide for patients with nonepileptic seizures.

Both individual and family therapies have been found useful in the treatment of patients with SSRDs and have resulted in reduced health care expenditures (Kaplan et al. 1994). Insight-oriented psychotherapy may have a role in the treatment of children with conversion disorder. Patients are encouraged to express their underlying emotions and to develop alternative ways to express their feelings of distress. Family therapy may be helpful in changing family members' views of a patient's physical impairment and helplessness, with the goal of reducing reinforcement of illness behavior. Family therapy may reveal important family stresses or dysfunctional family dynamics that are relevant in terms of the etiology of the child's symptoms. Family therapy has been shown to result in decreased somatization, reduced rates of relapse, and improvements in adaptive functioning (Dell and Campo 2011; Ibeziako and Bujoreanu 2011).

Psychopharmacology

Psychotropic medications are not indicated for treatment of SSRDs, although they may be beneficial for patients with co-occurring psychiatric disorders, such as anxiety or depression (Ibeziako et al. 2019; Kleinstäuber et al. 2014). Given that pediatric providers do prescribe these medications for physical symptoms, such as tricyclic antidepressants for pain or benzodiazepines for nausea, consultants should carefully review patients' medications for their effectiveness, wean patients off medications that are not effective, and reduce polypharmacy when possible (Ibeziako et al. 2019).

References

Abbey SE: Somatization and somatoform disorders, in The American Psychiatric Publishing Textbook of Psychosomatic Medicine. Edited by Levenson JL. American Psychiatric Publishing, 2005, pp 271–296

Allen LA, Woolfolk RL: Cognitive behavioral therapy for somatoform disorders. Psychiatr Clin North Am 33(3):579–593, 2010 20599134

American Academy of Child and Adolescent Psychiatry: Physical symptoms of emotional distress: somatic symptom and related disorders facts for families. December 2017. Available at: https://www.aacap.org/aacap/families_and_youth/facts_for_families/fff-guide/Physical_Symptoms_of_Emotional_Distress-Somatic_Symptoms_and_Related_Disorders.aspx. Accessed March 21, 2019.

American Psychiatric Association: Diagnostic and Statistical Manual of Mental Disorders, 5th Edition. Washington, DC, American Psychiatric Association, 2013

Barsky AJ: Clinical practice. The patient with hypochondriasis. N Engl J Med 345(19):1395–1399, 2001 11794173

Barsky AJ, Goodson JD, Lane RS, Cleary PD: The amplification of somatic symptoms. Psychosom Med 50(5):510–519, 1988 3186894

Bedard-Thomas KK, Bujoreanu S, Choi CH, et al: Perception and impact of life events in medically hospitalized patients with somatic symptom and related disorders. Hosp Pediatr 8(11):699–705, 2018 30327327

Boeckle M, Schrimpf M, Liegl G, Pieh C: Neural correlates of somatoform disorders from a meta-analytic perspective on neuroimaging studies. Neuroimage Clin 11:606–613, 2016 27182487

Bonvanie IJ, Kallesøe KH, Janssens KA, et al: Psychological interventions for children with functional somatic symptoms: a systematic review and meta-analysis. J Pediatr 187:272–281.e17, 2017 28416243

Burton C, Weller D, Marsden W, et al: A primary care Symptoms Clinic for patients with medically unexplained symptoms: pilot randomised trial. BMJ Open 2:e000513, 2012 22327629

Campo JV: Annual research review: functional somatic symptoms and associated anxiety and depression—developmental psychopathology in pediatric practice. J Child Psychol Psychiatry 53(5):575–592, 2012 22404290

Campo JV, Fritsch SL: Somatization in children and adolescents. J Am Acad Child Adolesc Psychiatry 33(9):1223–1235, 1994 7995788

Campo JV, Fritz G: A management model for pediatric somatization. Psychosomatics 42(6):467–476, 2001 11815681

Caplan R, Doss J, Plioplys S, et al: Pediatric Psychiatric Non-Epileptic Seizures: A Treatment Guide. New York, Springer International, 2017

Chabolla DR, Krahn LE, So EL, et al: Psychogenic nonepileptic seizures. Mayo Clin Proc 71(5):493–500, 1996 8628032

Dell ML, Campo JV: Somatoform disorders in children and adolescents. Psychiatr Clin North Am 34(3):643–660, 2011 21889684

DeMaso DR, Beasley PJ: The somatoform disorders, in Clinical Child Psychiatry, 2nd Edition. Edited by Kykylo WM, Kay JL. West Sussex, UK, Wiley, 2005, pp 471–486

Doss JL, Plioplys S: Pediatric psychogenic nonepileptic seizures: a concise review. Child Adolesc Psychiatr Clin N Am 27(1):53–61, 2018 29157502

Doss JL, Caplan R, Siddarth P, et al: Risk factors for learning problems in youth with psychogenic non-epileptic seizures. Epilepsy Behav 70(Pt A):135–139, 2017 28427021

Folks DG, Ford CV, Houck CA: Somatoform disorders, factitious disorders, and malingering, in Clinical Psychiatry for Medical Students. Edited by Stoudemire A. Philadelphia, PA, Lippincott Williams & Wilkins, 1998, pp 343–381

Folks DG, Feldman MD, Ford CV: Somatoform disorders, factitious disorders, and malingering, in Psychiatric Care of the Medical Patient, 2nd Edition. Edited by Stoudemire A, Fogel BS, Greenberg DB. New York, Oxford University Press, 2000, pp 459–476

Fritz GK, Fritsch S, Hagino O: Somatoform disorders in children and adolescents: a review of the past 10 years. J Am Acad Child Adolesc Psychiatry 36(10):1329–1338, 1997 9334545

Garber J, Walker LS, Zeman J: Somatization symptoms in a community sample of children and adolescents: further validation of the children's somatization inventory. Psychol Assess 3:588–595, 1991

Gureje O, Simon GE, Ustun TB, et al: Somatization in cross-cultural perspective: a World Health Organization study in primary care. Am J Psychiatry 154(7):989–995, 1997 9210751

Hart J, Björgvinsson T: Health anxiety and hypochondriasis: Description and treatment issues highlighted through a case illustration. Bull Menninger Clin 74(2):122–140, 2010 20545492

Ibeziako P, Bujoreanu S: Approach to psychosomatic illness in adolescents. Curr Opin Pediatr 23(4):384–389, 2011 21670681

Ibeziako P, DeMaso DR: The somatoform disorders, in Clinical Child Psychiatry, 3rd Edition. Edited by Klykylo WM, Kay JL. Indianapolis, IN, Wiley, 2012, pp 458–474

Ibeziako P, DeMaso DR: Growth, development, and behavior: somatic symptom and related disorders, in Nelson Textbook of Pediatrics, 20th Edition. Edited by Kliegman RM, Stanton BF, St. Geme J, et al. Philadelphia, PA, Elsevier, 2015, pp 135–137

Ibeziako P, Choi C, Randall E, et al: Bullying victimization in medically hospitalized patients with somatic symptom and related disorders: prevalence and associated factors. Hosp Pediatr 6(5):290–296, 2016 27073256

Ibeziako P, Brahmbhatt K, Chapman A, et al: Developing a clinical pathway for the somatic symptoms and related disorders in pediatric hospital settings. Hosp Pediatr 9(3):147–155, 2019 30782623

Kingma EM, Janssens KA, Venema M, et al: Adolescents with low intelligence are at risk of functional somatic symptoms: the TRAILS study. J Adolesc Health 49(6):621–626, 2011 22098773

Kleinstäuber M, Witthöft M, Steffanowski A, et al: Pharmacological interventions for somatoform disorders in adults. Cochrane Database Syst Rev (11):CD010628, 2014 25379990

Köteles F, Witthöft M: Somatosensory amplification: an old construct from a new perspective. J Psychosom Res 101:1–9, 2017 28867412

Kroenke K: Efficacy of treatment for somatoform disorders: a review of randomized controlled trials. Psychosom Med 69(9):881–888, 2007 18040099

Jamison RN, Walker LS: Illness behavior in children of chronic pain patients. Int J Psychiatry Med 22(4):329–342, 1992 1293062

Kaplan HI, Sadock BJ, Grebb JA: Somatoform disorders, in Kaplan and Sadock's Synopsis of Psychiatry: Behavioral Sciences/Clinical Psychiatry, 7th Edition. Baltimore, MD, Williams & Wilkins, 1994, pp 617–631

LaFrance WCJr, Baker GA, Duncan R, et al: Minimum requirements for the diagnosis of psychogenic nonepileptic seizures: a staged approach: a report from the International League Against Epilepsy Nonepileptic Seizures Task Force. Epilepsia 54(11):2005–2018, 2013 24111933

Malas N, Ortiz-Aguayo R, Giles L, et al: Pediatric somatic symptom disorders. Curr Psychiatry Rep 19(2):11, 2017 28188588

Malas N, Donohue L, Cook RJ, et al: Pediatric somatic symptom and related disorders: primary care provider perspectives. Clin Pediatr (Phila) 57(4):377–388, 2018 28840747

Maldonado JR, Spiegel D: Medical hypnosis, in Psychiatric Care of the Medical Patient, 2nd Edition. Edited by Stoudemire A, Fogel BS, Greenberg DB. New York, Oxford University Press, 2000, pp 73–90

Maldonado JR, Spiegel D: Conversion disorder, in Review of Psychiatry, Vol 20. Edited by Phillips K. Washington, DC, American Psychiatric Publishing, 2001, pp 95–128

Martel MM: Sexual selection and sex differences in the prevalence of childhood externalizing and adolescent internalizing disorders. Psychol Bull 139(6):1221–1259, 2013 23627633

Mayou R, Levenson J, Sharpe M: Somatoform disorders in DSM-V. Psychosomatics 44(6):449–451, 2003 14597678

Minuchin S, Rosman BL, Baker L: Psychosomatic families: anorexia nervosa in context. Cambridge, MA, Harvard University Press, 1978

Natalucci G, Faedda N, Calderoni D, et al: Headache and alexithymia in children and adolescents: what is the connection? Front Psychol Feb 1;9:48, 2018 29449820

Plioplys S, Doss J, Siddarth P, et al: A multisite controlled study of risk factors in pediatric psychogenic nonepileptic seizures. Epilepsia 55(11):1739–1747, 2014 25244006

Poikolainen K, Aalto-Setälä T, Marttunen M, et al: Predictors of somatic symptoms: a five year follow up of adolescents. Arch Dis Child 83(5):388–392, 2000 11040143

Shapiro CM: Alexithymia—a useful concept for all psychiatrists? J Psychosom Res 41(6):503–504, 1996 9032713

Shaw RJ, Spratt EG, Bernard RS, et al: Somatoform disorders, in Textbook of Pediatric Psychosomatic Medicine. Edited by Shaw RJ, DeMaso DR. Washington, DC, American Psychiatric Publishing, 2010, pp 121–139

Shaw RJ, Pao M, Holland JE, et al: Practice patterns revisited in pediatric psychosomatic medicine. Psychosomatics 57(6):576–585, 2016 27393387

Stoudemire A: Somatothymia. Psychosomatics 32:365–381, 1991 1961848

Stuart S, Noyes R Jr: Attachment and interpersonal communication in somatization. Psychosomatics 40(1):34–43, 1999 9989119

Thomson K, Randall E, Ibeziako P, et al: Somatoform disorders and trauma in medically admitted children, adolescents, and young adults: prevalence rates and psychosocial characteristics. Psychosomatics 55(6):630–639, 2014 25262040

Tsui P, Deptula A, Yuan DY: Conversion disorder, functional neurological symptom disorder, and chronic pain: comorbidity, assessment, and treatment. Curr Pain Headache Rep 21(6):29, 2017 28434123

Walker LS, Greene JW: The functional disability inventory: measuring a neglected dimension of child health status. J Pediatr Psychol 16(1):39–58, 1991 1826329

Walker LS, Beck JE, Garber J, et al: Children's Somatization Inventory: psychometric properties of the revised form (CSI-24). J Pediatr Psychol 34(4):430–440, 2009 18782857

Williams RA, Hollis HM: Health beliefs and reported symptoms among a sample of incarcerated adolescent females. J Adolesc Health 24(1):21–27, 1999 9890361

Wisniewski JJ, Naglieri JA, Mulick JA: Psychometric properties of a Children's Psychosomatic Symptom Checklist. J Behav Med 11(5):497–507, 1988 3236381

Wyllie E, Glazer JP, Benbadis S, et al: Psychiatric features of children and adolescents with pseudoseizures. Arch Pediatr Adolesc Med 153(3):244–248, 1999 10086400

10

Pediatric Pain

The International Association for the Study of Pain defines *pain* as "an unpleasant sensory and emotional experience associated with actual or potential tissue damage, or described in terms of such damage" (Merskey and Bogduk 1994, p. 209). Although the experience of pain is universal, each person's experience is subjective and may be shaped by past experiences. For consultants, pain behavior represents an important clinical dilemma in which psychosocial factors and physical illness interact to varying degrees to determine a patient's individual pain experience. It is important for consultants to understand this interaction so that the pediatric team can develop and implement focused treatments designed to relieve, remove, or reduce a patient's suffering.

Classification

There are several ways to classify pain, including systems based on quality, duration, or etiology. Pain may be described as being nociceptive, neuropathic, or related to sympathetic overactivity (see Table 10–1).

Pain occurs when partial destruction or injury to the tissues adjacent to nerve fibers results in the release of chemicals such as neuropeptides. The quality of the pain experienced is related to the type of nociceptor activated. Activation of the cutaneous Aδ receptors that are myelinated and of large diameter leads to a pricking pain sensation. Activation of the cutaneous C receptors, which are thin and unmyelinated, results in pain with a dull or burning sensation. Activation of muscle nociceptors results in pain that has an aching quality. Acute pain signals injury and promotes action to prevent any further damage and to enhance healing. Repeated injury to the nerve fibers may lead to a surge in nerve growth factor and sprouting of nerves in inappropriate locations, resulting in aberrant innervation and potentially lower pain thresholds.

Pain may be described as acute, recurrent, or chronic in nature. *Acute* pain generally refers to a discrete episode of pain with complete resolution. *Recurrent* pain refers to discrete episodes of pain that are generally of brief duration, with complete recovery between episodes. For example, recurrent abdominal pain is defined as three or more episodes of abdominal pain severe enough to affect a child's activities over a period longer than 3 months, generally with complete recovery between episodes (Fritz et al. 1997; Plunkett and Beattie 2005). *Chronic* pain persists on a daily basis for longer than what would generally be expected for healing of the underlying physical pathology. It may or may not be associated with tissue damage. Chronic pain is often associated with depressed mood and the restriction of functional and physical activities (Tran et al. 2015). Both emotional and physical factors generally play an important role in chronic pain.

In DSM-5, the role psychological factors can play in the onset, severity, exacerbation, or maintenance of pain as well as significant distress or functional impairment is recognized in the diagnosis of somatic symptom disorder with predominant pain (American Psychiatric Association 2013). This category of disorders is discussed in more detail in Chapter 9, "Somatic Symptom and Related Disorders."

Pediatric chronic pain is associated with many negative outcomes, including physical disability, increased rates of depression and anxiety, and decreased quality of life (Miller et al. 2018).

Table 10–1.   Classification of pain

Type of pain	Location of injury	Characterics
Nociceptive pain		
Visceral	Hollow organs (bowel, bladder)	Dull, crampy, heavy, crushing, poorly localized
Somatic	Skin, connective tissue, bone, muscle	Dull, heavy, crushing, sometimes worse with movement (bone pain)
Neuropathic pain/ neuralgia	Primary lesion or disturbance to peripheral or central nervous system	Burning, electrical tingling, pricking, shooting, stabbing, itching, cold Allodynia (pain resulting from mild stimulation of normal tissue) Hyperalgesia (greater than expected pain from noxious stimulation) Hyperalgia (persistence of pain at primary or remote site)
Pain exacerbated by sympathetic activity (complex regional pain syndrome)	Autonomic dysfunction Association with nerve injury	Burning, allodynia, paresthesia, hyperalgesia to cold Signs of autonomic dysfunction (cyanosis, mottling, hyperhidrosis, edema, cooling of extremity)

Epidemiology

Between 25% and 44% of children and adolescents report somatic complaints such as pain and headaches that are generally transient in nature, and approximately 25% of youth experience pain that persists for longer than 3 months (King et al. 2011). Ruskin et al. (2017) reported that chronic pain affects

11%–38% of children, with impairments in physical, emotional, and academic functioning. Headaches and limb pain are more frequently seen in the 11- to 13-year age range, whereas older adolescents are most likely to report headaches, chest pain, and abdominal pain. Approximately 10%–20% of children younger than 10 years report recurrent headaches, and the frequency of migraine increases significantly after puberty, particularly in adolescent girls (Hämäläinen and Masek 2003). Recurrent abdominal pain complaints have been reported in 10%–25% of school-age children and adolescents and account for 2%–4% of pediatric office visits. The gender ratio is equal in early childhood, but girls are more symptomatic in later childhood and adolescence (Fritz and Campo 2002). Symptoms of pain increase significantly in patients with underlying physical conditions. Approximately 25% of pediatric cancer patients report daily pain episodes, and pain is a common symptom in 60% of children with HIV (Galloway and Yaster 2000).

Developmental Factors

Background

Historically, there have been fears and misperceptions regarding the treatment of pain. These fears included concern about causing drug addiction, doing harm (e.g., respiratory depression), giving the impression of giving up, and hastening the demise of a physically ill child, as well as worry about diversion of medication to family members. Although young children may lack the vocabulary and sophistication to articulate their experiences of pain, they may demonstrate pain by social withdrawal or changes in their patterns of sleep, eating, and activity levels. Children as young as 18 months will make efforts to localize pain and seek reassurance from adult figures, and 2-year-old children are able to use specific words to indicate the presence of pain. As the understanding of pediatric pain has grown, there is now recognition of the need to proactively address pain across the entire age spectrum.

Cognitive Theories Related to Pain

Piagetian stages of cognitive development are helpful in understanding the developmental issues related to a child or adolescent's experience of pain (Gaffney et al. 2003).

Preoperational Phase

In the preoperational phase of development (ages 2–6 years), children are generally confused about the causes of pain and may view pain as a punishment for the real or imagined transgression of rules. They have a tendency toward magical thinking and may develop idiosyncratic explanations for their pain. Assessment of pain in this stage is complicated because young children do not have the ability to measure continuous qualities and tend to choose the end points of scales. Requests to imagine the "worst pain imaginable" are complicated because children in the preoperational phase cannot yet understand the abstract concept of possibility. In addition, they are generally not able to separate the physical and affective components of pain and differentiate pain from anxiety or fear until age 10–12 years. During this stage, children are not able to use self-generated coping strategies and tend to rely on their environment (i.e., the support of adults).

Concrete Operations Phase

By age 7–8 years, children have more developed abilities for measurement, assessment, and seriation (the ability to accurately place items in ascending or descending order). The ability to seriate physical qualities of pain develops before children are able to differentiate the associated emotional components of pain. Children's understanding broadens during this phase to include awareness of associated negative effects. The capacity for increasingly logical thought processes leads to a greater understanding of pain, although children may still equate pain with punishment. The ability to localize pain becomes more differentiated, and the ability to use self-initiated coping strategies such as distraction or guided imagery increases. Pain that limits school and physical activities may have particularly adverse effects at this stage because self-esteem is dependent on the child's ability to obtain mastery.

Formal Operations Phase

Children enter the phase of formal operations around ages 11–14 years. Adolescents develop an increased capacity for abstract thought and introspection and become more aware of the psychological aspects of pain and its protective function. They may be increasingly able to differentiate the emotional aspects of pain and make use of behavioral interventions to reduce pain symptoms. However, the adolescent's greater ability to focus on future events may lead to greater worries and concerns about the recurrence of pain and disease and potential disabilities.

Measurement of Pain

Use of Appropriate Measures

Pain is measured by self-report, observation, and/or physiological measures, which include changes in heart rate, blood pressure, sweating, and pupillary dilatation (Cowen et al. 2015). It is critical to use assessment measures that are developmentally appropriate. Because direct report is not feasible with infants and younger children, it is often necessary to rely on observational reports from family members or the pediatric team.

Self-Report Measures

Self-report measures are generally valid for children as young as 4–5 years. These measures are usually combined with parent observations. Self-report measures are limited by difficulties in discriminating between intensity and duration and between the physical and emotional components of pain. It is important to also ask about physical sensations (i.e., heat, burning, or skin sensitivity that occur in neuropathic pain) that may accompany pain complaints. The following self-report measures have been used (Leo 2003; see Figure 10–1).

Verbal Descriptor Scale

This scale requires the child to rate the pain experienced according to one of five to seven verbal descriptors, with a limited range of options offered. The child must have adequate verbal skills and ability to use this scale, and its use may not be appropriate in younger children.

Numeric Rating Scale

With the widely used numeric rating scale, the child is asked to rate his or her pain on an 11-point scale anchored at one end by no pain (or 0) and at the other by worst pain possible (or 10). These ratings are reliable and correlate well with other simple assessment measures. The child must have intact language and cognitive skills.

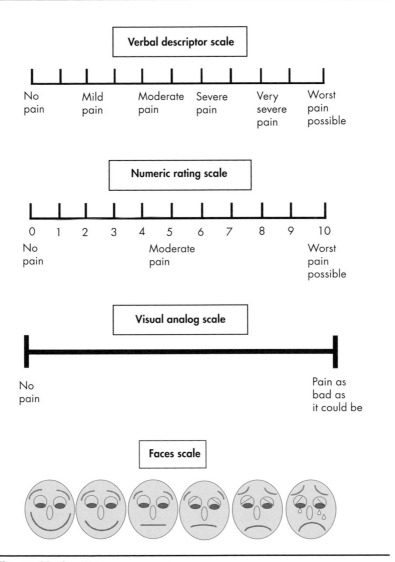

Figure 10–1. Pain assessment instruments.
Source. Reprinted from Leo RJ: "Evaluation of the Pain Patient," in *Concise Guide to Pain Management for Psychiatrists*. Washington, DC, American Psychiatric Publishing, 2003, p. 52. Copyright © 2003, American Psychiatric Publishing. Used with permission.

Visual Analog Scale

Similar to the numeric rating scale, this scale consists of a line with descriptive or numerical anchors on a continuum of pain intensity, similar to a Likert scale (Gaffney et al. 2003). The scale, anchored at one end by no pain (or 0) and at the other by worst pain possible (or 10), is presented to patients, who are asked to describe their current pain by making a mark across the line. This scale is valid and reliable for children age 8 years or older.

Faces Scale

This scale consists of six faces depicting different intensities of pain (Wong et al. 2001). It is a useful measure for children older than 6–8 years and is thought to be more direct and less complex than visual analog scales.

Pain Diary

Pain diaries may be used by older children and adolescents to report their pain experience at the time it occurs in order to avoid errors associated with retrospective recall. Pain diaries provide good baseline data prior to intervention and may include comments about functional ability, pain triggers, coping strategies, and medications used and their efficacy. Pain diaries may also be contrasted with parent reports of their child's pain.

Psychiatric Assessment

Psychiatric assessment may be requested when there is suspicion that the patient's symptoms and/or response to treatment have an emotional component that is problematic. When approaching such referrals, consultants should avoid the dichotomy between a physical and emotional etiology for the pain. Explanations of how emotional factors may exacerbate the child's experience of underlying physical pain are more successful in engaging patients and their families. It is important to validate the patient's experience of pain and to explore the impact the pain has had on all members of the family. Sociodemographic, medical, treatment, situational, and psychological variables are key to understanding a patient's response to pain (see Table 10–2).

Sociodemographic Variables

Pain responses have been noted to be associated with several sociodemographic variables, including the patient's age, gender, and ethnic background.

Table 10–2. Key elements in the psychiatric assessment of pediatric pain

Characteristics of pain

- Location/radiation

- Quality

- Intensity

- Duration and frequency (e.g., acute, recurrent, chronic, during procedures)

- Level of distress and assessment of the relationship of pain with severity of underlying etiology

Precipitating or exacerbating factors

- Eating

- Motion

- Menstrual cycle

- Stress

- Bright lights

- Lack of sleep/fatigue

Alleviating factors

- Distraction

- Vomiting

- Touch

- Bathing

- Heat

- Cold

Table 10–2.   Key elements in the psychiatric assessment of
pediatric pain *(continued)*

Use and efficacy of past and current treatment interventions

- Pharmacological

    - Types of medication used

    - Schedule of medications (e.g., scheduled vs. as-needed dosing)

    - Frequency of missed treatments (i.e., treatment adherence)

    - Reasons for missed treatments

    - Efficacy of previous treatment

    - Side effects of treatment

- Nonpharmacological

    - Physical therapy

    - Biofeedback

    - Guided imagery

    - Hypnosis

    - Distraction

Impact of pain

- Emotional (e.g., depression, anxiety, posttraumatic stress disorder)

- Family (e.g., disruption of work schedule, impact on marital relationship, impact on siblings, distraction from family conflict)

- Social and peer relationships

- Academic (e.g., absenteeism, placement in home teaching)

Family beliefs regarding pain

- Belief in single, undiagnosed primary medical cause for the pain

    - Investment in further medical workup

    - Unjustified concerns about potential medical illness

- Belief in role of environmental triggers

Table 10–2. Key elements in the psychiatric assessment of pediatric pain *(continued)*

Family beliefs regarding pain *(continued)*

• Belief in role of psychological factors

• Beliefs regarding pain control

  • Awareness of pharmacological strategies

  • Awareness of nonpharmacological approaches

  • Belief that child should rest and be excused from responsibilities during pain episodes

Family medical history

• Family history of unexplained somatic symptoms

• Pattern of reinforcement of illness behavior in the family

Reinforcement of pain behaviors

• Reinforcement by parents

  • Parents keep medical journals and diaries of symptoms

  • Parent stays home from work

• Increased attention or sympathy from family and/or friends

• Increased attention from medical providers

• Avoidance of school, social, or athletic stressor

Young children, for example, are more likely to experience distress during pain episodes or painful procedures partly because of their less mature coping skills (Schechter 2002). Firstborn children appear to have lower pain thresholds; this may be due in part to greater reinforcement of pain complaints that may occur with first-time parents. Girls, especially as adolescents, generally report lower pain tolerance and a higher frequency of pain complaints compared with boys, a finding hypothesized to be related to cultural and societal variables (Dahlquist and Switkin 2003). Culture and ethnicity play an important role in determining how much expression of pain is acceptable.

Medical Variables

Pain duration and predictability as well as disease severity influence the experience of pain. Prior negative experiences with painful procedures are associated with more patient distress. It appears to be the adverse nature of the prior experience rather than the number of pain episodes that is of greater significance. Sleep deprivation affects pain perception and may interfere with efforts to divert attention from pain sensations. Similarly, increased muscle tension or protective posturing secondary to pain may increase the child's experience of pain.

Treatment Variables

The choice and dosage of pain medications prescribed can influence the pain experience. Suboptimal dosing or the use of "as-needed" medication for breakthrough pain rather than scheduled dosing can contribute adversely to the pain experience. Forgetfulness, lack of supervision, or nonadherence due to the patient's or the family's reluctance to take medications may play significant roles. Consultants should inquire about current or past use of nonpharmacological interventions.

Situational Variables

Children who lack age-appropriate information about their illness and its treatment are more likely to experience distress. This is particularly true when children have little perceived control over the treatment. Children need adequate preparation for procedures whenever possible and should receive instruction in effective coping methods (e.g., distraction techniques). Pain tolerance is negatively affected when there are inconsistencies in the procedure expected or in the response by pediatric staff or parents. It is important to ensure that children have parental support during pain episodes and procedures.

Psychological Variables

Meaning of Pain

Children's knowledge, attitudes, and beliefs about their illness may influence their perception of pain and their response to treatment. Pain may be viewed as a punishment, as a challenge, or in some cases as a character-building experience. Pain that is perceived as having little benefit or that is associated with potential disfigurement or disability is likely to be less well tolerated (Schechter 2002). Similarly, a child with a diagnosis of cancer may interpret pain as an indication of disease progression or relapse and experience increased anxiety or depression.

Personality Characteristics

Personality characteristics affecting the child's response to pain include the tendency to withdraw from others in response to pain, the ability to seek support, and coping style. For example, children with low adaptability tend to report more distress during painful procedures, and those with negative thinking or a tendency to catastrophize tend to report more psychological distress and need for medication (Miller et al. 2018; Tran et al. 2015). Patients may be classified on the basis of their habitual tendency to approach or avoid new situations. Although there is no definitive coping style associated with adaptation to pain, the critical dimension appears to be whether the child has the freedom to use his or her own specific approach.

Stress

Pain is frequently correlated with stressful life events. School-related stressors (e.g., performance anxiety related to tests or sports), family stressors (e.g., death, abuse, divorce, new siblings), and stressors related to the illness (e.g., immobilization, disfigurement) might all play important roles in the development and/or exacerbation of pain.

Psychiatric Comorbidity

Psychiatric comorbidity is common and often overlooked in children with pain, in part because of the difficulties of making a psychiatric diagnosis in a physically ill child. Although depression may be secondary to the physical illness or its treatment, the presence of a depressive disorder increases the risk of developing chronic pain conditions. There is a strong relationship between pain and anxiety. Pain often results in symptoms of anxiety, and anxiety may decrease the pain threshold and increase the sensation of pain (Green and Kowalik 1994). The possibility of substance abuse is an important consideration in adolescents. Patients with chronic recurrent pain (e.g., sickle cell crises) may be at risk of developing a dependence on narcotic medication that begins with benign use but evolves into a pattern of drug-seeking behavior.

Family Influences

Parents play an important role in both mediating and promoting the child's experience of pain, and there is a tendency for pain to aggregate in families. Parents with a history of multiple chronic pain symptoms are more likely to have children with impairment and disability. Parents who are more somatically focused are more likely to take medications for physical symptoms and may encourage their child's own pain complaints. Consultants should explore the ways that parents wittingly or unwittingly might reinforce their child's pain behavior.

Secondary Gain

Pain symptoms may be promoted by secondary gain, which is the avoidance of a stressful or unpleasant situation. Pain behaviors may allow the child to remain home from school and avoid a stressful academic or social activity. Pain may provide the child with a legitimate excuse for dropping out of competitive sports. In families with high levels of dysfunction, pain may serve the function of diverting family attention away from a problematic conflict (e.g., marital problems) or provide a way for a parent to meet his or her own unresolved needs for attention through interactions with pediatric care providers or through sympathy and attention from friends and family members.

Principles of Pain Management

Formulation of the Problem

Principles of pain management are similar to those outlined for the treatment of somatic symptom disorders (see Chapter 9). The first step is for consultants to arrive at a developmental biopsychosocial formulation of the problem. In particular, consultants need to determine the roles that psychological factors and the physical illness itself play in the pain experience. This formulation should be communicated to the patient, family, and medical team. Consultants can use the steps outlined in Table 10–3 for implementing an integrated medical and psychiatric treatment program. Depending on the formulation of the pain experience, specific treatment recommendations fall into nonpharmacological and pharmacological categories.

Table 10–3. Guidelines for developing an integrated medical and psychiatric treatment approach to pediatric pain

1. Complete a psychiatric assessment

   • Use guidelines for the psychiatric assessment of pediatric pain (see Table 10–2)

   • Develop a developmental biopsychosocial formulation of the pain experience

   • Determine contributing roles of emotional factors and the physical illness

2. Convey the biopsychosocial formulation to the pediatric team

   • Remember that symptoms can be in significant excess of what would be expected from the physical findings that are present

   • Remember that physical findings may have accounted for early symptoms but may no longer be the etiology for the current symptoms

3. Convene an informing conference between the pediatrician and the family

   • Convey integrated medical and psychiatric findings to the family

   • Because the family has a medical model as their frame of reference, help reframe this understanding of symptoms into a developmental biopsychosocial formulation

4. Implement treatment interventions

   • Consider the following pharmacological interventions:
     • Nonsteroidal anti-inflammatory drug
     • Opioid
     • Antidepressant
     • Anticonvulsant
     • Antiarrhythmic
     • Clonidine
     • Psychostimulants
     • Antipsychotic
     • Anxiolytic
     • Topical anesthetic

Table 10–3.   Guidelines for developing an integrated medical and psychiatric treatment approach to pediatric pain *(continued)*

4.   Implement treatment interventions *(continued)*

•   Consider the following nonpharmacological interventions:

•   Physical therapy

•   Biofeedback

•   Relaxation

•   Guided imagery and hypnosis

•   Transcutaneous electrical nerve stimulation

•   Operant interventions

•   Family therapy

•   Individual psychotherapy

•   Rehabilitation model

Source.   Reprinted from Ibeziako PI, DeMaso DR: "The Somatoform Disorders," in *Clinical Child Psychiatry*, 3rd Edition. Edited by Klykylo W.M., Kay J.L. Indianapolis, IN, Wiley, 2012, pp. 458–474. Copyright © 2012, John Wiley. Used with permission.

Rehabilitation Model

A subset of patients may develop symptoms of chronic pain with severe impairment in their level of functioning. The ongoing experience of pain can result in a sensitization of the nervous system that produces physiological and neuroanatomical changes. Disuse may lead to further pain and disability. The term *pain-associated disability syndrome* has been used to describe this presentation (Bursch et al. 2003). Patients may experience a downward spiral of increasing disability and pain in which acute symptom-focused treatment is not found to be helpful. A rehabilitation or chronic illness model is required in which pain is accepted as a symptom that may not go away. This implies the decision to stop any further medical workup and instead focus on efforts to improve independent functioning and skill building to improve coping.

Adoption of a rehabilitation model frequently requires a paradigm shift on the part of the patient and family. Explanation of the fact that the pain is "real" may seem in conflict with a decision to stop making inquiries about the symptoms. It is important to explain how biological and psychological factors interact with the patient's social environment to influence pain and disability. Families may interpret the proposal to use nonpharmacological interventions as a statement that a child's pain complaints are only psychologically based. Specific goals of treatment are introduced that do not include the absence of pain. By contrast, progress is measured by changes in the child's level of adaptive functioning, including the ability to return to school and to resume normal social and recreational activities. The cost benefits of intensive interdisciplinary pediatric chronic pain rehabilitation programs have been demonstrated with respect to both health care costs and missed work on the part of parents (Evans et al. 2016).

Nonpharmacological Management

Several principles are useful when developing a treatment intervention for pediatric pain that incorporates nonpharmacological approaches.

- Pain is a subjective sensation, and it is important to believe the child's experience of pain.
- Developmentally appropriate measures should be used to assess pain and the child's response to treatment.
- It is important to try to avoid the dichotomy between organic and nonorganic pain by assuming that both factors may be relevant.
- Treatment should be multimodal and multidisciplinary in nature and incorporate both pharmacological and nonpharmacological approaches.
- Nonpharmacological interventions can be helpful even with pain for which emotional factors make little contribution to the pain experience.

Education

Parents and family members often require education about treatment approaches for chronic pain. It is important to help the family differentiate the appropriate response of sympathy and attention during an episode of acute pain from responses that reinforce chronic pain behaviors. Parents may mistakenly believe that the child should be allowed to rest during pain episodes. Excessive attention to the child's pain symptoms may inadvertently encourage the child to scan his or her body for somatic cues and reinforce somatic vigilance. Parents need to learn how to acknowledge their child's pain but at the same time encourage the use of distraction and other active coping strategies. Other common misconceptions include the belief in a single, as yet undiagnosed, cause of pain as well as an inaccurate understanding of the interplay with stress or other psychological factors. Parents require education about the appropriate use of analgesia and possible misconceptions about addiction. Education about the secondary effects of inactivity and muscle tension may be helpful.

Physical Therapy

Physical therapy is used to increase flexibility and mobility as well as endurance and stamina. Stretching and massage may reduce muscle tension, which is often a secondary cause of pain in patients with chronic pain. Physical therapy introduced in association with changes to the medication regimen, or following a nerve block, may allow the resumption of physical activities that have not been possible for many months, with the hope that these activities will be sustained after the block is discontinued (McCarthy et al. 2003).

Biofeedback

Biofeedback refers to the procedure in which physical parameters such as muscle tension or temperature are continuously monitored and fed back to the patient, who then attempts to alter the parameter. Although the measurement and control of physiological responses are usually not thought to be under voluntary control, biofeedback is based on the principle that it is possible to amplify and transform the response in such a way that it can be monitored and understood by the patient. Muscle tension and finger temperature are the most common physical functions measured in the treatment of pain. Biofeedback uses electrical equipment that allows the use of auditory and visual feedback from a physiological function (e.g., muscle contraction or relaxation). The patient's increased ability to monitor and control the muscle tension is then applied to controlling or altering the physiological process thought to cause the pain sensations (McGrath et al. 2003). For example, in the treatment of headaches associated with increased tension in the frontalis muscle, the patient is taught to reduce tension in this muscle. Biofeedback results in an increased sense of mastery and control for patients (ages 6 years and older), who are generally enthusiastic and receptive to this intervention.

Transcutaneous Electrical Nerve Stimulation

Transcutaneous electrical nerve stimulation (TENS) units are used for localized pain, complex regional pain syndromes, and postoperative pain (McCarthy et al. 2003). Electrodes are placed around the painful region, along peripheral nerve routes, or at spinal segments. Electrical stimulation of large afferent A nerve fibers by the TENS unit is believed to inhibit pain transmission to the spinal cord that ordinarily occurs via the smaller-diameter nerve fibers, with the result that the child feels tingling and vibrating sensations rather than aching pain. It is also believed that TENS units may activate the release of endogenous opioids. Patients are trained on the use of TENS units during physical therapy sessions and then wear the unit at home and during normal activities, including school.

Cognitive-Behavioral Therapy

Progressive Muscle Relaxation

Several methods of progressive muscle relaxation are used to distract patients from their pain and to reduce subjective pain intensity. In the tension relaxation method, the child is taught to constrict the muscles for 5–10 seconds and then relax specific muscle groups. This technique can be combined with suggestions of relaxation, heaviness, and warmth and images of relaxing situations. In the suggestion method, the child is given repeated suggestions of calmness, relaxation, heaviness, and warmth combined with pleasant imagery but without instructions to tense the muscles. With differential relaxation, the child learns to relax one part of the body while maintaining tension in other parts. For example, in the treatment of a migraine, the child learns to relax the jaw and shoulders but keeps tension in arms and trunks in order to be able to continue school activities.

Guided Imagery and Hypnosis

Guided imagery and hypnosis, described in Chapter 18, "Preparation for Procedures," are commonly used as part of a pain management intervention. The successful use of hypnosis for pain management has been reported in children receiving bone marrow aspiration and lumbar punctures as well as for postoperative pain and anxiety and chronic headache (Rogovik and Goldman 2007).

Behavior Modification

Behavior modification interventions are introduced when the target is not specifically the pain complaints but rather the associated pain behaviors, including the functional disability associated with the pain. Programs include incentives for improvements in functional ability and decreased attention to complaints of pain.

Psychotherapy

Individual psychotherapy can play an important role in helping change a child's erroneous cognitions about his or her ability to resume functioning. Encouragement of more adaptive coping strategies can become a focus of the therapy. It is helpful to explore potential sources of stress and gain understanding of the emotional factors that may perpetuate pain behaviors.

Family interventions are designed to help the family support healthy, functional behaviors and reduce support for pain behaviors. Evidence supports the use of family-based cognitive behavior therapy for patients with chronic pain (Sieberg and Manganella 2015). Treatment should also address family conflicts that may be causing stress for the child or interfering with efforts to cope with pain. Children with chronic pain may unconsciously use their symptoms to avoid stressful school or social situations or as a response to competitive athletic pressures. Parents similarly may receive secondary gain from their child's pain behavior—for example, by avoiding work or gaining increased closeness with their child. Illness behavior in general tends to promote or maintain maladaptive patterns of family interaction that need to be explored in family therapy. In addition, family members may experience feelings of frustration related to the disruption to family life caused by their child's pain. Families may harbor pessimistic feelings that no treatment will help with the pain, or they may fear the possibility of increased pain and disability. There may be strong feelings of anger directed toward the pediatric team. Therapy should be directed toward reducing feelings of anxiety and hopelessness and toward promoting active coping.

Mindfulness-Based Interventions

Mindfulness-based interventions are based on the premise that teaching patients to increase their awareness of and focus on the present in a nonjudgmental manner with acceptance of the situation can result in improved physical and emotional functioning (Ruskin et al. 2017). Patients with chronic pain are taught to approach rather than avoid painful sensations and to incorporate strategies such as thought diffusion and present-moment awareness. The expectation is that patients learn that although pain may be unavoidable, suffering and distress are optional. Although data on the use of mindfulness-based interventions in pediatric chronic pain are limited, increased pain acceptance was demonstrated in a sample of adolescents with chronic pain using mindfulness strategies (Ruskin et al. 2017). Mindfulness-based interventions have also resulted in improvements in quality of life, physical functioning, depression, and pain acceptance in adolescents with recurrent headaches (Hesse et al. 2015). Acceptance and commitment therapy (ACT) incorporates similar mindfulness strategies with the goal of acceptance rather than control of physical discomfort.

Pharmacological Management

Pharmacological measures include the use of nerve block procedures and epidurals to allow the child to begin physical therapy. Adjunctive pain medications and medications for anxiety or depression may also be required. By contrast, the decision may be made to wean patients from chronic, ineffective opioid regimens by using blinded pain cocktails. In this section, we summarize the common pharmacological agents used in the treatment of pediatric pain (Table 10–4).

When analgesic medications are being used, it is important to adopt a preventive approach to pain management by treating pain early and aggressively and by adhering to the following principles:

- Use scheduled rather than as-needed medications.
- Adopt an effective system for the assessment of pain and treatment response.
- Titrate one medication at a time.
- Initiate new medications at the lowest possible dosage.
- Slowly titrate every 3–7 days depending on medication and patient characteristics (e.g., age, prior experience with medications, other medications).

Table 10–4.   Pharmacological agents used to treat pediatric pain

Drug	Route	Pediatric dosing	Important side effects
Nonsteroidal anti-inflammatory drugs			
Aspirin	po	10–15 mg/kg every 4–6 hours	Antiplatelet effect, gastrointestinal upset, tinnitus, association with Reye's syndrome
Ibuprofen	po	5–10 mg/kg tid–qid	
Indomethacin	po/iv/pr	1–3 mg/kg bid–tid	
Acetaminophen	po/pr	20–30 mg/kg every 6 hours po 40–60 mg/kg every 6 hours pr	Hepatotoxic (with massive overdosage)
Opioids			Nausea, vomiting, constipation, itching, sedation, respiratory depression/arrest, urinary retention
Morphine	iv	0.1 mg/kg every 2–3 hours 0.02–0.03 mg/kg/hour for PCA	
Meperidine	iv	1.0–3.0 mg/kg every 3–4 hours	May cause tachycardia
Fentanyl	iv	1.0–3.0 µg/kg every 1–2 hours	May cause bradycardia
Codeine	po	0.5–1.0 every 4 hours	
Hydromorphone	iv	0.05–1.0 mg/kg every 3 hours	
Oxycodone	po	0.05–0.1 mg/kg every 4 hours	
Methadone	po/sc/im/iv	0.7 mg/kg/day divided Q4–6 hours	

Table 10–4.   Pharmacological agents used to treat pediatric pain (*continued*)

Drug	Route	Pediatric dosing	Important side effects
Antidepressants			
Amitriptyline	po	0.05–2 mg/kg/day	Anticholinergic side effects, autonomic side effects (orthostatic hypotension, sweating), electrocardiographic changes
Nortriptyline	po	0.05–2 mg/kg/day	Anticholinergic side effects, autonomic side effects (orthostatic hypotension, sweating), electrocardiographic changes
Venlafaxine	po	37.5–225 mg/day in divided doses (bid or tid)	Headache, initial anxiety, sustained hypertension
Duloxetine	po	30–60 mg/day increased to maximum of 120 mg/day	Hypertension, headache, palpitations, serotonin syndrome
Anticonvulsants			
Carbamazepine	po	15–30 mg/kg in divided doses (bid or tid)	Sedation, ataxia, dizziness, blood dyscrasias including aplastic anemia, hepatotoxicity
Sodium valproate	po	10–60 mg/kg in divided doses (bid or tid)	Sedation, blood dyscrasias, hepatotoxicity, weight gain, polycystic ovarian syndrome
Gabapentin	po	5–30 mg/kg in divided doses (tid or qid)	Somnolence, dizziness, ataxia, aggressive behavior

Table 10–4.   Pharmacological agents used to treat pediatric pain (*continued*)

Drug	Route	Pediatric dosing	Important side effects
Membrane stabilizers			
Lidocaine	iv	150 µg/kg/hour	Sedation, nausea
Mexiletine	po	10–15 mg/kg in divided doses (tid)	Sedation, fatigue, confusion, nausea, hypotension, diplopia, ataxia
Antihypertensive			
Clonidine	po/td/epidural infusion	0.05–0.2 µg/kg/hour	Sedation, hypotension, bradycardia, potential for rebound hypertension
Anxiolytics			
Lorazepam	po/im/iv	0.05 mg/kg/day tid–qid	Respiratory depression, drowsiness, disinhibition
Clonazepam	po	0.1–0.2 mg/kg/day bid–tid	
Antipsychotics			
Haloperidol	iv/im/po	0.05–0.15 mg/kg/day in divided doses (bid or tid)	Electrocardiographic changes, dystonic reactions, neuroleptic malignant syndrome, tardive dyskinesia
Chlorpromazine	po/im	2.5–6.0 mg/kg/day in divided doses (tid or qid)	

Table 10–4. Pharmacological agents used to treat pediatric pain *(continued)*

Drug	Route	Pediatric dosing	Important side effects
Antipsychotics			Increased heart rate, hypertension, aggressive behavior, insomnia, anorexia
Methylphenidate	po	0.3–2.0 mg/kg/day in divided doses (bid or tid)	
Dextroamphetamine	po	2.5–4.0 mg/kg/day in divided doses (bid or tid)	

Note.   bid=twice a day; im=intramuscular; iv=intravenously; po=orally; PCA=patient-controlled analgesia; pr=rectally; td=transdermally; qid=four times a day; sc=subcutaneous; tid=three times a day.
Source.   Adapted from Krane et al. 2003; Maunuksela and Olkkola 2003; Yaster et al. 2003.

- Titrate to end point of maximal significant pain relief (>50%) or intolerable side effects, or toxic serum level for tricyclic antidepressants or mexiletine.
- Continue chronic use only if significant pain relief, tolerable side effects, and increased patient activity and functioning occur.
- Introduce polypharmacy only if the first medication produces only partial pain relief and higher dosage produces side effects.
- Supplement medication treatment with nonpharmacological interventions.

Nonsteroidal Anti-inflammatory Drugs

The nonsteroidal anti-inflammatory drugs (NSAIDs), also referred to as *antipyretic analgesics*, include a large group of medications that are often first-line choices for all classes of pain. They are used in the treatment of rheumatoid arthritis, dental pain, bone pain, muscle pain, and menstrual cramps. They are particularly useful in trauma where swelling and inflammation play a role in producing pain. The mechanism of action involves inhibition of the cyclooxygenase and lipoxygenase enzyme pathways, resulting in decreased production of the prostaglandins (specifically thromboxanes and leukotrienes) that result in inflammation and pain. Effects on platelet aggregation, gastric mucosa, and renal parenchyma bleeding may limit their use. NSAIDS have the benefit of not causing dependence or respiratory depression.

Acetaminophen

Acetaminophen, which is one of the most commonly prescribed analgesics for mild to moderate pain, appears to inhibit the cyclooxygenase enzyme pathway in the central nervous system. Given that it does not inhibit tissue prostaglandin synthesis or platelet aggregation, acetaminophen has no significant anti-inflammatory effect. There are no gastrointestinal or renal side effects analogous to the NSAIDs. Taken in excess, acetaminophen does have the potential to cause hepatotoxicity. Unlike the NSAIDS, the use of acetaminophen is not associated with Reye's syndrome.

Opioids

Opioid medications (or narcotics) act centrally by binding with the central nervous system's μ opioid receptors. These receptors are subdivided into the

α_1 receptors, which cause supraspinal analgesia, and the α_2 receptors, which cause respiratory depression, inhibition of gastrointestinal motility, and spinal analgesia. Opioid drugs mimic the action of endogenous opioids to inhibit the release of pain neurotransmitters. Opioids produce analgesia, respiratory depression, euphoria, and physical dependence. Data support the safety and effectiveness of opioids in the treatment of infants, children, and adolescents with moderate to severe pain (Yaster et al. 2003).

Opioids are classified on the basis of their strength and their duration of action. Short-acting opioids include fentanyl, morphine, and meperidine, and long-acting opioids include methadone, codeine, and oxycodone. Codeine and oxycodone are commonly used for moderate pain in association with NSAIDs. Morphine, meperidine, and fentanyl are more effective for severe pain. Because of its relatively brief duration of action, fentanyl is useful for short, painful procedures.

Patient-controlled analgesia (PCA) is a pain control system that uses a computerized pump to deliver pain medication at predetermined dosages when the patient pushes a button (Ferrante et al. 1990). PCA has been found to be effective in children as young as 1 year (Yaster et al. 2003). PCA results in immediate pain relief and provides the child with a greater sense of control over his or her pain. It has been used for postsurgical recovery, cancer pain, flares of inflammatory diseases, sickle cell crises, and burn pain in children as young as 6 or 7 years.

Side effects common to all opioids include decreased gastrointestinal motility with constipation and nausea; itching; sedation; respiratory slowing; and, at high dosages, respiratory arrest (Table 10–5). Because the immature blood-brain barrier is permeable to morphine, children younger than 3 months require 25% of the traditional dosage. Physical dependence occurs with all opioids within 7 days and may result in patients having to be weaned, with a reduction in dosage by 10%–20% per day.

Antidepressants

As noted previously, there is a clear relationship between pain and depression. Tricyclic antidepressants (TCAs) and serotonin-norepinephrine reuptake inhibitors (SNRIs) have been used as adjuncts in the pharmacological treatment of pain, with most of the data derived from studies of adult patients (Ansari

Table 10–5.   Management of side effects of opioids

Side effect	Treatment intervention	Route	Dosage	Side effects of treatment
Nausea, vomiting	Metoclopramide	iv	1–2 mg/kg	Sedation, fatigue, confusion, headache, extrapyramidal symptoms
	Promethazine	iv, im	0.25–0.5 mg/kg qid	Blurred vision, confusion, urinary difficulties, dry mouth, nervousness
	Dolasetron	po, iv	1.8 mg/kg (100 mg maximum)	Diarrhea, headache
	Odansetron	po	>12 years, 16 mg/day <12 years, 12 mg/day	Headache, dizziness, agitation, fever, pruritus, fatigue, diarrhea, constipation
		iv	0.1–0.15 mg/kg (16 mg maximum)	
	Lorazepam	po, iv	2–6 mg/day bid or tid	Ataxia, dizziness, drowsiness, slurred speech
Constipation	Docusate sodium	po	>12 years, 50–360 mg/day <12 years, 50–150 mg/day	Stomach/intestinal cramps, allergic reactions
	Milk of magnesia	po	80 mEq single dose	Diarrhea, polydipsia, stomach cramps
	Lactulose	po	10 g in 120 mL of water	Diarrhea, stomach cramps, gas
	Senna	po	>12 years, 15 mg/day <12 years, 5–10 mg/day	Electrolyte and fluid imbalance, nausea/vomiting, stomach cramps

Table 10–5. Management of side effects of opioids (*continued*)

Side effect	Treatment intervention	Route	Dosage	Side effects of treatment
Constipation (*continued*)	Bisacodyl	po	>12 years, 10–15 mg single dose 6–12 years, 5 mg single dose	Diarrhea, cramps
	Magnesium citrate	po	80 mEq single dose	Diarrhea, stomach cramps
Pruritus	Diphenhydramine	po, iv	12.5–25 mg qid	Drowsiness, delirium, thickening of bronchial secretions
	Hydroxyzine	po, iv	>6 years, 50–100 mg/day <6 years, 50 mg/day	Drowsiness, thickening of bronchial secretions
	Fexofenadine	po	>12 years, 60 mg bid <12 years, 30 mg bid	Headache, coughing
Sedation	Adjust dose Change opioid Adjust schedule to normalize sleep–wake cycle Avoid other sedating medications Change route of administration			

Note. bid=twice a day; iv=intravenously; po=orally; qid=four times a day; tid=three times a day.

2000; Carter and Sullivan 2002; Krane et al. 2003). Although there has been interest in the use of selective serotonin reuptake inhibitors, they have generally not been found to be as effective in pain treatment, with the exception of one trial of citalopram to treat recurrent abdominal pain in pediatric patients (Campo et al. 2004).

Tricyclic Antidepressants

Although TCAs have been found to be superior to placebo in the treatment of pain in adult patients, a recent Cochrane review did not find strong evidence for their use in pediatric patients (Cooper et al. 2017). Evidence suggests that TCAs have a direct analgesic effect that is separate from their efficacy in treating depression or insomnia. Different mechanisms have been suggested, including increased availability of serotonin, endogenous opioid peptide release, and a direct action on opioid receptors (Gray et al. 1998). TCAs may also potentiate the action of opioids, allowing a reduction in chronic opioid requirements. The effect of TCAs on pain reduction and improved sleep is more rapid (3–7 days) at lower dosages (0.1–0.2 mg/kg/day) than is expected in the treatment of depression.

Amitriptyline is one of the most widely studied TCAs and has been found to be effective in a wide range of pediatric pain syndromes, including migraine, peripheral neuropathies, phantom limb pain, fibromyalgia, and pain related to the invasion of nerves by tumors. Studies have emphasized the helpfulness of even low dosages as well as benefit from the drug's sedation. Nevertheless, there is no theoretical or empirical basis to suggest that amitriptyline has any unique efficacy in pain management compared with other TCAs. Where sedation is problematic or the patient is particularly susceptible to anticholinergic side effects, imipramine and nortriptyline are alternative considerations.

TCAs may have anticholinergic side effects, including dry mouth, constipation, blurred vision, urinary retention, confusion, and delirium. Autonomic side effects include orthostatic hypotension, profuse sweating, palpitations, tachycardia, and high blood pressure. Electrocardiographic changes include flattened T waves; prolonged QT, QRS, and PR intervals; and depressed ST segments. Electrocardiographic monitoring is recommended at baseline and after the patient has been stabilized at a therapeutic dosage (see Chapter 17, "Pharmacological Approaches and Considerations").

Serotonin-Norepinephrine Reuptake Inhibitors

There continues to be interest in the SNRIs, including venlafaxine and duloxetine, which some authors have suggested are at least as effective as the TCAs and with fewer side effects (Goldstein et al. 2004). Venlafaxine has been used in the treatment of adults with headache, neuropathic pain, fibromyalgia, diabetic peripheral neuropathy, and reflex sympathetic dystrophy (Kiayias et al. 2000). Unfortunately, a Cochrane review in adult patients found little compelling evidence to support the use of venlafaxine in neuropathic pain (Gallagher et al. 2015). Placebo effects were noted to be high in several studies, and the authors cautioned about side effects, including fatigue, somnolence, nausea, and dizziness. In addition, although isolated case reports have found duloxetine to be helpful in treating pediatric pain, no randomized trials support these findings (Kachko et al. 2011).

Anticonvulsants

Carbamazepine, clonazepam, and phenytoin have been widely used in the treatment of migraine and neuropathic pain, and divalproex sodium has been used for migraine prophylaxis. Newer agents such as topiramate and lamotrigine have been used for diabetic neuropathy and trigeminal neuralgia. Anticonvulsants have certain drawbacks, including the potential to cause behavioral changes and the requirement for serum level monitoring because of their narrow therapeutic window (see Chapter 17, "Psychopharmacological Approaches and Considerations"). A Cochrane review found no evidence to support or refute the use of antiepileptic drugs to treat chronic noncancer pain in children and adolescents (Cooper et al. 2017). Table 10–6 lists the anticonvulsants used for pain management.

Gabapentin is one of the most promising agents used to treat neuropathic pain associated with postherpetic neuralgia, post-poliomyelitis neuropathy, complex regional pain syndrome, phantom limb pain, and diabetic/HIV neuropathy (Krane et al. 2003). Gabapentin has fewer side effects and fewer drug interactions than other anticonvulsants and does not require serum level monitoring. Gabapentin appears to be helpful in reducing spontaneous paroxysmal pain with burning and lancinating quality as well as allodynia to cold and tactile stimuli.

Table 10–6. Anticonvulsants used for pain management

Drug	Mechanism of action	Pharmacology	Adverse effects	Clinical applications
Carbamazepine	Inhibits norepinephrine uptake Prevents repeated discharges in neurons Blocks sodium channels	Slow absorption Protein bound Hepatic metabolism Urinary excretion $t_{1/2} = 10–20$ hours	Sedation, nausea, diplopia, vertigo, hematological abnormalities, jaundice, oliguria, hypertension, acute left ventricular heart failure Need to monitor complete blood count and liver function tests	Diabetic neuropathy Trigeminal neuralgia
Oxcarbazepine	Prevents repeated discharges in neurons Binds to sodium channels Increases potassium conductance	Metabolized to 10-monohydroxy metabolite with $t_{1/2} = 9$ hours	Dizziness, somnolence, diplopia, fatigue, ataxia, nausea, abnormal vision, hyponatremia	Trigeminal neuralgia Neuropathic pain syndromes
Topiramate	Blocks sodium channels Inhibits calcium channels Potentiates GABAergic inhibition	Rapid oral absorption $t_{1/2} = 21$ hours 70% eliminated unchanged in urine	Kidney stones, somnolence, dizziness, ataxia, paresthesias, nervousness, abnormal vision, weight loss, cognitive slowing	Migraine headaches Neuropathic pain Diabetic neuropathy

Table 10–6. Anticonvulsants used for pain management *(continued)*

Drug	Mechanism of action	Pharmacology	Adverse effects	Clinical applications
Gabapentin	Possible increase in total brain concentration of GABA	Not metabolized Not protein bound Renal excretion $t_{1/2}$ = 5–7 hours	Somnolence, dizziness, ataxia, fatigue, concentration difficulties, gastrointestinal disturbance, nystagmus, pedal edema	First-line drug for pain management Complex regional pain syndrome Postherpetic neuralgia Diabetic neuropathy Phantom limb pain Multiple sclerosis Possible use for inflammatory pain
Lamotrigine	Blocks sodium channels Inhibits glutamate release Modulates calcium and potassium currents	Complete oral absorption 98% bioavailability $t_{1/2}$ = 24 hours Hepatic metabolism Drug-drug reactions with other anticonvulsants	Dizziness, nausea. headache, ataxia, diplopia, blurred vision, somnolence, Stevens-Johnson syndrome	Complex regional pain syndrome Trigeminal neuralgia Spinal cord injury Multiple sclerosis Central poststroke pain

Table 10–6. Anticonvulsants used for pain management *(continued)*

Drug	Mechanism of action	Pharmacology	Adverse effects	Clinical applications
Levetiracetam	Reduces high-voltage calcium currents Opposes inhibition of GABA Affects potassium conductance	Rapid oral absorption $t_{1/2}$=7–11 hours Renal excretion No hepatic metabolism	Somnolence, asthenia, dizziness, depression, nervousness	Migraine prophylaxis Postherpetic neuralgia Neuropathic pain
Pregabalin	GABA analogue Increases neuronal GABA concentration	90% oral bioavailability $t_{1/2}$=6 hours 99% excreted unchanged in urine	Dizziness, somnolence, headache	Diabetic neuropathy Postherpetic neuralgia
Zonisamide	Blocks sodium and calcium channels, facilitates serotonin and dopamine transmission Increases GABA release	100% oral bioavailability $t_{1/2}$=60 hours Renal excretion	Somnolence, ataxia, anorexia, difficulty with concentration, agitation, headache, Stevens-Johnson syndrome	Neuropathic pain Migraine headaches

Note.   GABA=γ-aminobutyric acid; $t_{1/2}$=drug half-life.
Source.   Adapted from Hayes K: "Adjuvant Treatments," in *The Massachusetts General Hospital Handbook of Pain Management*, 3rd Edition. Edited by Ballantyne JC. Philadelphia, PA, Lippincott Williams & Wilkins, 2006, pp. 127–140. Copyright © 2006, Lippincott Williams & Wilkins. Adapted with permission from Wolters Kluwer Health, Inc.

Membrane Stabilizers

Membrane-stabilizing agents have been used to enhance the efficacy of opioids, antidepressants, and anticonvulsants. Lidocaine and mexiletine are thought to act through a sodium channel–binding mechanism. Lidocaine is used as an adjunct medication for mucositis pain related to chemotherapy agents, refractory cancer pain, and neuropathies and to predict the potential efficacy of mexiletine. In a lidocaine test for tolerance, lidocaine is administered over 30 minutes by continuous infusion with close electrocardiographic and blood pressure monitoring. The infusion is stopped if the patient develops drowsiness or dysarthria or intolerable side effects such as tinnitus, dysphoria, dysrhythmias, or seizures. A reduction in pain during the lidocaine test suggests that mexiletine, the oral analogue of lidocaine, may be useful in longer-term treatment of the patient's pain symptoms (Krane et al. 2003). Mexiletine's most common side effects are nausea, vomiting, sedation, confusion, diplopia, and ataxia. Verapamil has been used to treat migraines and cluster headaches.

Antihypertensive Agent

Clonidine, an α_2-adrenergic agonist, has been used in the treatment of diabetic neuropathy and postherpetic neuralgia. Intrathecal clonidine has also been used to reduce muscle spasms in patients with spinal cord injuries. Clonidine may work both peripherally and centrally by increasing conduction of potassium. Clonidine is generally considered a second-line drug in pain management after antidepressants and anticonvulsants, but it does have some unique advantages, such as its transdermal route of administration. Its sedative effect may also be advantageous. Side effects of clonidine include hypotension and sedation. Abrupt cessation may result in rebound hypertension and nervousness.

Psychostimulants

Psychostimulant medications are believed to have antinociceptive properties that may be mediated by norepinephrine, serotonin, dopamine, or endogenous opioid mechanisms. Indications for psychostimulants include reduction of drowsiness caused by narcotic medications as well as the potential to reduce the dosage of narcotics without diminution of the analgesic effect. Methylphenidate and dextroamphetamine have been found to be safe and effective adjuncts to opiate analgesia and have also been used in the treatment of spasmodic torticollis, spastic colon, and headaches.

Antipsychotic Agents

Antipsychotic agents have been used in the treatment of many chronic pain syndromes, including cancer, arthritis, migraine, neuropathy, and phantom limb pain. The mechanism of action is unknown, but these medications may have a local anesthetic action in spinal nerves. Chlorpromazine and haloperidol have been used to treat nausea associated with the use of opiates or pain. However, ondansetron, a $5\text{-}HT_3$ receptor antagonist, is still the first-line treatment for opioid-induced nausea and vomiting.

Anxiolytic Agents

Benzodiazepines do not have any direct analgesic action but may be useful in treatment of pain by reducing comorbid symptoms of anxiety and insomnia. Benzodiazepines may also decrease pain by reducing muscle spasm. When prescribed at adequate dosages, anxiolytics cause anterograde amnesia, which may be useful as a premedication to alleviate anticipatory anxiety. Short-term use of benzodiazepines can be effective in postoperative pain and sickle cell crises. Hydroxyzine similarly may have an application in the augmentation of opioids in sickle cell crises.

Topical Anesthetics

EMLA, a formulation of lidocaine and prilocaine under an occlusive dressing, has been used to provide anesthesia to a skin depth of 2–4 mm to reduce pain from needle procedures. EMLA needs to be applied 1 hour prior to the procedure to provide anesthesia. Tetracaine applied as gel or cream has a more rapid onset of action than EMLA and causes vasodilatation, which may be an advantage during blood draws. Vapocoolant spray has also been used to reduce the pain from injections. Capsaicin, derived from chili peppers, depletes substance P in small afferent neurons, and it has been used for diabetic neuropathy and postherpetic neuralgia. Capsaicin requires regular and multiple daily applications for a 3- to 4-week period. Its application may be limited by a burning sensation necessitating pretreatment with lidocaine cream.

Cannabis-Based Medicines

There is growing interest in the use of cannabis-based medicines (CBMs) in the management of chronic pain, with estimates of rates of use as high as 12%–15% in pain clinics (Ware et al. 2003). However, although CBMs are considered safe and moderately effective, early studies have shown no benefits compared with codeine. In a meta-analysis of 43 randomized controlled trials of adult patients, Aviram and Samuelly Leichtag (2017) reported moderate to high quality of evidence for the efficacy of CBMs for treatment of patients with chronic pain, in particular those with cancer and neuropathic pain. CBMs appear to have the strongest effects when used by inhalation. CBMs administered orally are more likely to result in gastrointestinal side effects. Nugent et al. (2017), in a separate meta-analysis, reported risks of cognitive side effects, psychotic symptoms, and cannabis use disorder and concluded that evidence-based nonpharmacological and nonopioid therapies are the preferred therapies to treat chronic pain.

References

American Psychiatric Association: Diagnostic and Statistical Manual of Mental Disorders, 5th Edition. Arlington, VA, American Psychiatric Association, 2013

Ansari A: The efficacy of newer antidepressants in the treatment of chronic pain: a review of current literature. Harv Rev Psychiatry 7(5):257–277, 2000 10689591

Aviram J, Samuelly Leichtag G: Efficacy of cannabis-based medicines for pain management: a systematic review and meta-analysis of randomized controlled trials. Pain Physician 20(6):E755–E796, 2017 28934780

Bursch B, Joseph MH, Zeltzer LK: Pain-associated disability syndrome, in Pain in Infants, Children and Adolescents, 2nd Edition. Edited by Schechter NL, Berde CB, Yaster M. Philadelphia, PA, Lippincott Williams & Wilkins, 2003, pp 841–848

Campo JV, Perel J, Lucas A, et al: Citalopram treatment of pediatric recurrent abdominal pain and comorbid internalizing disorders: an exploratory study. J Am Acad Child Adolesc Psychiatry 43(10):1234–1242, 2004 15381890

Carter GT, Sullivan MD: Antidepressants in pain management. Curr Opin Investig Drugs 3(3):454–458, 2002 12054096

Cooper TE, Heathcote LC, Clinch J, et al: Antidepressants for chronic non-cancer pain in children and adolescents. Cochrane Database Syst Rev 8:CD012535, 2017 28779487

Cowen R, Stasiowska MK, Laycock H, Bantel C: Assessing pain objectively: the use of physiological makers. Anesthesia 70(7);828–847, 2015 25772783

Dahlquist LM, Switkin MC: Chronic and recurrent pain, in Handbook of Pediatric Psychology, 3rd Edition. Edited by Roberts MC. New York, Guilford, 2003, pp 198–215

Evans JR, Benore E, Banez GA: The cost-effectiveness of intensive interdisciplinary pediatric chronic pain rehabilitation. J Pediatr Psychol 41(8):849–856, 2016 26514643

Ferrante FM, Ostheimer GW, Covino BG: Patient-Controlled Analgesia. Boston, MA, Blackwell Scientific, 1990

Fritz GK, Campo JV: Somatoform disorders, in Child and Adolescent Psychiatry: A Comprehensive Textbook, 3rd Edition. Edited by Lewis M. Philadelphia, PA, Lippincott Williams & Wilkins, 2002, pp 847–858

Fritz GK, Fritsch S, Hagino O: Somatoform disorders in children and adolescents: a review of the past 10 years. J Am Acad Child Adolesc Psychiatry 36(10):1329–1338, 1997 9334545

Gaffney A, McGrath PJ, Dick B: Measuring pain in children: developmental and instrument issues, in Pain in Infants, Children and Adolescents, 2nd Edition. Edited by Schechter NL, Berde CB, Yaster M. Philadelphia, PA, Lippincott Williams & Wilkins, 2003, pp 128–141

Gallagher HC, Gallagher RM, Butler M, et al: Venlafaxine for neuropathic pain in adults. Cochrane Database Syst Rev (8):CD011091, 2015 26298465

Galloway KS, Yaster M: Pain and symptom control in terminally ill children. Pediatr Clin North Am 47(3):711–746, 2000 10835999

Goldstein DJ, Lu Y, Detke MJ, et al: Effects of duloxetine on painful physical symptoms associated with depression. Psychosomatics 45(1):17–28, 2004 14709757

Gray AM, Spencer PS, Sewell RD: The involvement of the opioidergic system in the antinociceptive mechanism of action of antidepressant compounds. Br J Pharmacol 124(4):669–674, 1998 9690858

Green WH, Kowalik SC: Psychopharmacologic treatment of pain and anxiety in the pediatric patient. Child Adolesc Psychiatr Clin N Am 3:465–483, 1994

Hämäläinen M, Masek BJ: Diagnosis, classification, and medical management of headache in children and adolescents, in Pain in Infants, Children and Adolescents, 2nd Edition. Edited by Schechter NL, Berde CB, Yaster M. Philadelphia, PA, Lippincott Williams & Wilkins, 2003, pp 707–718

Hayes K: Adjuvant treatments, in The Massachusetts General Hospital Handbook of Pain Management, 3rd Edition. Edited by Ballantyne JC. Philadelphia, PA, Lippincott Williams & Wilkins, 2006, pp 127–140

Hesse T, Holmes LA, Kennedy-Overfelt V, et al: Mindfulness-based intervention for adolescents with recurrent headaches: a pilot feasibility study. Evidence-Based Complementary and Alternative Medicine 2015:508958, 10.1155/2015/508958, Epub 2015

Ibeziako PI, DeMaso DR: The somatoform disorders, in Clinical Child Psychiatry, 3rd Edition. Edited by Klykylo WM, Kay JL. Indianapolis, IN, Wiley, 2012, pp 458–474

Kachko L, Ben Ami S, Liberman A, et al: Duloxetine contributing to a successful multimodal treatment program for peripheral femoral neuropathy and comorbid 'reactive depression' in an adolescent. Pain Res Manag 16(6):457–459, 2011 22184557

Kiayias JA, Vlachou ED, Lakka-Papadodima E: Venlafaxine HCl in the treatment of painful peripheral diabetic neuropathy. Diabetes Care 23(5):699, 2000 10834432

King S, Chambers CT, Huguet A, et al: The epidemiology of chronic pain in children and adolescents revisited: a systematic review. Pain 152(12):2729–2738, 2011 22078064

Krane FJ, Leong MS, Golianu B, et al: Treatment of pediatric pain with nonconventional analgesics, in Pain in Infants, Children and Adolescents, 2nd Edition. Edited by Schechter NL, Berde CB, Yaster M. Philadelphia, PA, Lippincott Williams & Wilkins, 2003, pp 225–240

Leo RJ: Evaluation of the pain patient, in Concise Guide to Pain Management for Psychiatrists. Washington, DC, American Psychiatric Publishing, 2003, pp 35–62

Maunuksela E-L, Olkkola KT: Nonsteroidal anti-inflammatory drugs in pediatric pain management, in Pain in Infants, Children and Adolescents, 2nd Edition. Edited by Schechter NL, Berde CB, Yaster M. Philadelphia, PA, Lippincott Williams & Wilkins, 2003, pp 171–180

McCarthy CF, Shea AM, Sullivan P: Physical therapy management of pain in children, in Pain in Infants, Children and Adolescents, 2nd Edition. Edited by Schechter NL, Berde CB, Yaster M. Philadelphia, PA, Lippincott Williams & Wilkins, 2003, pp 434–448

McGrath PJ, Dick B, Unruh AM: Psychologic and behavioral treatment of pain in children and adolescents, in Pain in Infants, Children and Adolescents, 2nd Edition. Edited by Schechter NL, Berde CB, Yaster M. Philadelphia, PA, Lippincott Williams & Wilkins, 2003, pp 303–316

Merskey H, Bogduk N (eds): Classification of Chronic Pain: Descriptions of Chronic Pain Syndromes and Definitions of Pain Terms, 2nd Edition. Seattle, WA, IASP Press, 1994, pp 209–214

Miller MM, Meints SM, Hirsh AT: Catastrophizing, pain, and functional outcomes for children with chronic pain: a meta-analytic review. Pain 159(12):2442–2460, 2018 30015710

Nugent SM, Morasco BJ, O'Neil ME, et al: The effects of cannabis among adults with chronic pain and an overview of general harms: a systematic review. Ann Intern Med 167(5):319–331, 2017 28806817

Plunkett A, Beattie RM: Recurrent abdominal pain in childhood. J R Soc Med 98(3):101–106, 2005 15738551

Rogovik AL, Goldman RD: Hypnosis for treatment of pain in children. Can Fam Physician 53(5):823–825, 2007 17872743

Ruskin DA, Gagnon MM, Kohut SA, et al: A mindfulness program adapted for adolescents with chronic pain: feasibility, acceptability, and initial outcomes. Clin J Pain 33(11):1019–1029, 2017 28328699

Schechter NL: The development of pain perception and principles of pain control, in Child and Adolescent Psychiatry: A Comprehensive Textbook, 3rd Edition. Edited by Lewis M. Philadelphia, PA, Lippincott Williams & Wilkins, 2002, pp 404–413

Sieberg CB, Manganella J: Family beliefs and interventions in pediatric pain management. Child Adolesc Psychiatr Clin North Am 24(3):631–645, 2015 26092744

Tran ST, Jastrowski Mano KE, Hainsworth KR, et al: Distinct influences of anxiety and pain catastrophizing on functional outcomes in children and adolescents with chronic pain. J Pediatr Psychol 40(8):744–755, 2015 25840447

Ware MA, Doyle CR, Woods R, et al: Cannabis use for chronic non-cancer pain: results of a prospective survey. Pain 102(1–2):211–216, 2003 12620613

Wong DL, Hockenberry-Eaton M, Wilson D, et al: Wong's Essentials of Pediatric Nursing, 6th Edition. St. Louis, MO, Mosby, 2001

Yaster M, Kost-Byerly S, Maxwell LG: Opioid agonists and antagonists, in Pain in Infants, Children and Adolescents, 2nd Edition. Edited by Schechter NL, Berde CB, Yaster M. Philadelphia, PA, Lippincott Williams & Wilkins, 2003, pp 181–224

11

Fabricated or Induced Illness Symptoms

Factitious disorder was placed among the DSM-5 somatic symptom and related disorders because somatic symptoms predominate and are most often
encountered in medical settings (American Psychiatric Association 2013).
Factitious disorder imposed on self (FDIOS) generally occurs in early adulthood
in the context of falsified or induced physical/psychological symptoms that
are evident even in the absence of obvious external rewards (Yates and Feldman 2016). By contrast, *factitious disorder imposed on another* (FDIOA), the
focus of this chapter, poses a rare but challenging problem in the pediatric setting that requires careful vigilance on the part of consultants.

Background and Diagnostic Criteria

The term *Munchausen by proxy* (MBP) was first used in 1977 to describe an
extreme form of child abuse in which children were unnecessarily treated for
pediatric conditions that were falsified by their caregivers (Meadow 2002). A
long-cited review described MBP as 1) illness in a child that is simulated or

305

produced by a parent or someone acting *in loco parentis*; 2) presentation of the child for medical assessment and care, usually persistently, often resulting in multiple medical procedures; 3) denial of knowledge by the perpetrator as to the etiology of the child's illness; and 4) abatement of the child's acute symptoms and signs when the child is separated from the perpetrator (Rosenberg 1987). Two types of perpetrators of MBP were noted: 1) active inducers (i.e., those who actively induced symptoms of illness in their children) and 2) doctor addicts (i.e., those who actively focused on obtaining medical treatment for nonexistent illnesses and had a pattern of false reporting of history and symptoms) (Libow and Schreier 1986).

Some years later, the diagnosis of factitious disorder by proxy emerged in DSM-IV-TR to replace MBP, and then this diagnosis was subsequently changed in DSM-5 to factitious disorder imposed on another (American Psychiatric Association 2000, 2013). FDIOA is considered a variant of child maltreatment called "medical child abuse," in which children receive unnecessary and harmful or potentially harmful medical care from their caretaker (Yates and Bass 2017). FDIOA is rare disorder, with an annual incidence that ranges from 0.4 to 2.0 per 100,000 (Denny et al. 2001; McClure et al. 1996). Nonetheless, it is a troubling disorder, one that causes children to face significant potentially disabling morbidities along with mortality rates ranging from 6% to 7.6% (Sheridan 2003; Yates and Bass 2017).

The DSM-5 diagnosis of FDIOA requires the following criteria to be met: 1) the individual carries out falsification of physical or psychological symptoms, or induction of injury or disease, in another, associated with identified deception; 2) the individual presents another individual (victim) to others as ill, impaired, or injured; 3) the deceptive behavior is evident even in the absence of obvious external awards; and 4) the behavior is not better explained by another mental disorder, such as delusional disorder or another psychotic disorder (American Psychiatric Association 2013). The perpetrator, not the victim, receives the diagnosis, with the victim generally given an abuse diagnosis.

Clinical Features

Victim Characteristics

Girls and boys appear to be equally victimized, with the majority of children being 5 years or younger, although the age range does extend into adolescence.

The time between symptom/sign onset and diagnosis ranges from 7 to 15 months (Denny et al. 2001). Older children are more likely to collude with their parents regarding the presentation, and over time it is not unusual for victims to develop their own independent symptoms consistent with FDIOS.

The clinical presentation of victims covers a wide spectrum of physical illnesses that involve most pediatric specialties (Table 11–1). In a meta-analysis of 451 FDIOA cases, multiple symptoms were found in at least three organ systems and as many as seven different systems (Sheridan 2003). Methods of falsification can include symptom exaggeration and distortion as well as false reporting and inducement of symptoms. Alteration of laboratory specimens may take multiple forms, including simulated bloody diarrhea, hypoglycemia, and infection. Falsification of medical records, interference with intravenous lines, poisoning, overmedicating, suffocation, and starvation have all been reported (Bass and Glaser 2014). In one study, 23% of children had gastrointestinal symptoms (i.e., vomiting, failure to thrive, reflux, esophagitis, diarrhea, pseudo-obstruction, abdominal pain), 30% had recurrent seizures, 20% had repeated episodes of apnea, 13% had abnormal serum insulin levels, and 10% had been diagnosed with rare autoimmune or genetic disorders (Ayoub 2006). In this same study, children also presented with feigned bleeding difficulties and poisoning.

Besides facing the consequences of unnecessary and potentially harmful pediatric procedures and surgery, victims can suffer long-lasting psychological trauma adversely impacting attachment, self-esteem, and interpersonal relationships (Ayoub 2010). Interrupted school performance with lower levels of academic achievement, decreased participation in athletic activities, social isolation, and assumption of a sick role are common, as are high rates of oppositionality, inattention, lying, and problematic social relationships (Bass and Glaser 2014). Victims are at higher risk as adolescents to develop FDIOS. In addition to the significant mortality rates noted earlier, the rates of sibling illness and sibling death are both elevated, at 61% and 25%, respectively (Sheridan 2003).

Perpetrator Characteristics

A systematic review of 796 cases found that over 95% of perpetrators were female and the victim's mother (Yates and Bass 2017). The majority were married (75.8%), with a mean age at the child's presentation of 27.6 years, and

Table 11–1. Examples of falsified or induced physical signs/ symptoms potentially found in factitious disorder imposed on another (FDIOA)

Respiratory manifestations	Apnea
	Nonaccidental suffocation
	Asthma
	Bronchopulmonary dysplasia
	Cystic fibrosis
	Chest pain
Gastrointestinal manifestations	Vomiting
	Abdominal pain
	Bleeding
	Chronic diarrhea
	Failure to thrive
Infectious manifestations	Fever
Neurological manifestations	Seizures
	Loss of consciousness
Hematological manifestations	Anemia
	Bleeding
Dermatologic manifestations	Erythema
	Vesiculations
	Lacerations
	Skin pigmentation
	Puncture wounds
Renal manifestations	Hematuria
	Proteinuria
	Urinary tract infection

Table 11–1. Examples of falsified or induced physical signs/ symptoms potentially found in factitious disorder imposed on another (FDIOA) *(continued)*

Renal manifestations *(continued)*	Renal calculi
	Renal failure
Ophthalmic manifestations	Hemorrhagic conjunctivitis
	Keratitis
	Nystagmus
	Periorbital cellulitis
Allergic manifestations	Rash
	Food allergy

45.6% were in a healthcare-related profession. Over half of the perpetrators exhibited pathological lying that often started in adolescence and emerged at times of increased life stress (Yates and Bass 2017). They were often perceived as knowledgeable and caring, with a familiarity about the medical system, and seemed to enjoy the relationship with their child's pediatric care providers. Many had their own history of exaggerated or fabricated physical or emotional illnesses, including factitious and somatic symptom disorders, along with higher rates of obstetric complications (Bools et al. 1993; Yates and Bass 2017). High rates of psychiatric treatment, diagnoses of depression or person-ality disorder, and higher rates of substance abuse have been reported (Ayoub 2010). Psychological evaluations have found high rates of narcissistic and an-tisocial personality disorders as well as an increased risk of childhood physical and sexual abuse histories, early family disruption and loss, and other unresolved psychological trauma histories (Yates and Bass 2017).

Fewer than 7% of perpetrators of FDIOA were found to be the father (Sheridan 2003). Male partners of perpetrators tend to be minimally involved in their children's care, although some have been noted to be demanding and overbearing. The marital relationship is generally poor and in some cases ap-pears to be based on a mutual involvement in the child's illness. The fathers tend to support and collude with their wives even in the face of clear evidence of medical child abuse. In families where fathers are estranged or separated, fathers tend to be marginalized and uninvolved with their children, although they are more open to acknowledging the role of the mother in their child's victimization.

Etiology

Most theories regarding the etiology of FDIOA focus on the psychopathology of the perpetrator. It is hypothesized that the perpetrator is motivated by the need for attention or recognition, particularly from health care providers, and/or has a need to covertly deceive authority figures. Psychodynamic theories postulate a history of early trauma or loss in the perpetrator, usually related to maternal rejection. Many perpetrators seem to crave and thrive on the relationship with their child's doctors, which is characterized as being intense and often lacking the usual professional-parent boundaries (Ayoub and Alexander 1998). There is some evidence supporting the intergenerational transmission of abnormal illness behavior in mothers who perpetrate FDIOA (Bass and Glaser 2014). Disorders of attachment have also been postulated to explain factitious illness, with higher rates of insecure attachment in the perpetrator (Bass and Glaser 2014).

Differential Diagnosis

Parental Behavior

There is a spectrum of parental behavior that can occur in the context of a child presenting with apparent factitious symptoms that extends from overanxious parenting on the one end to FDIOA on the other (Table 11–2). Understanding these behaviors and the underlying motivations are important in determining the presence of FDIOA. For example, the term *hypochondriasis by proxy* has been used to describe less severe instances in which parental anxiety results in an exaggerated perception of the child as being ill (Roth 1990). These parents may make repeated requests for pediatric evaluations and create difficulties for the health care providers with their failure to be reassured by negative findings. However, this is thought to be a different situation from parents who engage in the characteristic behaviors associated with FDIOA, in which the motive is more that of serving their own psychological needs. It is also impor-

Table 11–2. Parental behaviors and motivations in the context of apparent fabricated or induced illness symptoms

Category of parental behavior	Motivation of parent
Help seeking—needs assistance	Parent who is overwhelmed and seeks out medical care to gain additional physical and logistical support
Severe anxiety (hypochondriasis by proxy)	Parent with an exaggerated perception of his or her child's ill health based on extreme anxiety
Delusional	Parent with psychotic illness whose delusions include the belief that his or her child is ill
Overanxious	Parent with an exaggerated perception of his or her child's ill health based on extreme anxiety
Neglect/failure to thrive/abuse	Parent who is unable to cope or feed; parent who directly harms child
False allegations	Parent who makes false allegations of abuse for the primary purpose of obtaining custody or of harming his or her spouse
Keeping child dependent and at home	Parents who keep their children home unnecessarily for minor physical illness with the goal of serving their own dependency needs
Factitious disorder imposed on another	Parent who intentionally falsifies the child's history and symptoms and/or directly induces physical illness

tant to differentiate behavior by parents who keep their child home for minor physical complaints as a result of their own dependency needs (Ayoub and Alexander 1998).

Malingering

Malingering has been described as intentional "pretending" to be sick that is motivated by external incentives like avoiding work, school, or other negative situations or for financial gain. The discrepancy between claimed distress or disability and the medical findings, as well as the motivation, is often obvious. In the pediatric setting, this difficulty is generally seen in adolescents as opposed to the much younger children being victimized by FDIOA. There may be adolescents who have experienced FDIOA and who now present with FDIOS. These adolescents may also have an element of malingering in their avoidance of tasks or events they see as negative or threatening, particularly if their behaviors are reinforced by their parents.

Factitious Disorder Imposed on Self

The essential feature of FDIOS is the falsification of medical or psychological signs and symptoms in oneself that is associated with identified deception (American Psychiatric Association 2013). In contrast to malingering, there is no obvious reward in the deception. FDIOS is more likely to present in adolescents who were victims of FDIOA when they were younger or in those who have had parents who have modeled physical illness and/or encouraged their illness falsification.

Somatic Symptom Disorder

Somatic symptom disorder describes a pattern of multiple, recurring, clinically significant somatic complaints associated with disproportionate and persistent thoughts about the seriousness of the symptoms (see Chapter 9, "Somatic Symptom and Related Disorders"). The distinction between somatic symptom disorder and FDIOS/FDIOA is based on the degree of volitional choice and consequences that occur in the latter (Bass and Glaser 2014).

Assessment

The diagnosis of FDIOA is challenging and often overlooked in the pediatric setting because the working assumption is that "parents want the best for their children." In this context, intentional deception on the part of a parent is not a common consideration. Alternatively, faced with the inability to establish a satisfactory medical expansion for a patient's symptoms, a frustrated pediatric team may be led to a premature FDIOA diagnosis. Such confusion is particularly likely to occur with conditions in which "gold standard" diagnostic tests are not available, such as Lyme disease and mitochondrial disease.

A thorough and careful multidisciplinary assessment should be conducted when FDIOA is suspected (Table 11–3). As the majority of these assessments occur in the inpatient hospital setting, steps must be taken to ensure the safety of the child, including one-to-one nursing and/or exclusion of the parents if there are concerns about medical child abuse. This can be complicated when the diagnosis is not yet established, given the risk of parents requesting a premature medical discharge. In these cases, it is important to quickly involve the relevant child protective services (CPS) agency such that, if necessary, it can move to temporarily remove custody from the parents (see Chapter 4, "Legal and Forensic Issues").

Although visitation may be helpful for the child for psychological reasons, care must be taken to closely supervise the contact between the child and parents, since there is potential for the child to be revictimized in the context of these visits, even within the structure of the hospital setting. Some experts have gone so far as to recommend that no contact occur until a forensic evaluation has been completed and a treatment plan is in place and progress on the part of the parent has been demonstrated (Lasher and Sheridan 2004).

Authenticity of the Medical History

It is the obligation of the pediatric team to establish the diagnosis of FDIOA (see Table 11–4). This requires a thorough review of all past medical records, including discussion of the case with current and past pediatric providers and the primary care physician, to determine whether there are inconsistencies in the child's presentation or prior suspicions of FDIOA. Relevant school and legal records should be reviewed. Sibling records should also be evaluated, since falsification of illness in siblings is often seen in FDIOA. Given the risk of false allegations of FDIOA, it is critical for the pediatric team to ensure a meticulous medical diagnostic evaluation to determine whether there is underlying physical illness accounting for the symptoms. This does not rule out the possibility of amplification or overreporting of symptoms of genuine illness. Illness fabrication is generally proven by circumstantial rather than direct evidence— for example, information from different sources may reveal discrepancies in the medical history (patterns of exaggeration or fabrication of medical symptoms or symptoms that are inconsistent with the expected presentation of a given illness or disorder) or the overreporting of symptoms to different pediatric providers.

Table 11–3. Multidisciplinary team members with role in assessment of factitious disorder imposed on another

Team member	Role
Physician	Pediatric evaluation of child
	Review of current and past medical records
	Coordination of medical treatment
Nurse	Direct observation of interactions between parent and child
Social worker	Liaison between family and medical team
	Liaison with child protective services agencies
	Coordination of outpatient services
Consultant (psychiatrist/ psychologist)	Psychiatric evaluation of parents
	Psychiatric evaluation of the child
	Psychological support to parents and child
	Consultation to the medical team
Child protection consult team	Consultation on child medical abuse from neglect/abuse experts regarding reporting requirements for and management of medical child abuse
Legal consult/risk management	Consultation on legal issues including data collection, parental rights, reporting requirements, and hospital policies
Ethics consult, where indicated	Consultation on issues related to parental and patient rights
Community agencies	**Role**
Child protective services	Medical child abuse investigation
	Custody and placement of the child
Law enforcement, where indicated	Criminal prosecution of the parents

Table 11–4. Components of the assessment of factitious disorder imposed on another

History	Review of all past available medical records
	Consultation with current and past medical providers
	Establish authenticity of reported personal and family history
	Review past medical history of siblings and parents with primary care physicians
Examination	Pediatric evaluation of the child
	Psychiatric evaluation of the child
	Psychiatric evaluation of the parent(s)
Observation	One-to-one nursing observation
	Observation of discrepancies between parent report of symptoms and actual behavior
	Observation of changes in symptoms and behaviors coinciding with visits by parents
Investigation	Meticulous pediatric diagnostic evaluation
	Verification of source of all laboratory specimens
	Toxicology screening
	Collection of physiological data including vital signs, oxygen saturation, and video EEG monitoring
	Covert video surveillance where indicated and available
Management	Documentation of baseline symptoms and behaviors
	Discontinuation of unnecessary medications
	Evaluation and treatment of any new medical symptoms
	Potential exclusion of parents based on consultation with child protective services agencies
	Regular multidisciplinary meetings including child protective services agencies where indicated

Table 11–4.   Components of the assessment of factitious disorder imposed on another *(continued)*

Management *(continued)*	Medical rehabilitation treatment with involvement of physical therapy and occupational therapy where indicated
	Liaison and collaboration with family members when possible
	Informing conference with parents

Involvement of Child Protective Services Agencies

CPS agencies should be involved early in cases of suspected FDIOA to assist with issues related to custody, placement, and long-term treatment plans. It may be necessary to educate the child protective service caseworkers if they do not have the necessary knowledge of and experience with this condition. These agencies are also responsible for authorizing the exchange of medical information when the child has been placed in protective custody. Any inconsistencies in the medical history should be reported to CPS agencies to assist in their evaluation, which will include interviews with extended family members, teachers, and other childcare providers.

Psychiatric Evaluation of the Parent

The consultant's psychiatric evaluation of the parent aims to develop a biopsychosocial formulation and establish the presence or absence of psychiatric disorders in order to inform the pediatric team's overall understanding of the clinical presentation. Consultants should be alert to assessing the potential for psychosis or suicidality to emerge when the parent is confronted about the diagnosis. It is important to disclose the limits of confidentiality in this evaluation and to obtain consent from the parent.

While the aforementioned characteristics of FDIOA perpetrators have been described, it is important for consultants to keep in mind that there is no established specific diagnostic profile. As previously mentioned, these parents are often found to fabricate other details of their personal history, appear to enjoy contact with pediatric providers, and may have their own independent histories of FDIOA or FDIOS. In cases of established FDIOA, consultants can help assess the level of a parent's ability and willingness to acknowledge her or his behavior and her or his ability to participate in future treatment aimed at family reunification.

Psychiatric Evaluation of the Child

The consultant's psychiatric evaluation of the child also aims to develop a biopsychosocial formulation and establish the presence or absence of psychiatric disorders. Consultants should particularly be attuned to developmental appropriateness of the relationship between the parent and child, which is commonly problematic. FDIOA victims often have preexisting psychological issues that entail difficulties with attachment and separation, including a highly involved and protective relationship with the perpetrator. Consent to conduct an evaluation should be given by the parent or the CPS agency in cases where the child has been taken into temporary custody. Establishing a therapeutic relationship with the child early in the course of the multidisciplinary evaluation can be helpful because there is often significant disabling distress for the child should the allegations of FDIOA be confirmed and the child temporarily removed from the parent's custody.

Legal Issues

Informing Meeting

When strong consensus has been reached about a diagnosis of FDIOA, it is necessary for the family to be notified about the conclusions in a process referred to as confronting the perpetrator (Bools et al. 1993). An informing conference, led by the primary physician, is convened in which the medical data supporting the diagnosis are presented to the parent(s). This meeting is commonly followed by an involuntary transfer of custody, with the child either remaining in the hospital or being placed in a foster care home (see Chapter 4, "Legal and Forensic Issues"). If there are concerns about the patient's safety and/or the reactions of the parents, arrangements can be made prior to the meeting to ensure that CPS workers and/or law enforcement officers are available.

During this time, consultants should offer mental health support to both the child and the parent(s). In cases in which the parent acknowledges the abuse and is willing to engage in treatment, family reunification may prove to be an option. However, it is far more common for the initial response of the parents to be the denial of the allegations. Placement of the child with other family relatives is not recommended. All decisions regarding custody and placement are made by the CPS agency, with the pediatric team providers involved in the case generally being required to provide expert testimony and recommendations regarding medical and psychiatric treatment.

Covert Video Surveillance

Although controversial, the use of covert video surveillance in the inpatient setting has been used to help with the diagnosis of FDIOA and as evidence in criminal prosecution proceedings (Foreman 2005). Covert video surveillance has been used both to establish and to refute FDIOA. It is important to have standard protocols to ensure the safety of the child from possible harmful behaviors perpetrated by the parents during covert video surveillance as well as a system to inform the parents about the surveillance (Galvin et al. 2005).

False Allegations

There have been a number of high-profile acquittals of parents incarcerated on charges of FDIOA (Dyer 2004). This is more likely to occur in children with co-occurring complex pediatric conditions (Petska et al. 2017). These children often have neurological impairment and functional limitations such that their care and treatment require the involvement of multiple specialists and complicated treatment regimens. There are several advocacy groups that have been organized in response to false allegations. These issues deserve serious consideration given the potential risks to the child of unnecessary or traumatic separation from their parent, as well as the premature ending of medical treatment or diagnostic investigation to establish a medical etiology. False allegations can lead to potential liability in medical malpractice claims against the hospital and medical providers.

Amid concern about liability, consultants should remember that the mandatory child abuse reporting requirements state that mandated reporters shall not be liable in any civil or criminal actions for filing a report as long as the filing was made in good faith and was not frivolous. It is also important to keep in mind that hospitals have been sued on behalf of victims of FDIOA for failing to uncover the abuse in a timely manner and thereby exposing the victims to unnecessary investigations or treatment.

Treatment

On the basis of three principles (i.e., acknowledgment of the perpetration, psychiatric stability, and treatment of substance abuse), a three-phase treatment for families with FDIOA has been described (Ayoub 2006, 2010). In the first phase, treatment is focused on exploring the victimization of the parents and its relationship to parental attitudes and actions toward their children. The goal is to reduce isolation and diminish cognitive distortions in parents as well as explore how the marital relationship may have contributed to and perpetuated the child's abuse. In the second phase, treatment focuses on reworking the relationship of the child with the family and a redefinition of the child's identity from that of being ill to one of embracing wellness. This includes communication between the parent(s) and the child about the medical child abuse. In the final phase, the goal is stabilization and normalization of healthy relationships over time, increased contact between the parent and child, and increased responsibility in caretaking roles, with supervision.

Treatment of the Parents

Treatment of parents who perpetrate FDIOA is complicated, especially when there is denial of the abuse and continued deception. However, psychiatric treatment should be offered to the parents and may be court ordered if there is a future plan for family reunification. However, it is important to take note of the high rates of recidivism even following confrontation about the abuse and subsequent psychiatric treatment (Bools et al. 1993). Treatment for fathers is a central component to the success of intervention with mothers, especially if the couple is intact. Fathers who continue to support the denial of FDIOA significantly reduce the odds for successful treatment in mothers (Ayoub 2010). Fathers should be encouraged to take on an active role in the family, particularly if they have previously abdicated this role. Many of these fathers will need education and training in basic parenting skills. Comorbid psychiatric issues in the fathers—for example, substance abuse or domestic violence—are important to address if present.

Treatment of the Child

Psychotherapy should be provided to child victims of FDIOA. Goals include developing safety and social skills, reducing self-blame, embracing wellness, developing autonomy, understanding and managing family conflicts and loyalties, and reframing peer relationships (Ayoub 2010). Common issues are denial of illness falsification, anger directed toward the medical team, collusive family members, continued adoption of the sick role, and posttraumatic stress symptoms. Psychopharmacological interventions should be used as indicated by the presence of a specific psychiatric disorder and its indicated psychotropic medications.

Unfortunately, the prognosis is often poor. Many victims of FDIOA have long-term mental health issues, including FDIOS, conversion disorder, and posttraumatic stress disorder. Predictors associated with poor psychiatric outcome include victimization that lasted more than 2 years, delayed permanent placement, unsupervised contact with their mothers, contact with mothers who had received insufficient treatment, and contact with fathers who are unable to care for them because of dependency on mothers (Ayoub 2010). Complications of FDIOA include chronic complications of unnecessary medical investigations and treatment, permanent disfigurement, academic delays due to absenteeism, delays in social development due to a lack of opportunities to engage with peers, problems with low self-esteem, and higher rates of mortality (Shaw et al. 2008).

Family Reunification

Family reunification should be attempted only if there is a strong expectation of success, which requires some acknowledgment by the parents about their behavior (Ayoub 2010). When attempted, reunification should start first with very closely monitored parental visitation, and the high risk of subsequent abuse should be kept in mind. Family therapy should be offered as part of the reunification process, with limited research showing success (Sanders 1996). Generally, predictors associated with poor outcome in family reunification include parental history of severe childhood abuse, persistent denial of abusive behavior, refusal to accept help, severe personality disorder, mental handicap, and alcohol/drug abuse (Ayoub 2010). The persistence of denial of FDIOA by the parent perpetrator in the face of a finding by the court is justification for denial of contact and placement. If denial continues, then termination of parental rights with fathers as well as mothers is generally recommended (Ayoub 2010).

References

American Psychiatric Association: Diagnostic and Statistical Manual of Mental Disorders, 4th Edition, Text Revision. Washington, DC, American Psychiatric Association, 2000

American Psychiatric Association: Diagnostic and Statistical Manual of Mental Disorders, 5th Edition. Arlington, VA, American Psychiatric Association, 2013

Ayoub C: Munchausen by proxy, in Mental Disorders for the New Millennium, Vol 3: Biology and Function. Edited by Plante TG. Westport, CT, Praeger Press, 2006, pp 173–193

Ayoub CC: Munchausen by proxy, in Textbook of Pediatric Psychosomatic Medicine. Edited by Shaw RJ, DeMaso DR. Washington, DC, American Psychiatric Publishing, 2010, pp 185–198

Ayoub CC, Alexander R: Definitional issues in Munchausen by proxy. AM Prof Soc Abuse Child Advis 11:7–10, 1998

Bass C, Glaser D: Early recognition and management of fabricated or induced illness in children. Lancet 383(9926):1412–1421, 2014 24612863

Bools CN, Neale BA, Meadow SR: Follow up of victims of fabricated illness (Munchausen syndrome by proxy). Arch Dis Child 69(6):625–630, 1993 8285772

Denny SJ, Grant CC, Pinnock R: Epidemiology of Munchausen syndrome by proxy in New Zealand. J Paediatr Child Health 37(3):240–243, 2001 11468037

Dyer C: Review of child care cases finds few instances that raise "serious doubt." BMJ 329(7477):1256, 2004 15564241

Foreman DM: Detecting fabricated or induced illness in children. BMJ 331(7523): 978–979, 2005 16254277

Galvin HK, Newton AW, Vandeven AM: Update on Munchausen syndrome by proxy. Curr Opin Pediatr 17(2):252–257, 2005 15800422

Lasher L, Sheridan M: Munchausen by Proxy: Identification, Intervention and Case Management. New York, The Haworth Press, 2004

Libow JA, Schreier HA: Three forms of factitious illness in children: when is it Munchausen syndrome by proxy? Am J Orthopsychiatry 56(4):602–611, 1986 3789106

McClure RJ, Davis PM, Meadow SR, Sibert JR: Epidemiology of Munchausen syndrome by proxy, non-accidental poisoning, and non-accidental suffocation. Arch Dis Child 75(1):57–61, 1996 8813872

Meadow R: Different interpretations of Munchausen syndrome by proxy. Child Abuse Negl 26(5):501–508, 2002 12079086

Petska HW, Gordon JB, Jablonski D, Sheets LK: The intersection of medical child abuse and medical complexity. Pediatr Clin North Am 64(1):253–264, 2017 27894448

Rosenberg DA: Web of deceit: a literature review of Munchausen syndrome by proxy. Child Abuse Negl 11(4):547–563, 1987 3322516

Roth D: How "mild" is mild Munchausen syndrome by proxy? Isr J Psychiatry Relat Sci 27(3):160–167, 1990 2265997

Sanders M: Narrative family therapy with Munchausen by proxy: a successful treatment case. Fam Syst Health 14:315–329, 1996

Shaw RJ, Dayal S, Hartman JK, DeMaso DR: Factitious disorder by proxy: pediatric condition falsification. Harv Rev Psychiatry 16(4):215–224, 2008 18661364

Sheridan MS: The deceit continues: an updated literature review of Munchausen Syndrome by Proxy. Child Abuse Negl 27(4):431–451, 2003 12686328

Yates G, Bass C: The perpetrators of medical child abuse (Munchausen Syndrome by Proxy)—a systematic review of 796 cases. Child Abuse Negl 72:45–53, 2017 28750264

Yates GP, Feldman MD: Factitious disorder: a systematic review of 455 cases in the professional literature. Gen Hosp Psychiatry 41:20–28, 2016 27302720

12

Solid Organ Transplantation

Solid organ transplantation has evolved from the first successful kidney transplant more than 60 years ago to become an established part of pediatric care, as evidenced in today's common use of kidney, liver, heart, lung, pancreas, intestine, and vascular composite allograph transplants. Significant improvements in surgical techniques and advances in immunosuppressive medication regimens have led to vastly improved outcomes and long-term survival.

The shortage of organ donors to meet the nation's demand for organs, along with the increased attention to total medical expenditures associated with these high-risk interventions, has led to heightened scrutiny of the suitability of candidates in need of transplantation (Cousino et al. 2018; Schnitzler et al. 2018; Thomson et al. 2018). Understanding posttransplant nonadherence is of great importance because the failure to follow lifelong immunosuppressive agent regimens results in organ rejection and loss of life.

In this context, psychiatric consultants are increasingly being embedded within transplant hospital programs to create integrated behavioral health care partnerships that provide direct clinical service to patients, consultation and mental health education to transplant care teams, and care coordination when indicated (Samsel et al. 2017). In these partnerships, consultants participate in the screening assessment of potential transplant recipients as well as assessment of posttransplant adjustment and health-related quality of life. In doing so, consultants are well positioned to respond to concerns from the patient, family, and transplant care team regarding informed consent, ethical dilemmas, developmental considerations, adherence, psychiatric comorbidity, pain management, and procedural anxiety.

Overview of Solid Organ Transplantation

Established in 1984 under the U.S. Department of Health and Human Services, the United Network for Organ Sharing (UNOS) is the private nonprofit organization that manages the nation's organ transplant system (see https://unos.org). UNOS operates the national Organ Procurement and Transplantation Network (OPTN), which is responsible for the fair and equitable allocation and distribution of organs on the basis of specific criteria that include organ type, tissue match, blood type, length of time on the waiting list, geographic location, and immune status (see https://optn.transplant.hrsa.gov). Every transplant hospital program, organ procurement organization, and transplant histocompatibility laboratory in the United States is an OPTN member, as are voluntary health organizations, such as the National Kidney Foundation; general public members, such as ethicists and donor family members; and medical professional or scientific organizations, such as the American Society for Transplantation.

With nearly 115,000 patients of all ages currently waiting for a transplant, the greatest limiting factor in organ transplantation remains the significant shortage of donated organs. In 2018, 1,955 patients ≤18 years of age were waiting for an organ and 1,899 received lifesaving solid organ transplants (https://unos.org/data/transplant-trends/#waitlists_by_age). Although the waiting times for children and adolescents were less than the waiting times for adults, in 2011–2014, children and adolescents did have significant median waiting times for transplantation, from a low of 72 days for as an adolescent waiting for a heart to a high of 936 days for a preschooler waiting for a kidney, with an overall median wait for any organ of just over 1 year.

On the basis of 2008–2015 data, kidney (>96%) transplants had the highest 5-year survival rates, followed by liver (85%–93%) and heart (80%–89%) transplants, then intestinal (64%–82%) and lung (49%–75%) transplants, which had the lowest 5-year survival rates (Table 12–1).

Table 12–1.   Survival rates for solid organ transplants performed: 2008–2015

Organ	Child age (years)	1-year survival (%)	3-year survival (%)	5-year survival (%)
Kidney	1–5	98.3	97.1	96.0
	6–10	99.5	99.1	99.1
	11–17	99.8	98.8	96.9
Heart	1–5	92.4	87.1	81.4
	6–10	92.3	89.7	89.3
	11–17	96.8	92.3	80.0
Liver	1–5	94.3	89.3	85.4
	6–10	96.3	93.5	93.5
	11–17	95.2	92.6	86.6
Lung	1–5	73.7	67.2	NC[1]
	6–10	89.3	84.1	74.7
	11–17	86.2	62.3	48.6
Intestine	1–5	87.3	72.2	63.7
	6–10	93.5	85.0	82.3
	11–17	82.6	73.9	65.0

[1]Graft survival not computed because $N < 10$.

Source.   Organ Procurement and Transplantation Network, https://optn.transplant.hrsa.gov/data/view-data-reports/national-data.

Pretransplant Psychiatric Assessment

Pretransplant assessments are used to identify psychiatric issues that need to be addressed before and after transplantation (Table 12–2). They serve an important role in enhancing patient care by helping maximize the transplant care team's understanding of patients' strengths and vulnerabilities as well as through identification of any problematic psychopathology that may be associated with subsequent problematic posttransplant adjustment and/or treatment nonadherence. Although there are no absolute psychiatric contraindications in pediatric transplantation, it is important for consultants to identify candidates with active alcohol or substance use, severe psychopathology, patterns of poor medical adherence, other problematic health care behaviors, and/or very poor social support (Cahn-Fuller and Parent 2017). These findings require careful review and discussion with the entire transplant care team with regard to suitability, feasibility, and timing of transplantation.

Adjusting to life after pediatric transplantation can be challenging. Important factors in need of consideration include transitioning from hospital to home, returning to physical activity, improving feeding and nutrition, reentering school, managing potential cognitive deficits, and enhancing health-related quality of life (Brosig et al. 2014). Measures of parent and family functioning have been associated with important health-related factors, such as treatment adherence, readiness for discharge, and number of hospitalizations (Cousino et al. 2017). In light of this, it is helpful for consultants to identify factors that have the potential to interfere with a family's ability to provide adequate emotional and social support. This is particularly relevant in younger transplant recipients, for whom the burden of the pediatric care falls most heavily on the family.

Beginning the Pretransplant Assessment

Clarify Assessment Expectations

The transplant care team should clearly explain to the patient and family that the pretransplant psychiatric assessment is an important component of determining suitability for transplantation. It can be explained to the patient and family that the team is concerned about both the physical and the psychosocial health of the patient and that both are critical to successful transplantation. As part of this, it is helpful for the transplant physician(s) to state explicitly that the psychiatric consultant is a member of the transplant care team and that information from the assessment will be shared with the team. It should also be clarified with the patient and family that the ultimate decision-making responsibility regarding transplantation lies with the entire transplant care team and not with the consultant alone.

Table 12–2. Pediatric pretransplant psychiatric assessment

Understanding of illness and expectations of transplant

- Understanding of illness

- Understanding of surgery process

- Understanding of posttransplant treatment expectations

- Cognitive issues affecting comprehension of illness and treatment (cognitive impairment, intellectual disability, stage of cognitive development)

- Motivation for transplant

- Anxieties about transplant surgery

- Attitude toward transplant donor

- Attitude toward having a transplanted organ (e.g., gender/ethnicity of the donor)

- Anxiety about posttransplant treatment

- Posttransplant goals

Previous hospital experiences

- Prior history of traumatic medical experiences

- Prior history of procedural anxiety

- Prior history of difficulties with pain management

- Coping styles during stressful procedures

Treatment adherence

- Past history of treatment adherence (e.g., medications, appointments, laboratory tests, diet, exercise)

- Family support for treatment

- Family availability to provide supervision of treatment

- Presence of family conflict or disagreement affecting treatment

Relationship with medical providers

- Relationship of family with medical providers (e.g., trust, confidence, anger, feeling of entitlement)

- Previous experiences with medical providers

Table 12–2. Pediatric pretransplant psychiatric assessment *(continued)*

Family issues

- Family psychiatric illness
- Family history of alcohol or substance use
- Marital conflict
- History of domestic violence
- Involvement with child protective service agencies
- Presence of social support
- Work issues (e.g., work schedule, work flexibility)
- Financial issues (e.g., financial resources, insurance coverage)

Past psychiatric history

- Psychiatric comorbidity
- History of outpatient psychiatric treatment
- History of psychiatric medications
- History of psychiatric hospitalizations
- History of risk-taking behaviors

Substance use history

- History of alcohol, substance, and nicotine use
- Previous history of substance use treatment
- Legal problems related to substance use

Anticipate Family Reactions

As a member of the transplant care team, the psychiatric consultant is in a position to frame his or her role as a source of patient support throughout the transplant process and as someone who can assist the family with developmental issues, behavioral health concerns, management of pain and anxiety, and/or general wellness. The consultant is positioned to play an important role in facilitating communication between the family and the transplant care team and should be alert to helping the family process their reactions to and help them "make meaning" of the child's life-threatening illness. This is important because parents facing their child's transplantation commonly report increased stress and emotional symptoms, including posttraumatic stress symptoms (Cousino et al. 2017).

Provide Feedback

It is important for the psychiatric consultant to provide his or her formulation and recommendations to the transplant care team. This should include not only a written report but also a face-to-face meeting to allow for discussion of issues and recommendations raised. The consultant's feedback also should be communicated directly to the patient and family. In cases where communication is problematic, the consultant may consider working with the transplant care team to develop a written family contract related to psychosocial concerns to help minimize any potential confusion or misinterpretation on the part of the patient and the family. This contract may include techniques to assist the child in preparation for painful and stressful procedures, recommendations for mobilizing family supports and resources, and/or interventions to address factors that may prejudice the transplant outcome.

Be Alert to Developmental Issues

It is important to assess the patient's level of cognitive and emotional development and to anticipate the relevant developmental vulnerabilities that may affect the transplant process. For example, preschool-age children with immature cognitive abilities may interpret invasive procedures as a punishment for perceived past misbehavior and may be unable to comprehend abstract concepts such as the finality and irreversibility of death. Developmental issues in adolescence include possible concerns about medication side effects, including growth retardation, hirsutism, breast enlargement, weight gain, and/or delayed development of secondary sex characteristics. Children and adolescents may need advice on ways to explain their transplant when they return to school so that they are prepared to respond to possible queries and misconceptions from their peers.

Consider Neurodevelopmental Assessments

Formal assessment of neurodevelopmental functioning should be considered because many patients with end-stage renal, liver, and cardiac diseases have cognitive and academic delays associated with their illnesses (DeMaso 2004). For example, patients with hepatic encephalopathy may present with a constellation of symptoms that includes cognitive impairment, confusion, disorientation, and affective dysregulation (DiMartini et al. 2005). Complex congenital heart disease lesions are associated with significant cognitive, developmental, and neurological abnormalities (DeMaso 2004; DeMaso et al. 2017). Such cognitive and developmental difficulties may affect the patient's ability to understand the transplant process or follow the lifelong treatment requirements.

Understanding and Expectations of Transplantation

The psychiatric consultant should assess the understanding and expectations of the transplant with both the patient and the family. It is important to determine whether the patient and family are competent to give assent and consent for the transplant. The consultant should be aware that both cognitive and emotional issues can interfere with family members' abilities to assimilate the large amount of information given to them and fully understand the implications of the proposed transplant. Prior to the psychiatric assessment, the family will have already met with the transplant care team and have received a thorough explanation of the transplant process. The consultant should assess the patient and family's understanding of and response to this information as well as their motivation to undergo transplantation and participate in the long-term medical care that will be required.

Psychiatric Comorbidity

The finding that pretransplant emotional functioning appears to correlate with posttransplant emotional functioning emphasizes the importance of identifying comorbid psychosocial problems prior to transplantation (DeMaso et al. 2004). Body image and self-esteem concerns are common in children with chronic physical illnesses and take on particular relevance in adolescents, for whom peer issues and social acceptance are of special importance (Wallander and Thompson 1995). Given the stresses inherent throughout the transplant process, identification of psychiatric disorders prior to transplantation can afford consultants the opportunity to be helpful in treating, mitigating, or even preventing problems after transplantation (Cousino et al. 2017; DeMaso et al. 2004).

Treatment Adherence

Adherence to prescribed treatment regimens, including cooperation with necessary procedural interventions, remains one of the most frustrating and problematic areas of transplant medicine (see Chapter 14, "Treatment Adherence"). Poor adherence has repeatedly been linked to morbidity and mortality in pediatric recipients. Significant correlates of nonadherence after transplantation include adolescence, lower family cohesion, greater parental distress, greater child distress, and poorer behavioral functioning (Dew et al. 2009). Nonadherence to clinic appointments and test nonadherence (13 recipients per 100 per year) have been more common in pediatrics than nonadherence to immunosuppression (6 recipients per 100 per year) (Dew et al. 2009). In this context, consultants should inquire, especially with an adolescent, about overall patterns of adherence related to health care and lifestyle beyond that of simple medication-taking adherence.

Family Factors

High rates of caregiver distress and psychiatric illness, particularly depression and posttraumatic stress symptoms, have been identified prior to (and after) transplantation (Cousino et al. 2017). As mentioned earlier in this chapter, there are associations between family functioning and child-related health factors, such as adherence, number of medication barriers, and number of hospitalizations (Cousino et al. 2017). As such, consultants should be attuned to the level of family functioning in tandem with the level of understanding and expectations regarding the patient's illness and subsequent treatment. Consultants should assess the family's available social support network. Because transplantation results in frequent medical appointments, unexpected complications, lengthy hospitalizations, and invasive procedures that are disruptive to family functioning, inquiring about the potential impact of the transplantation on parents' work-life balance can be helpful in identifying potential issues prior to transplantation.

The likelihood of a successful transplant outcome is increased if there is trust and respect between the family and the transplant care team. If the family perceives that their concerns are not being considered, there may be feelings of anxiety or anger that undermine the family's confidence in the team and result in the family potentially "acting out" through critical aspects of the treatment. The psychiatric consultant can play a significant role through on-going assessment and support for a strong working partnership between parents and the team (see Chapter 16, "Family Interventions").

Knowledge of a family's previous pediatric care experiences, such as an inpatient hospitalization, can help identify potential areas of difficulty for the upcoming transplant. For example, children who have had to deal with multiple invasive and painful procedures or who have experienced excessive pain or anxiety during an earlier hospitalization may be at particular risk for having these difficulties during the transplant process (see Chapter 2, "Coping and Adaptation in Physically Ill Children"). Conversely, the pretransplant evaluation may identify particularly successful coping strategies used during previous hospitalizations that may be helpful throughout the transplant process.

Alcohol and Substance Use

Although less prevalent than among adult transplant candidates, alcohol and substance use is an important risk factor to consider for adolescent candidates. Pretransplant histories of alcohol or other substance use disorders, as well as a family history of substance use disorders, are associated with a greater risk of posttransplant substance abuse. These same factors have been shown to be associated with greater postoperative complications, more hospital admissions, and lower quality of life after transplantation (Shapiro et al. 1995). In the presence of substance abuse, consultants should attempt to estimate the patient's potential for rehabilitation as well as his or her risk for relapse. Transplant hospital programs commonly require a defined period of abstinence that may range from 6 to 24 months prior to listing the individual for transplant.

Assessment of Living Donors

From 1987 to 2015, more than 140,000 living donor (LD) transplants occurred: 95% of these transplants were kidney; 4% were liver; and < 1% were lung, intestine, or pancreas (Gruessner and Gruessner 2018). Survival rates for patients receiving LD transplants, compared with patients receiving deceased donor transplants, were significantly higher only in kidney transplants, with the best long-term results in LD liver transplants being in pediatric recipients (Gruessner and Gruessner 2018). Despite significant improvements in surgical techniques, there has been a decline of more than 20% in all kinds of pediatric LD donor transplants.

The rate of perioperative mortality and morbidity for kidney LDs are about 0.03% and 10%, respectively (Gohds 2010), with long-term mortality rate in liver LDs being comparable (Muzaale et al. 2012). LDs have been found to have low rates of depression, anxiety, or substance use problems following transplantation, although heightened feelings of guilt along with concerns about responsibility have been reported for donors when the recipient died (Butt et al. 2017). Although it is rare to refuse a donor on psychosocial grounds unless there is severe psychopathology or doubt about donor competence to give informed consent, careful psychiatric assessment of the donor remains the recommendation. This assessment should establish whether the LD is fully informed and able to provide consent, and the assessor should be alert to any evidence of family coercion (see Table 12–3).

Transplant Process

The transplant process can be conceptualized as an interconnected series of phases of varying durations consisting of decision and preparation, listing and waiting, surgery and hospitalization, and posttransplant adjustment. Each phase has characteristic challenges that must be faced by the patient, family, and transplant team.

Decision and Preparation

The pretransplant assessment affords consultants the opportunity to assist families in adjusting to the need for and decision to go forward with an organ transplant. Parents commonly request assistance with ways to inform and prepare their child for the transplant. Most transplant hospital programs have educational material regarding transplantation that is routinely given to patients and their families. This material is often a combination of factual information and narrative stories from successful transplant recipients as exemplified in the Boston Children's Hospital's Transplant Experience Journal (DeMaso et al. 2019). Some programs offer potential new organ recipients the opportunity to meet directly with patients and parents who have successfully undergone transplantation. The consultant should be aware of these resources and should know of the availability of child life specialists who can provide ongoing support.

Using their knowledge of child development and of the transplant process, consultants are well positioned to help prepare patients. In contrast to

Table 12–3.   Elements of psychiatric assessment of the living organ donor

- Relationship of donor to potential recipient
- Quality of relationship between donor and potential recipient
- Donor understanding of transplant process and its effects (e.g., loss of kidney)
- Motivation of donor (e.g., ambivalence, feelings of guilt, family pressure)
- Presence of social support
- Financial resources
- Psychiatric comorbidity
- Likely reactions to the event of organ rejection
- Risks (e.g., sexual activity, drug use) of communicable disease

many parents' expectations, children generally do well with frank and open discussion of the need and reasons for transplant surgery. In younger patients, preparation begins with the parents being educated about the importance of being open, honest, and age-appropriate about the child's illness and treatment. Although parents can elect to initially speak with their child alone, most choose to have a transplant team physician(s) join them for the informing and preparation discussion.

Listing and Waiting

Listing for a transplant occurs after parents have given consent (and older adolescents have given assent) for the surgery. Listing generally heralds a period of enormous anxiety on the part of the patient and the family while they anticipate a donor organ becoming available. The wait between listing and surgery is unpredictable and can extend from weeks to even months. During this period, the patient remains at risk for acute medical decompensation as a result of events that include infection, stroke, and progressive organ dysfunction. Rates of delirium are elevated in patients waiting for transplant and may be overlooked unless the patient is carefully monitored. There is always the lingering and often unspoken fear that a donor will not be identified in time to save the child's life.

Psychosocial stressors often characterize the waiting period. Parents may have strong feelings of guilt related to the knowledge that another child needs to die in order for their child to have a chance to live. There may be concerns regarding competition for organs as well as anger about the process of organ allocation. Patients may be hospitalized at transplant programs that are located far away from their home community. It is not unusual for families to be temporarily separated during the waiting period. These events can lead to significant emotional distress and potential conflict between parents as well as creating a situation in which the healthy siblings' emotional needs become neglected. Siblings can develop feelings of anxiety and resentment toward their ill sibling. Unfortunately, unwelcome financial costs and burdens are common.

Pediatric ventricular assist devices (VADs) increasingly have been used as a bridge for patients who are waiting for heart transplantation but who are becoming more ill because of progressive heart failure. The use of VADs has decreased mortality in these children; in a study by Blume et al. (2018), nearly 50% of patients with VADs underwent transplantation within 6 months, with an overall mortality of 19%. Currently, just over 50% of patients supported by VADs are able to leave the hospital during their transplant wait. Major adverse events, including bleeding, infection, and stroke are more frequent in the first 3 months of VAD implantation (Blume et al. 2018). Less frequently, VADs become a "destination treatment" for patients for whom organ transplant is not an option. Patients in this category require a similarly rigorous presurgical assessment given the constraints and risks of life on a VAD.

Surgery and Hospitalization

When families receive the call telling them that a donor has been found, the news is often greeted with a mixture of relief and anxiety. Although the family is relieved that their child's life may be saved, they are acutely anxious about the surgery. After a common "honeymoon" period of elation following the transplant, the patient and family slowly begin to face the realities of living with a new chronic physical illness. They may be disappointed to find the need for continued isolation from school and/or a slow recovery after the surgery. The psychiatric consultant can provide the patient and family with the therapeutic opportunity to tell their story and in doing so better understand the process, which promotes their resiliency.

The time immediately following the transplant surgery is when patients and families have the most interest in the child's donor and may make requests to find out more about the donor's identity. Feelings of sadness or guilt may arise in parents as their own child becomes more stable. Although some recipients have found it helpful to write an anonymous letter of thanks to the donor's family, others have expressed distress over the perceived obligation to write and the inadequacy of the thank you (Poole et al. 2011).

In the immediate postoperative period or during any rehospitalization, consultants must be on continual alert for acute disabling mental status changes. The postsurgical recovery may be quite variable, with the potential for a number of acute serious medical events. Delirium, with its fluctuating consciousness, confusion, and sleep disruptions, may be the result of sepsis, electrolyte imbalances, residual effects of general anesthesia, hypoxic episodes, immunosuppressants, and/or analgesic medications (see Chapter 5, "Delirium").

Posttransplant Adjustment

In order to increase their effectiveness in working with patients, families, and the transplant care team, the consultant should have an up-to-date biopsychosocial formulation of posttransplant adjustment that integrates the medical issues, emotional adjustment, and academic functioning of each patient (Spieth and Harris 1996).

Pediatric Issues

Despite the significant advances in immunosuppressive regimens, consultants should keep in mind that patients are embarking on lifelong immunosuppressive medications that are required to modulate their immune system response to the donor organ. Consultants will find patients following transplants in one of three phases of immunosuppression: 1) induction, to prevent acute rejection immediately after transplant; 2) maintenance, to provide long-term suppression; and 3) antirejection, to treat acute rejection either after the initial transplant or at a subsequent follow-up. Currently, most transplant programs use a triple-drug regimen that includes the second-generation calcineurin inhibitor tacrolimus, the antiproliferative agent mycophenolic acid, and a corticosteroid (Holt 2017). In general, higher dosages of maintenance immunosuppressive agents are used early after transplantation, and then the dosages are gradually reduced over the first year to minimize toxicity. The triple-drug regimens are often reduced over time to double- or single-drug regimens depending on the patient's clinical course (Holt 2017). Consultants should remain alert to changes in mental status (e.g., symptoms of delirium, anxiety, or depression) because they may reflect organ failure and/or the immunosuppressive medications and their side effects. Although not exhaustive, Table 12–4 outlines common immunosuppressive agents and their side effects.

Despite improvements in overall graft function and survival rates after transplantation, cardiovascular, neurological, renal, and gastrointestinal (GI) system complications can lead to significant morbidity. Common cardiovascular complications include hypertension, dyslipidemia, coronary artery disease from new-onset diabetes mellitus and renal failure, left ventricular hypertrophy, arrhythmias, and heart failure (Sen et al. 2019). Neurological complications (which occur in more than 30% of recipients), neurotoxicity of immunosuppressive agents, seizures, cerebrovascular events, opportunistic infections, and central pontine myelinosis also occur (Pizzi and Ng 2017). Recipients can develop both acute kidney injury and chronic kidney disease. Occurring in almost 40% of recipients, GI complications can include infection, mucosal injury or ulceration, perforation, biliary tract disease, pancreatitis, GI malignancies, and posttransplant lymphoproliferative disorder (PTLD; Sen et al. 2019). With an overall incidence of 1%–3%, the risk for PTLD is directly associated with the intensity of the immunosuppressive regimen, such that treatment of PTLD begins with the reduction of immunosuppressive agents and the addition of antibody therapy, usually with rituximab, an anti-CD_{20} antibody (Sen et al. 2019).

The first year after transplantation is characterized by close medical follow-up to monitor for potential organ rejection and medical complications. It is a period of frequent appointments, regular biopsies and procedures, and multiple medication changes. It is also generally a time of heightened anxiety as the patient is gradually reintroduced into peer and academic settings and the parents slowly relinquish their heightened supervisory roles. Assuming all is going well, entrance into the second year generally heralds a reduction in the intensity and frequency of medical monitoring as well as a lessening of special attention and treatment for the patient.

In general, medical issues improve over the course of the first posttransplant year, allowing recipients to gradually assume (or reassume) activities that are developmentally on target. For instance, youth who are no longer on di-

Table 12–4. Side effects of selected immunosuppressive agents

Medication	Potential side effects
Corticosteroids	
Methylprednisolone, prednisone, prednisolone	*Central nervous system:* increased intracranial pressure with papilledema (pseudotumor cerebri), seizures, vertigo, headache, psychosis, hypomania, mood lability, depression, cognitive impairment
	Gastrointestinal: peptic ulcer, pancreatitis, abdominal distention, ulcerative esophagitis
	Endocrine: menstrual irregularities, Cushingoid state, growth suppression, diabetes mellitus
	Dermatological: impaired wound healing, thin fragile skin, petechiae, facial erythema, increased sweating
	Ophthalmic: posterior subcapsular cataracts, increased intraocular pressure, glaucoma, exophthalmos
	Electrolyte disturbances: sodium retention, fluid retention, congestive heart failure, hypertension
	Musculoskeletal: muscle weakness, steroid myopathy, loss of muscle mass, osteoporosis, vertebral compression fractures, aseptic necrosis of femoral and humeral heads, pathologic fracture
Calcineurin inhibitors	
Cyclosporine	*Central nervous system:* tremor, restlessness, headache, acute confusional state, psychosis, speech apraxia, cortical blindness, seizures, coma
	Gastrointestinal: diarrhea, nausea, vomiting, abdominal discomfort
	Renal: renal dysfunction
	Cardiovascular: hypertension
	Hematological: lymphoma, leukopenia
	Endocrine: gynecomastia
	Dermatological: hirsutism, gum hyperplasia, acne

Table 12–4.   Side effects of selected immunosuppressive agents *(continued)*

Medication	Potential side effects
Calcineurin inhibitors (*continued*)	
Tacrolimus	*Central nervous system:* tremor, restlessness, headache, insomnia, vivid dreams, hyperesthesias, agitation, cognitive impairment, dysarthria, delirium, focal neurological abnormalities, speech disturbances, hemiplegia, cortical blindness, seizures, coma, leukoencephalopathy (demyelination in parieto-occipital region)
	Gastrointestinal: diarrhea, nausea, vomiting, abdominal pain
	Cardiovascular: chest pain, hypertension
	Hematological: anemia, leukopenia
	Endocrine: Cushing's syndrome, diabetes mellitus
	Dermatological: acne, alopecia, exfoliative dermatitis, hirsutism, skin discoloration
IMDH inhibitors	
Mycophenolate mofetil	*Central nervous system:* agitation, convulsion, delirium, depression, emotional lability, hallucinations, neuropathy, paresthesia, psychosis, somnolence, vertigo
	Gastrointestinal: anorexia, dysphagia, gastrointestinal hemorrhage, gingivitis, gum hyperplasia, jaundice, liver damage, mouth ulceration, nausea, vomiting
	Cardiovascular: angina pectoris, arrhythmias, congestive heart failure, palpitation, postural hypotension, pulmonary hypertension, syncope
	Renal: acute kidney failure, hematuria, urinary frequency, urinary incontinence, urinary retention
	Endocrine: Cushing's syndrome, diabetes mellitus, hypothyroidism, parathyroid disorder
	Hematological: coagulation disorder, ecchymosis, pancytopenia

Table 12–4.   Side effects of selected immunosuppressive agents *(continued)*

Medication	Potential side effects
IMDH inhibitors *(continued)*	
Mycophenolate mofetil *(continued)*	*Dermatological:* acne, alopecia, hirsutism, pruritus, rash, skin carcinoma, sweating, rash
	Respiratory: apnea, asthma, epistaxis, hemoptysis, hiccup
	Special senses: abnormal vision, deafness, tinnitus
Azathioprine	*Gastrointestinal:* nausea, vomiting, diarrhea, abdominal discomfort, hepatotoxicity, veno-occlusive disease
	Hematological: leukopenia, thrombocytopenia, lymphoma
	Dermatological: rash, alopecia
Inhibitors of late T-cell function	
Sirolimus	*Central nervous system:* anxiety, confusion, depression, dizziness, emotional lability, hypesthesia, hypotonia, insomnia, neuropathy, paresthesia, somnolence
	Gastrointestinal: anorexia, dysphagia, flatulence, gastritis, gum hyperplasia, ileus, abnormal liver function tests, mouth ulceration
	Renal: bladder pain, dysuria, hematuria, nocturia, urinary incontinence, urinary retention
	Cardiovascular: atrial fibrillation, congestive heart failure, hemorrhage, syncope, tachycardia, venous thromboembolism
	Hematological: ecchymosis, leukocytosis, lymphadenopathy, thrombotic thrombocytopenic purpura (hemolytic-uremic syndrome)
	Endocrine: Cushing's syndrome, diabetes mellitus
	Dermatological: hirsutism, pruritus, skin hypertrophy, skin ulcer, sweating
	Musculoskeletal system: arthrosis, bone necrosis, leg cramps, myalgia
	Special senses: abnormal vision, cataract, conjunctivitis, deafness, ear pain, otitis media, tinnitus

Table 12–4. Side effects of selected immunosuppressive agents *(continued)*

Medication	Potential side effects
Mononclonal antibodies	
Muromonab-CD3 (OKT3)	*Central nervous system:* agitation, aphasia, cerebral edema, cerebral herniation, cerebrovascular accident, central nervous system infection or malignancy, cranial nerve VI palsy, encephalitis, hyperreflexia, involuntary movements, intracranial hemorrhage, impaired cognition, myoclonus, status epilepticus, stupor, transient ischemic attack, vertigo
	Gastrointestinal: bowel infarction
	Cardiovascular: cardiovascular collapse, hemodynamic instability
	Renal: delayed graft function, renal insufficiency or renal failure, occasionally in association with cytokine release syndrome
	Hematological: aplastic anemia, disseminated intravascular coagulation, neutropenia, pancytopenia
	Dermatological: erythema, flushing, Stevens-Johnson syndrome, urticaria
	Special senses: blindness, blurred vision, deafness, diplopia, otitis media, nasal and ear stuffiness, papilledema

Note. IMDH = inosine monophosphate dehydrogenase.

alysis have more time for age-appropriate physical and social activities. Similarly, heart transplant recipients are able to be home rather than in the hospital receiving continuous intravenous medications and/or mechanical circulatory support. Improvements in physical health after transplantation are associated with reduced hospitalizations, shorter lengths of stay, and decreased reliance on medications, all of which can facilitate improvements in emotional, family, and academic functioning.

Emotional Adjustment

Although the physical functioning of transplant recipients improves following surgery, the results regarding emotional adjustment are more mixed. This variability in psychological functioning is likely reflective of limited research, particularly the paucity of longer-term or longitudinal follow-up studies. Adjustment may also vary with the type of transplant. Although a majority of youngsters have healthy emotional functioning following heart transplantation, approximately 30% present with significant emotional difficulties (DeMaso et al. 2004; Uzark et al. 2012; Wray and Radley-Smith 2006). Children with liver and lung transplants have been found to have psychosocial functioning similar to that of the healthy population despite significant differences in physical functioning (Alonso et al. 2003; Hirshfeld et al. 2004). Kidney transplantation has been associated with improved overall emotional health, but there may be persistent difficulties with peer relationships and treatment adherence (Bursch and Stuber 2005).

Pretransplant psychological dysfunction in either the child or the family has been correlated with poor posttransplant adjustment in heart transplant recipients (DeMaso et al. 2004). Conversely, patients with higher levels of perceived support, adaptive functioning, and quality of life prior to transplantation have improved rates of posttransplant survival (Trzepacz and DiMartini 1992). Children whose sense of self has been based on having a chronic physical illness may have significant difficulties leaving the sick role behind and adjusting to the new expected healthy role after transplantation (DiMartini et al. 2005).

Although there is no current synthesized empirical evidence, expert consensus and opinion support consultants in their use of psychotherapy and/or psychopharmacology in the treatment of comorbid psychiatric disorders, particularly anxiety, depressive, and/or trauma-related disorders, in youth who have undergone transplantation. The consultant should review psychotropic medications for interactions with the patient's current immunosuppressive regimen and discuss the medications directly with the managing transplant care physician(s) prior to prescribing. It is worth noting that the significant dose-related impact of corticosteroids on mood lability and depression should also be considered by consultants because the displayed disabling emotions may be transitory in nature and due to the immunosuppressive dose regimen (e.g., an increase in corticosteroids for an acute rejection episode) as opposed to a more ingrained co-occurring primary depressive or anxiety disorder.

In cases of mild to moderate psychiatric severity, the transplant care team may be willing to assume the primary medication management with support from the psychiatric consultant. For those patients with severe psychiatric disorders, the consultant will either need to assume primary management of the psychotropic medication or refer to a specialty psychiatry setting.

Consultants must also remain vigilant for nonadherence throughout the transplant process. It is one the most common reason for late rejection, suggesting that even the potential for a fatal outcome may not protect patients from failing to take their medications as directed. Reassessment for factors contributing to the lack of treatment is critical (see Chapter 14).

Academic Functioning

Patients with chronic renal and liver disease, particularly those whose disease had an early onset, have been found to have delays in cognitive and motor functioning. Although improvement is seen after transplantation, patients continue to have cognitive performance deficits in executive functioning, verbal fluency, and language compared with healthy controls (Joshee et al. 2018). Longer-term studies of pediatric liver transplant recipients have shown that patients have a higher prevalence of cognitive and academic delays with learning problems (Sorensen et al. 2011). Although many children are found to function within the normal range on most measures of cognitive functioning following heart transplantation, cognitive difficulties that may predate transplantation must be considered (Chinnock et al. 2008; Todaro et al. 2000). Together, these findings outline the importance of psychiatric consultants investigating the academic functioning of all transplant recipients, particularly those with known or suspected central nervous system vulnerabilities.

Conclusion

Solid organ transplantation is a common and widely accepted medical treatment option for children and adolescents who formerly would not have survived their illness (Bernard et al. 2010). Because of the steady and consistent improvements in outcomes for pediatric transplant recipients in childhood, many of these individuals may anticipate long-term survival into adulthood. The integration of psychiatric consultants has emerged in this context to help transplant recipients understand and help address the cognitive and emotional difficulties that they face and to enhance the focus on health and wellness for both patients and family members.

References

Alonso EM, Neighbors K, Mattson C, et al: Functional outcomes of pediatric liver transplantation. J Pediatr Gastroenterol Nutr 37(2):155–160, 2003 12883302

Bernard RS, Fisher MK, Shaw RJ: Organ transplantation, in Textbook of Pediatric Psychosomatic Medicine. Edited by Shaw RJ, DeMaso DR. Washington, DC, American Psychiatric Publishing, 2010, pp 329–342

Blume ED, VanderPluym C, Lorts A, et al; Pedimacs Investigators: Second annual Pediatric Interagency Registry for Mechanical Circulatory Support (Pedimacs) report: pre-implant characteristics and outcomes. J Heart Lung Transplant 37(1):38–45, 2018 28965736

Brosig C, Pai A, Fairey E, et al: Child and family adjustment following pediatric solid organ transplantation: factors to consider during the early years post-transplant. Pediatr Transplant 18(6):559–567, 2014 24923434

Bursch B, Stuber M: Pediatrics, in The American Psychiatric Publishing Textbook of Psychosomatic Medicine. Edited by Levenson JL. Washington, DC, American Psychiatric Publishing, 2005, pp 761–786

Butt Z, Dew MA, Liu Q, et al: Psychological outcomes of living donors from a multicenter prospective study: results from the Adult-to-Adult Living Donor Liver Transplantation Cohort Study 2 (A2ALL-2). Am J Transplant 17:1267–1277, 2017 27865040

Cahn-Fuller KL, Parent B: Transplant eligibility for patients with affective and psychotic disorders: a review of practices and a call for justice. BMC Med Ethics 18(1):72, 2017 29216883

Chinnock RE, Freier MC, Ashwal S, et al: Developmental outcomes after pediatric heart transplantation. J Heart Lung Transplant 27(10):1079–1084, 2008 18926397

Cousino MK, Rea KE, Schumacher KR, et al: A systematic review of parent and family functioning in pediatric solid organ transplant populations. Pediatr Transplant 21(3):e12900, 2017 28181361

Cousino MK, Schumacher KR, Rea KE, et al: Psychosocial functioning in pediatric heart transplant recipients and their families. Pediatr Transplant 22(2):e13110, 2018 29316050

Dew MA, Dabbs AD, Myaskovsky L, et al: Meta-analysis of medical regimen adherence outcomes in pediatric solid organ transplantation. Transplantation 88(5):736–746, 2009 19741474

DeMaso DR: Pediatric heart disease, in Handbook of Pediatric Psychology in School Settings. Edited by Brown RT. Hillsdale, NJ, Lawrence Erlbaum, 2004, pp 283–297

DeMaso DR, Douglas Kelley S, Bastardi H, et al: The longitudinal impact of psychological functioning, medical severity, and family functioning in pediatric heart transplantation. J Heart Lung Transplant 23(4):473–480, 2004 15063408

DeMaso DR, Calderon J, Taylor GA, et al: Psychiatric disorders in adolescents with single ventricle congenital heart disease. Pediatrics 139(3):e20162241, 2017 28148729

DeMaso DR, Marcus N, Kinnamon C, et al: Experience Journals: Transplant. 2019. Available at: http://www.experiencejournal.com/transplant. Accessed January 1, 2019.

Dew MA, Dabbs AD, Greenhouse JB, et al: Meta-analysis of medical regimen adherence outcomes in pediatric solid organ transplantation. Transplantation 88(5):736–746, 2009 19741474

DiMartini AF, Mew MA, Trzepacz PT: Organ transplantation, in The American Psychiatric Publishing Textbook of Psychosomatic Medicine. Edited by Levenson JL. Washington, DC, American Psychiatric Publishing, 2005, pp 675–700

Gohds AJ: Living kidney donation: the outcomes for donors. In J Organ Transplant Med 1(2):63–71, 2010 25013567

Gruessner RW, Gruessner AC: Solid-organ transplants from living donors: cumulative United States experience on 140,156 living donor transplants over 28 years. Transplant Proc 50(10):3025–3035, 2018 30577162

Hirshfeld AB, Kahle AL, Clark BJ 3rd, et al: Parent-reported health status after pediatric thoracic organ transplant. J Heart Lung Transplant 23(9):1111–1118, 2004 15454179

Holt CD: Overview of immunosuppressive therapy in solid organ transplantation. Anesthesiol Clin 35(3):305–380, 2017

Joshee P, Wood AG, Wood ER, et al: Meta-analysis of cognitive functioning in patients following kidney transplantation. Nephrol Dial Transplant 33(7):1268–1277, 2018 28992229

Muzaale AD, Dagher NN, Montgomery RA, et al: Estimates of early death, acute liver failure, and long-term mortality among live liver donors. Gastroenterology 142(2):273–280, 2012 22108193

Pizzi M, Ng L: Neurologic complications of solid organ transplant. Neurol Clin 35(4):809–823, 2017 28962815

Poole JM, Shildrick M, De Luca E, et al: The obligation to say 'Thank you': heart transplant recipients' experience of writing to the donor family. Am J Transplant 11(3):619–622, 2011 21342451

Samsel C, Ribeiro M, Ibeziako P, DeMaso DR: Integrated behavioral health care in pediatric subspecialty clinics. Child Adolesc Psychiatr Clin N Am 26(4):785–794, 2017 28916014

Schnitzler MA, Skeans MA, Axelrod DA, et al: OPTN/SRTA 2016 annual data report: economics. Am J Transplant 18(Suppl 1):464–503, 2018 29292607

Sen A, Callisen H, Libricz S, Patel B: Complications of solid organ transplantation: cardiovascular, neurologic, renal, and gastrointestinal. Crit Care Clin 35(1):169–186, 2019 30447778

Shapiro PA, Williams DL, Foray AT, et al: Psychosocial evaluation and prediction of compliance problems and morbidity after heart transplantation. Transplantation 60(12):1462–1466, 1995 8545875

Sorensen LG, Neighbors K, Martz K, et al; Studies of Pediatric Liver Transplantation (SPLIT) and Functional Outcomes Group (FOG): Cognitive and academic outcomes after pediatric liver transplantation: Functional Outcomes Group (FOG) results. Am J Transplant 11(2):303–311, 2011 21272236

Spieth LE, Harris CV: Assessment of health-related quality of life in children and adolescents: an integrative review. J Pediatr Psychol 21(2):175–193, 1996 8920152

Strouse TB, Wolcott DL, Skotzo CE: Transplantation, in Textbook of Consultation-Liaison Psychiatry. Edited by Rundell JR, Wise MG. Washington, DC, American Psychiatric Press, 1996, pp 641–670

Thomson K, McKenna K, Bedard-Thomas K, et al: Behavioral health care in solid organ transplantation in a pediatric setting. Pediatr Transplant 22(5):e13217, 2018 29744988

Todaro JF, Fennell EB, Sears SF, et al: Review: cognitive and psychological outcomes in pediatric heart transplantation. J Pediatr Psychol 25(8):567–576, 2000 11085760

Trzepacz PT, DiMartini A: Survival of 247 liver transplant candidates. Relationship to pretransplant psychiatric variables and presence of delirium. Gen Hosp Psychiatry 14(6):380–386, 1992 1473708

Uzark K, Griffin L, Rodriguez R, et al: Quality of life in pediatric heart transplant recipients: a comparison with children with and without heart disease. J Heart Lung Transplant 31(6):571–578, 2012 22381209

Wallander JL, Thompson RJ: Psychosocial adjustment of children with chronic physical conditions, in Handbook of Pediatric Psychology, 2nd Edition. Edited by Roberts MC. New York, Guilford, 1995, pp 124–141

Wray J, Radley-Smith R: Longitudinal assessment of psychological functioning in children after heart or heart-lung transplantation. J Heart Lung Transplant 25(3):345–352, 2006 16507430

Pediatric Cancer, Stem Cell Transplantation, and Palliative Care

Pediatric Cancer

Although children make up less than 1% of all cancers diagnosed in the United States, more than 10,000 new cancer cases will be diagnosed each year in children younger than 15 years, with nearly 1,200 deaths (American Cancer Society 2018). After accidents, cancer remains the second-leading cause of death in this age group. Nonetheless, the overall outlook for childhood cancer has improved dramatically compared with 50 years ago, when these same illnesses were often considered incurable. The 5-year relative survival rate for all pediatric cancers has now reached 83%, although this rate varies by cancer type, patient age, and other characteristics (American Cancer Society 2018) (Table 13–1). The Children's Oncology Group, a National Cancer Institute–supported clinical trials collaborative, has brought together children's hospitals, universities, and cancer centers from around the world to make and continue to make the innovative advances that characterize pediatric cancer treatment today (see www.childrensoncologygroup.org).

Standards of Psychosocial Care

The significant psychosocial impact of pediatric cancer on the child and family over the course of treatment and beyond is well established and widely un-

Table 13–1.   Overview of childhood cancers (ages 0–14 years) distribution and 5-year survival rates

Type of cancer	Distribution of childhood cancers (%)	5-year survival rate (%)
Childhood leukemia	29	86
Acute lymphoblastic leukemia	¾ of total leukemia	91
Acute myeloid leukemia	¼ of total leukemia	65
Brain and other central nervous system tumors (excluding benign tumors)	26	73
Neuroblastoma	6	79
Wilms' tumor	5	93
Non-Hodgkin lymphoma	5	91
Hodgkin lymphoma	3	98
Rhabdomyosarcoma	3	70
Retinoblastoma	2	95
Osteosarcoma	2	70
Ewing sarcoma	1	78

Source.   Data from American Cancer Society 2018.

derstood (Kazak et al. 2015). This impact is particularly noteworthy on a family's early child-rearing years because the mean age at diagnosis is 6 years, with an average duration of treatment of 1–3 years (American Cancer Society 2018). The Psychosocial Standards of Care Project for Childhood Cancer (PSCPCC), a multidisciplinary group of professionals from psychology, psychiatry, and social work, has outlined evidence- and consensus-based standards of care for the pediatric psychosocial care of children with cancer and their families (Wiener et al. 2015a).

These standards illustrate the important role that psychiatric consultants have in providing biopsychosocial assessments that in turn generate effective intervention strategies that enhance the resiliency of young patients and their families facing cancer (Table 13–2). Being attuned to the correlates of adjustment in childhood physical illness (see Chapter 2, "Adaptation and Coping in Physically Ill Children"), consultants are well positioned to facilitate clear and effective communication between the family and oncology team while addressing problematic physical sequelae, cognitive dysfunction, and/or psychosocial adjustment.

Yearly screening of the long-term survivors of pediatric cancers is a recommended PSCPCC standard (Wiener et al. 2015a). For screening, consultants may consider using either the Psychosocial Assessment Tool or the Distress Thermometer, both of which have been identified as evidence-based screening approaches for pediatric cancer (Kazak et al. 2015). The Psychosocial Assessment Tool is a parent report measure based on the Pediatric Preventive Psychosocial Health Model, a public health approach to identifying families at universal, targeted, and clinical levels of risk across multiple domains (e.g., family resources, family problems, social support) (Kazak et al. 2012). The Distress Thermometer is a brief measure that allows the rating of patient distress on a 1–10 analog scale by multiple respondents (patients, parents, and staff) (Haverman et al. 2013; Patel et al. 2011). Screening that is a family-centered part of overall oncology care can be an important first step in accessing psychosocial care quickly and efficiently (Kazak et al. 2015).

Physical Sequelae

There are numerous physical sequelae of cancer: those that are a direct effect of the specific cancer, those related to side effects of its treatment, or a combination of both. General effects including nausea, vomiting, anorexia, fatigue, malaise, weight loss, physical limitations, and/or pain are almost universal. The direct physical manifestations depend to a large degree on the location of the cancer. Leukemia, for example, involves the bone marrow, and patients generally present with signs of anemia, bleeding, or infection. By contrast, solid organ tumors cause damage by local growth or metastases (Shah and Wayne 2015). The effects of brain tumors depend on their size and location, such that patients may experience headaches, vomiting, personality changes, or neurological symptoms (Warren 2015). Patients can develop acute mental status changes consistent with delirium related to the direct effects of their cancers as well as their treatment. Surgical treatment may include amputation and enucleation for specific tumors.

Table 13–2.   Pediatric psychosocial standards

Standard of care	Quality of evidence	Strength of recommendation
1. Youth with cancer and their family members should routinely receive systematic assessments of their psychosocial health care needs.	High	Strong
2. Patients with brain tumors and others at high risk for neuropsychological deficits as a result of cancer treatment should be monitored for neuropsychological deficits during and after treatment.	High	Strong
3. Long-term survivors of child and adolescent cancers should receive yearly psychosocial screening for 1) adverse educational and/or vocational progress and social and relationship difficulties; 2) distress, anxiety, and depression; and 3) risky health behaviors.	Moderate to High	Strong
4. Adolescent and young adult survivors and their parents should receive anticipatory guidance on the need for lifelong follow-up care by the time treatment ends; this guidance should be repeated at each follow-up visit.	Low to Moderate	Strong
4. Youth with cancer and their family members should have access to psychosocial support and interventions throughout the cancer trajectory and access to psychiatry as needed.	High	Strong

Table 13–2.   Pediatric psychosocial standards *(continued)*

Standard of care	Quality of evidence	Strength of recommendation
5. Pediatric oncology families are at high risk for financial burden during cancer treatment, with associated negative implications for quality of life and parental emotional health. • Assessment of risk for financial hardship should be incorporated at time of diagnosis for all pediatric oncology families. Domains of assessment should include risk factors for financial hardship during therapy, including preexisting low-income or financial hardship, single parent status, distance from treating center, anticipated long/intense treatment protocol, and parental employment status. • Targeted referral for financial counseling and supportive resources (including both governmental and charitable supports) should be offered on the basis of results of family assessment. • Longitudinal reassessment and intervention should occur throughout the cancer treatment trajectory and into survivorship or bereavement.	Moderate	Strong
6. Parents and caregivers of children with cancer should have early and ongoing assessment of their mental health needs. Access to appropriate interventions for parents and caregivers should be facilitated to optimize parent, child, and family well-being.	Moderate	Strong
7. Youth with cancer and their family members should be provided with psychoeducation, information, and anticipatory guidance related to disease, treatment, acute and long-term effects, hospitalization, procedures, and psychosocial adaptation. Guidance should be tailored to the specific needs and preferences of individual patients and families and be provided throughout the trajectory of cancer care.	Moderate	Strong

Table 13–2. Pediatric psychosocial standards *(continued)*

Standard of care	Quality of evidence	Strength of recommendation
8. Youth with cancer should receive developmentally appropriate preparatory information about invasive medical procedures.	Low	Strong
All youth should receive psychological intervention for invasive medical procedures.	High	Strong
9. Children and adolescents with cancer should be provided opportunities for social interaction during cancer therapy and into survivorship following careful consideration of the patient's unique characteristics, including developmental level, preferences for social interaction, and health status. The patient, parent(s), and a psychosocial team member (e.g., designee from child life, psychology, social work, or nursing) should participate in this evaluation at time of diagnosis, throughout treatment, and when the patient enters survivorship; it may be helpful to include school personnel or additional providers.	Moderate	Strong
10. Siblings of children with cancer are a psychosocially at-risk group and should be provided with appropriate supportive services. Parents and professionals should be advised about ways to anticipate and meet siblings' needs, especially when siblings are unable to visit the hospital regularly.	Moderate	Strong

Table 13–2.   Pediatric psychosocial standards *(continued)*

Standard of care	Quality of evidence	Strength of recommendation
11. In collaboration with parents, school-age youth diagnosed with cancer should receive school reentry support that focuses on providing information to school personnel about the patient's diagnosis and treatment, implications for the school environment, and recommendations to support the child's school experience. Pediatric oncology programs should identify a team member with the requisite knowledge and skills who will coordinate communication between the patient/family, school, and the health care team.	Low	Strong
12. Adherence should be assessed routinely and monitored throughout treatment.	Moderate	Strong
13. Youth with cancer and their families should be introduced to palliative care concepts to reduce suffering throughout the disease process regardless of disease status. When necessary, youth and families should receive developmentally appropriate end-of-life care (which includes bereavement care after the child's death).	Moderate	Strong
14. A member of the health care team should contact the family after a child's death to assess family needs, to identify negative psychosocial sequelae, to continue care, and to provide resources for bereavement support.	Moderate	Strong

Table 13–2.   Pediatric psychosocial standards *(continued)*

Standard of care	Quality of evidence	Strength of recommendation
15. Open, respectful communication and collaboration among medical and psychosocial providers, patients, and families is essential to effective patient- and family-centered care. Psychosocial professionals should be integrated into pediatric oncology care settings as integral team members and be participants in patient care rounds and meetings.	Moderate	Strong
Pediatric psychosocial providers should have access to medical records, and relevant reports should be shared among care team professionals, with psychological report interpretation provided by psychosocial providers to staff and patients/families for patient care planning. Psychosocial providers should follow documentation policies of the health system where they practice in accordance with ethical requirements of their profession and state and federal laws.	Low	Strong
Pediatric psychosocial providers must have specialized training and education and be credentialed in their discipline to provide developmentally appropriate assessment and treatment for children with cancer and their families. Experience working with children with serious, chronic illness is crucial, as is ongoing relevant supervision or peer support.	Low	Low

Source.   Adapted from Wiener L, Kazak AE, Noll RB, et al.: "Standards for the Psychosocial Care of Children With Cancer and Their Families: An Introduction to the Special Issue." *Pediatric Blood & Cancer* 62 (suppl 5):S419–S424, 2015. Copyright © 2015, John Wiley & Sons. Used with permission.

Pain is nearly universal and may be due to the direct effects of the cancer, treatment procedures, and/or medication side effects (Flowers and Birnie 2015; Shah and Wayne 2015). Responding to pain can become further complicated when patients minimize their pain complaints as a result of their association of pain with clinic visits, procedures, and/or hospitalizations as well as a means to avoid creating concern in their parents. Psychiatric consultants play an important role in the assessment and subsequent management of pain (Zeltzer and Krane 2015; see Chapter 10, "Pediatric Pain").

The side effects of chemotherapy can include infection, bleeding, anemia, hair loss, nausea and vomiting, malaise, mouth sores, anorexia, and pain as well as functional limitations (Shah and Wayne 2015). Additional problems include growth delays, short stature, renal dysfunction, endocrine abnormalities, and neurotoxicity. The adverse effects of chemotherapy, such as cardiotoxicity with the anthracyclines or pulmonary toxicity with bleomycin, may prove problematic. Side effects of radiation include skin irritation, loss of appetite, diarrhea, headache, and the possibility of secondary malignancies. Cranial radiation in particular may cause acute anorexia, confusion, and somnolence as temporary, reversible effects, but late effects on memory and cognition may be both irreversible and progressive. There can also be interactions between chemotherapy and radiation, such as cranial irradiation–related hearing loss with cisplatin. Loss of fertility and delays in sexual maturation can result from irradiation and chemotherapy.

Cognitive Dysfunction

Cancer-related cognitive dysfunction affects one-third or more of pediatric cancer survivors. The dysfunction is characterized by decline in Full Scale IQ and/or impairment in core functional domains of attention, vigilance, working memory, executive function, processing speed, or visual motor integration (Castellino et al. 2014; Daly and Brown 2015). It can manifest months and even years after treatment for brain tumors, acute lymphoblastic leukemia, or tumors involving the head and neck (Castellino et al. 2014). Risk factors include young age at diagnosis, treatment with cranial irradiation, use of parenteral or intrathecal methotrexate, female sex, and preexisting comorbidities. Although limiting use and reducing doses or volume of cranial irradiation and intensifying chemotherapy have improved survival and reduced the severity of cognitive dysfunction, problems in core domains of attention, processing speed, working memory, and visual-motor integration can remain and compromise quality of life and academic performance (Castellino et al. 2014; Daly and Brown 2015). Self-monitoring skills and peer relationships can be compromised as well.

The PSCPCC established as a care standard that patients with brain tumors and others at high risk for neuropsychological deficits as a result of cancer treatment should be monitored for cognitive deficits during and after treatment (Annett et al. 2015). Strategies to intervene in cognitive dysfunction have included educational interventions (e.g., school remediation or reintegration programs, cognitive-behavioral therapy) and pharmacological treatments (e.g., stimulants for attention) (Castellino et al. 2014; Daly and Brown 2015).

Psychosocial Adjustment

Pediatric cancer is a life stressor with understandably high levels of psychosocial distress across multiple areas impacting child and family functioning through its treatment (Kazak et al. 2015). The PSCPCC psychosocial standard of care found consistent and strong evidence for the following: 1) both children and families experience increased distress, poorer quality of life, and difficulties in psychosocial functioning immediately after and during the months following cancer diagnosis; 2) stressors and experiences that predate the diagnosis of cancer in a child are associated with functioning after diagnosis; 3) families at socioeconomic risk have more difficulties with respect to access to care and barriers to treatment; and 4) perceived support from family members and others is related to psychosocial functioning and reduced distress across the course of treatment (Kazak et al. 2015).

Expert consensus and opinion support consultants in their use of psychotherapy and/or psychopharmacology in the treatment of youth with pediatric cancer and co-occurring psychiatric disorders, particularly anxiety, depressive, and/or trauma-related disorders (Bursch and Forgey 2013; Dejong and Fombonne 2006; Kersun and Kazak 2006; Pao and Kazak 2015; Portteus et al. 2006). As a rule, psychotropic medications should be reviewed for interactions with a patient's current cancer treatment regimen as well as discussed directly with the managing oncologist prior to prescribing. In patients with psychiatric problems with mild to moderate severity, the oncologist may be willing to assume the primary medication management with consultation and support from the psychiatric consultant. For those patients with severe psychiatric disorders, consultants will generally need to assume primary management of the psychotropic medication(s) or refer the patient to a specialty psychiatry setting.

Even for parents who are resilient and well-functioning, the stressor of cancer can cause transient and marked distress, with a slow return to a new changed "normal" that includes the reality of the illness (Kearney et al. 2015). Parents' struggles with their own emotional issues can disrupt the cancer treatment, adversely impact parenting for the ill child and siblings, and threaten family functioning and stability over time. This led to the PSCPCC standard that parents (and caregivers) of children with cancer should have early and ongoing mental health assessment and appropriate interventions that optimize family well-being (Kearney et al. 2015).

Different family tasks are associated with different stages in a child's cancer treatment, as shown in Table 13–3. Transitions between these phases require flexibility on the part of the family. In the early phases of diagnosis and treatment, most families have a tendency to pull inward, with the goals of increasing cohesion and mobilizing resources and support. In time, after the family has integrated the illness into the daily routine, the need for increased cohesion may diminish, and the family may focus on efforts to resume normal developmental tasks and resolve conflicts between the needs of the patient and those of other family members. In the rehabilitation phase, there may often be a paradoxical increase in psychological symptoms as pent-up emotions surface and the financial, interpersonal, and emotional difficulties incurred during the acute phase can now be addressed.

Siblings may exhibit symptoms of anxiety, depression, and/or posttraumatic stress as well as disruptions in their academic and social functioning. Most difficulties improve over the first year after diagnosis, although there is the potential for resurfacing of these problem with declines in health or death of the ill child (Gerhardt et al. 2015). In an effort to not lose sight of the healthy children in the family, the PSCPCC has highlighted siblings of children with cancer as a psychosocially at-risk group that should be provided appropriate supportive services (Gerhardt et al. 2015).

Table 13–3. Family tasks associated with specific stages of pediatric cancer

Stage of cancer treatment	Family tasks
Diagnosis	Temporary reassignment of family roles
	Shifts in power and responsibilities
	Engaging family and social support
Acute	Adapting to physical changes in child
	Grieving loss of family life prior to diagnosis
	Balancing treatment demands with family routine
Rehabilitation after initial treatment	Restoration of previous roles and responsibilities
	Reentry into school
	Reintegration with peers
	Adaptation to the functional limitations of the child
	Living with the uncertainty of relapse
Long-term survivor	Living with long-term disabilities caused by illness
	Mourning of losses such as fertility or career goals
	Adjusting to financial restrictions
	Living with the uncertainty of relapse
Relapse	Further readjustment of roles
	Anticipatory grief
Terminal	Integrating and accepting the imminent loss of the child
	Anticipating permanent change in family structure
	Anticipating potential loss or alteration of parental role
	Planning for life after death of the child

Stem Cell Transplantation

Stem cell transplant (SCT) can be referred to as a bone marrow transplant, peripheral blood stem cell transplant, or umbilical cord blood transplantation, depending on the source of the cells that are transplanted. SCT is used to treat hematological malignancies that originate in hematopoietic cells, such as leukemia and lymphoma, in which eradication of the disease requires ablation of the bone marrow (Abraham and Fry 2015; Stuber 2010; Valardi and Locatelli 2016). It may also be used as a rescue treatment when the intensity of the chemotherapy or radiation required to eliminate (*salvage*) aggressive or metastatic disease destroys the bone marrow (Valardi and Locatelli 2016). The transplant process involves a patient being treated with such intensity of chemotherapy and total body irradiation that the ability of the bone marrow to create blood cells is destroyed (*conditioning*). The patient is then *rescued* with an infusion of hematopoietic cells using an intravenous drip. The infused cells may be the patient's own bone marrow cells (autologous transplant), related or unrelated donor bone marrow (allogeneic transplant), peripheral blood cells, or stem cells from umbilical cord blood (Abraham and Fry 2015; Stuber 2010; Valardi and Locatelli 2016).

Between the ablation and engraftment of transplanted hematopoietic cells, the patient is unable to produce red cells, white cells, or platelets. The resulting immunosuppression requires protective isolation from environmental microbes through use of sterile rooms, equipment, toys, and clothes as well as reduction in visitors. Although use of granulocyte-stimulating factor has substantially decreased the amount of time patients are severely immunosuppressed, isolation remains a difficult time for patients and their families.

SCT has improved the survival rate for many children with hematological malignancies. According to the Stem Cell Therapeutic Outcomes Database, from 2008 through 2012, acute lymphoblastic leukemia survival probability estimates for first complete remission were 94.2% for ages 0–10 years and 85.6% for ages 11–20 years at 1 year after transplant and 85.5% and 76.9% at 3 years after transplant from human leukocyte antigen (HLA)–identical siblings. By comparison, from unrelated donors, the estimates were 82.4% and 73.9% at 1 year and 72% and 62.6% at 3 years (Health Resources and Services Administration 2019). Acute myelogenous leukemia survival probability estimates for first complete remission were 83.1% for ages 0–10 years and 79.7% for ages 11–20 years at 1 year after transplant and 71.0% and 62.4% at 3 years from HLA-identical siblings compared with 66.0% and 72.8% at 1 year and 58.7% and 60.3% at 3 years from unrelated donors (Health Resources and Services Administration 2019).

The patient's exposure to high levels of chemotherapy and radiation places him or her at high risk for the same physical sequelae, cognitive dysfunction, and psychosocial adjustment problems as described in the previous section on pediatric cancer. If the patient has an allogeneic transplant, there is the added physical risk of graft-versus-host disease, in which the transplanted hematopoietic cells attempt to reject the rest of the patient's body. Infections, hypothyroidism, cataracts, and bone or joint complications, as well as learning disabilities and psychological problems, are seen in more than a quarter of survivors in the first 10 years following transplant (Stuber 2010; Valardi and Locatelli 2016). The previously described psychosocial standards by the PSCPCC are applicable to these patients, possibly to an even greater degree, given the potentially more extreme stress involved in undergoing bone marrow transplant, which often follows failure of a first-line pediatric cancer treatment (Lahaye et al. 2017; Wiener et al. 2015a).

Psychiatric consultants can provide valuable input and guidance regarding mental health issues to the SCT team through sequential biopsychosocial assessments that highlight adjustment strength and vulnerabilities for individual patients and their families (see Chapter 2). Psychotherapy and/or psychopharmacology interventions can be helpful to these youngsters and their families. Polypharmacy is the rule during SCT. In addition to the chemotherapeutic agents used during the conditioning phase of treatment, patients are frequently prescribed antiemetic medications, narcotic analgesics, and high-dosage corticosteroids or immunosuppressants to prevent the development of graft-versus-host disease. Significant physical side effects include nausea, vomiting, mucositis, and sedation, and in many cases side effects may be cumulative as a result of the need to use several agents simultaneously. The addition of psychotropic medications should be reviewed for interactions with the patient's current treatment regimen and discussed with the managing oncologist.

Palliative Care

Goals of Palliative Care

Palliative care has become an essential aspect of pediatric care for children and adolescents who have life-threatening conditions or need end-of-life care (National Hospice and Palliative Care Organization 2009; Section on Hospice and Palliative Medicine and Committee on Hospital Care 2013). It aims to relieve suffering, improve quality of life, facilitate informed decision-making, and assist in care coordination between clinicians and across sites of care. Recognized in 2006 by the American Board of Medical Specialties, hospice and palliative medicine is the field of medicine that aims to improve quality of care and reduce distress for patients facing serious life-threatening illnesses (Section on Hospice and Palliative Medicine and Committee on Hospital Care 2013).

Palliative care is not provided in lieu of traditional care; rather, it can occur concurrently with disease-modifying therapies from initial diagnosis to later in treatment, when traditional care may become secondary to palliative care (Hirst 2011). There is wide range of pediatric conditions, including those that are life-threatening, those in which early death is inevitable, those in which the condition is progressive, and illness with irreversible conditions, that can benefit from palliative care (National Hospice and Palliative Care Organization 2009) (Table 13–4).

Psychiatric consultants and formally trained palliative care medicine specialists have shared expertise in emphasizing quality of life and identifying comfort as a primary goal in palliative care (Brown and Sourkes 2010). For patients with complex or severe psychiatric issues (e.g., depression, anxiety, delirium), psychiatric consultants bring unique expertise in being able to ensure that care standards for childhood psychiatric disorders are met (Muriel et al. 2016). This stepped-care approach in collaborative behavioral health care is analogous to the goals of integrated behavioral health care in primary care pediatrics (see Chapter 1, "Pediatric Consultation-Liaison Psychiatry").

End-of-Life Strategies for the Consultant

Dying is defined as the end stage of an illness when treatment is no longer thought to offer the possibility of a cure. At this point, the focus for the oncology

Table 13–4. Diagnostic categories that can benefit from palliative care

Life-threatening conditions for which curative treatment may be feasible but can fail, where access to palliative care services may be beneficial alongside attempts at life-prolonging treatment and/or if treatment fails

- Advanced or progressive cancer or cancer with a poor prognosis

- Complex and severe congenital or acquired heart disease

- Trauma or sudden severe illness

- Extreme prematurity

Conditions where early death is inevitable and where there may be long periods of intensive treatment aimed at prolonging life, allowing participation in normal activities, and maintaining quality of life (e.g., life-limiting conditions)

- Cystic fibrosis

- Severe immunodeficiencies

- HIV infection

- Chronic or severe respiratory failure

- Renal failure (non–transplant candidates)

- Muscular dystrophy, myopathies, neuropathies

- Severe short gut, TPN-dependent

Progressive conditions without curative treatment options, where treatment is exclusively palliative after diagnosis and may extend over many years

- Progressive severe metabolic disorders (e.g., metachromatic leukodystrophy, Tay-Sachs disease, severe mitochondrial disorders)

- Certain chromosomal disorders, (e.g., trisomy 13 and 18)

- Severe osteogenesis imperfect subtypes

- Batten disease

Table 13–4.   Diagnostic categories that can benefit from palliative care *(continued)*

Irreversible but nonprogressive conditions with complex health care needs leading to complications and likelihood of premature death

• Severe cerebral palsy

• Prematurity with residual multiorgan dysfunction or severe chronic pulmonary disability

• Multiple disabilities following brain or spinal cord infectious or anoxic or hypoxic insult or injury

• Severe brain malformations (e.g., holoprosencephaly, anencephaly)

Note.   TPN = total parenteral nutrition.
Source.   Reprinted with permission from National Hospice and Palliative Care Organization: "Standards of Practice for Pediatric Palliative Care and Hospice." 2009. Available at: www.nhpco.org/sites/default/files/public/quality/Ped_Pall_Care%20_Standard.pdf.pdf.   2009. Accessed on March 26, 2019.

or SCT team becomes that of comfort and care. Although sudden death in pediatric cancer is relatively rare, it can occur in aggressive treatment regimens such as those involved in bone marrow transplant. Although many children die in the hospital, there has been an increasing trend toward patients returning home during the terminal stages of their illness. This is further reflected in an increasing trend for hospitals to provide a specialized bereavement room in the hospital that creates a home-like atmosphere for the dying child and family.

End-stage cancers present many challenges for both the family and the oncology team. Most oncology treatment centers have developed comprehensive palliative care protocols in which attention is paid to the physical, psychosocial, and spiritual interventions that are specifically aimed at alleviating patient suffering. During the terminal phase, families may become more directly involved in their child's day-to-day care. Care changes from the oncology or SCT team's usual emphasis on cure to that of maximizing the quality of life, lessening pain, and assisting family members in preparing for their child's death.

Consultants who are well grounded in a developmental understanding of death can be enormously helpful in facilitating the grief process in children and families as well as the oncology or SCT team. Children with a life-threatening illness often possess an advanced understanding of death relative to their healthy same-age peers. These conceptions of death generally correspond with the progression through four sequential stages of cognitive development (Table 13–5) (Brown and Sourkes 2010).

During infancy and early childhood, the ages corresponding to those of the *sensorimotor stage*, children have little, if any, understanding of death and rather equate it as a separation from caregivers. Between 2 and 6 years, during the *preoperational phase* of development, children begin to develop an awareness of death but do not recognize it as being an inevitable outcome for all living things, the concept of universality. In addition, children at this stage lack the concept of reversibility, meaning that they are unable to understand the permanence of death. Young children also have limited comprehension of the concept of causality and may use magical thinking—for example, perceiving themselves as being responsible for negative events simply based on the fact that events coincide closely in time with their own thoughts or actions. During the *concrete operations* state, between ages 6 to 12 years, children have a greater capacity for logical thinking and can understand objective causes of death. They also grasp the concept of nonfunctionality, meaning that all functions of the living physical body cease to exist at the time of death. Moving into adolescence, during the *formal operational stage* of development, the capacity for abstract reasoning and the experience of death become more similar to those of adults— for example, with a focus on existential issues such as afterlife.

A child's death represents a reversal in the natural order of life in which parents have the expectation that they will outlive their children. Reactions to a child's death fall along a spectrum from normal or variants of normal to problematic or disordered as shown in Table 13–6. Family members may develop profound and enduring symptoms of sadness, guilt, somatic symptoms, sleep difficulties, and anger as well as significant family dysfunction and marital difficulties. In some cases, parents may overlook the needs of their surviving children, creating feelings of abandonment and emotional isolation. Siblings, too, are strongly affected during the dying process and may present with somatic symptoms, separation anxiety, school phobia, and poor school performance.

The principles detailed in the following subsections may help inform the work of psychiatric consultants with families of dying children (American Academy of Pediatrics 2000; DeMaso et al. 1997).

Table 13–5.   Development of the death concept

Stage	Age	Death concept
Sensorimotor	Birth to 2 years	No concept of death
Preoperational	2–6 years	Magical thinking
Concrete operational	6–12 years	Attainment of
		• Universality
		• Irreversibility
		• Causality
		• Nonfunctionality
Formal operational	12 years to adulthood	Increasing abstract reasoning

Source.   Reprinted from Brown MR, Sourkes B: "Pediatric Palliative Care," in *Textbook of Pediatric Psychosomatic Medicine.* Edited by Shaw RJ, DeMaso DR. Washington, DC, American Psychiatric Publishing, 2010, pp. 245–257. Copyright © 2010, American Psychiatric Publishing. Used with permission.

Mention Grief as Process

Grief is a process that classically falls into three stages that may occur over weeks or months to years: 1) shock and denial, 2) protest and anguish, and 3) mourning and restitution. Children tend to "dose" themselves in their mourning (i.e., a young child can be crying one minute then be right back into play the next). Understanding, grieving, commemorating, and moving on are important bereavement tasks. Consultants can emphasize the importance of parents taking care of themselves as a way of helping their other children. Consultants can recommend support from friends, pediatricians, religious leaders, hospice programs, support groups, and psychotherapy.

Be Open and Honest

Children benefit by knowing at an age-appropriate level about their own or their sibling's illness or death. Some families may be concerned that their children may be too young and that hearing about death may be too painful and

Table 13–6.   Common grief manifestations in family members following the death of a child

Normal/variant	Problematic/disordered[a]
Shock, numbness	Long-term denial and avoidance of feelings
Crying	Repeated crying spells
Sadness	Disabling depression and suicidal ideation
Anger	Persistent anger
Feeling guilty	Believing self to be guilty
Transient unhappiness	Persistent unhappiness
Keeping concerns inside	Social withdrawal
Increased clinging	Separation anxiety
Disobedience	Oppositional or conduct disorder
Lack of interest in school	Decline in school performance
Transient sleep disturbance	Persistent sleep problems
Physical complaints	Adoption of physical symptoms of the deceased child
Decreased appetite	Eating disorder
Temporary regression	Disabling or persistent regression
Being good or bad	Being much too good or bad
Belief that the deceased is still alive	Persistent belief that the deceased is still alive
Relates better to friends than to adults	Promiscuity or delinquent behavior
Behavior lasts days to weeks	Behavior last weeks to months

[a]Should prompt investigation by medical and nursing staff with probable mental health referral.
Source.   Adapted with permission from American Academy of Pediatrics, Committee on Psychosocial Aspects of Child and Family Health: "The Pediatrician and Childhood Bereavement." *Pediatrics* 105(2):445–447, 2000. Copyright © 2000, American Academy of Pediatrics.

increase their worry. However, children and adolescents generally know or suspect what is going on, and open and honest discussion may reduce feelings of isolation from the rest of the family as well as correct irrational worries. Consultants can tell the family that the goal in telling the patient or siblings is to help them gain family support by opening communication within the family as well as to provide an opportunity to facilitate grief.

Be Age Appropriate

As mentioned earlier, the manifestation of grief varies according to the developmental level of the child. Consultants can educate the family about the child's developmental level and the expected responses to death.

Explain the Illness and Death

Consultants can help families and medical staff members tailor explanations to the child's developmental age. For instance, death can be explained to young children as "the body stops working." It can be helpful to draw on past experiences of loss (e.g., other family members or even pets). Euphemisms (e.g., death is like being asleep) should be avoided, particularly with younger children, who may concretely respond to such analogies.

Remember That Showing Feelings Is Normal and Helpful

It is reassuring for parents to know that they can let their children see their own feelings of sadness and anger. It is part of the child's learning experience in dealing with loss. By contrast, parent withdrawal may cause fear and may be experienced as another loss. Consultants can provide parents with permission to express their own grief in the context of their interactions with their children.

Be Alert to Behavior Changes

As noted earlier regarding siblings, behavioral changes are common. Consultants can advise the family to continue normal family routines and discipline as much as possible. Permission can also be given to use family, friends, and relatives for support and help during this time of loss.

Discuss the Funeral

The funeral gives family members an opportunity for connecting or grieving with each other as well as an opportunity to commemorate. Even young children can participate. It is helpful for the young child to know that there is someone nearby who can support him or her (i.e., close enough to put a hand on the shoulder). It is helpful to prepare and structure a younger child's involvement in the funeral process. This may include limiting the amount of time at the funeral, allowing special or private time, or bringing something for the child to do.

Conclusion

Centers and programs providing care to children and families facing pediatric cancers, requiring stem cell transplantation, and/or needing palliative care are increasingly implementing and providing collaborative behavioral health care models that mange the whole patient. Working within these models, consultants have the ability and opportunity to deliver their services in subspecialty care settings that effectively integrate multiple disciplines to deliver high-quality, evidence-based, family-centered health care.

References

Abraham A, Fry TJ: Medical aspects of transplantation, in Pediatric Psycho-Oncology, 2nd Edition. Edited by Wiener LS, Pao M, Kazak AE, et al. New York, Oxford University Press, 2015, pp 141–147

American Academy of Pediatrics, Committee on Psychosocial Aspects of Child and Family Health: The pediatrician and childhood bereavement. Pediatrics 105(2):445–447, 2000 10654974

American Cancer Society: Cancer Facts and Figures 2018. Atlanta, GA, American Cancer Society, 2018

Annett RD, Patel SK, Phipps S: Monitoring and assessment of neuropsychological outcomes as a standard of care in pediatric oncology. Pediatr Blood Cancer 62(suppl 5):S460–S513, 2015 26700917

Brown MR, Sourkes B: Pediatric palliative care, in Textbook of Pediatric Psychosomatic Medicine. Edited by Shaw RJ, DeMaso DR. Washington, DC, American Psychiatric Press, 2010, pp 245–257

Bursch B, Forgey M: Psychopharmacology for medically ill adolescents. Curr Psychiatry Rep 15(10):395, 2013 23963629

Castellino SM, Ullrich NJ, Whelen MJ, et al: Developing interventions for cancer-related cognitive dysfunction in childhood cancer survivors. J Natl Cancer Inst 106(8):dju186, 2014 25080574

Daly BP, Brown RT: Cognitive sequelae of cancer treatment, in Pediatric Psycho-Oncology, 2nd Edition. Edited by Wiener LS, Pao M, Kazak AE, et al. New York, Oxford University Press, 2015, pp 165–176

Dejong M, Fombonne E: Depression in paediatric cancer: an overview. Psychooncology 15(7):553–566, 2006 16355435

DeMaso DR, Meyer EC, Beasley PJ: What do I say to my surviving children? J Am Acad Child Adolesc Psychiatry 36(9):1299–1302, 1997 9291733

Flowers SR, Birnie KA: Procedural preparation and support as a standard of care in pediatric oncology. Pediatr Blood Cancer 62 (suppl 5):S694–S723, 2015 26700922

Gerhardt CA, Lehmann V, Long KA, et al: Supporting siblings as a standard of care in pediatric oncology. Pediatr Blood Cancer 62(Suppl 5):S750–S804, 2015 26700924

Haverman L, van Oers HA, Limperg PF, et al: Development and validation of the distress thermometer for parents of a chronically ill child. J Pediatr 163(4):1140–6.e2, 2013 23910979

Health Resources and Services Administration: Stem cell therapeutic outcomes database, U.S. patient survival report (2008–2012). Rockville, MD, Health Resources and Services Administration, 2019. Available at: https://bloodcell.transplant.hrsa.gov/research/transplant_data/us_tx_data/survival_data/survival.aspx. Accessed March 26, 2019.

Hirst JM: The psychiatrist's role on the pediatric palliative care team. Psychiatric Times, October 7, 2011. Available at: www.psychiatrictimes.com/delirium/psychiatrists-role-pediatric-palliative-care-team. Accessed March 26, 2019.

Kazak AE, Brier M, Alderfer MA, et al: Screening for psychosocial risk in pediatric cancer. Pediatr Blood Cancer 59(5):822–827, 2012 22492662

Kazak AE, Abrams AN, Banks J, et al: Psychosocial assessment as a standard of care in pediatric oncology. Pediatr Blood Cancer 62 (suppl 5):S426–S459, 2015

Kearney JA, Salley CG, Muriel AC: Standards of psychosocial care for parents of children with cancer. Pediatr Blood Cancer 62 (suppl 5):S632–S683, 2015 26700921

Kersun LS, Kazak AE: Prescribing practices of selective serotonin reuptake inhibitors (SSRIs) among pediatric oncologists: a single institution experience. Pediatr Blood Cancer 47(3):339–342, 2006 16007589

Lahaye M, Aujoulat I, Vermylen C, et al: Long-term effects of haematopoietic stem cell transplantation after pediatric cancer: a qualitative analysis of life experiences and adaptation strategies. Front Psychol 8:704, 2017 28539897

Muriel AC, Wolfe J, Block SD: Pediatric palliative care and child psychiatry: a model for enhancing practice and collaboration. J Palliat Med 19(10):1032–1038, 2016 27551812

National Hospice and Palliative Care Organization: Standards of practice for pediatric palliative care and hospice. Alexandria, VA, National Hospice and Palliative Care Organization, 2009. Available at: www.nhpco.org/sites/default/files/public/quality/Ped_Pall_Care%20_Standard.pdf.pdf. Accessed on March 26, 2019.

Pao M, Kazak AE: Anxiety and depression, in Pediatric Psycho-Oncology, 2nd Edition. Edited by Wiener LS, Pao M, Kazak AE, et al. New York, Oxford University Press, 2015, pp 105–118

Patel SK, Mullins W, Turk A, et al: Distress screening, rater agreement, and services in pediatric oncology. Psychooncology 20(12):1324–1333, 2011 20925136

Portteus A, Ahmad N, Tobey D, et al: The prevalence and use of antidepressant medication in pediatric cancer patients. J Child Adolesc Psychopharmacol 16(4):467–473, 2006 16958571

Section on Hospice and Palliative Medicine and Committee on Hospital Care: Pediatric palliative care and hospice care commitments, guidelines, and recommendations. Pediatrics 132:966–972, 2013 28448256

Shah NN, Wayne AS: Leukemias and lymphomas, in Pediatric Psycho-Oncology, 2nd Edition. Edited by Wiener LS, Pao M, Kazak AE, et al. New York, Oxford University Press, 2015, pp 3–10

Stuber M: Pediatric oncology, in Textbook of Pediatric Psychosomatic Medicine. Edited by Shaw RJ, DeMaso DR. Washington, DC, American Psychiatric Press, 2010, pp 231–244

Valardi A, Locatelli F: Hematopoietic stem cell transplantation, in Nelson Textbook of Pediatrics, 20th Edition. Edited by Kliegman RM, Stanton BF, St. Geme J, et al. Philadelphia, PA, Elsevier, 2016, pp 1062–1073

Warren KE: Tumors of central nervous system, in Pediatric Psycho-Oncology, 2nd Edition. Edited by Wiener LS, Pao M, Kazak AE, et al. New York, Oxford University Press, 2015, pp 39–46

Wiener L, Kazak AE, Noll RB, et al: Standards for the psychosocial care of children with cancer and their families: an introduction to the special issue. Pediatr Blood Cancer 62(suppl 5):S419–S424, 2015a 26397836

Wiener L, Pao M, Kazak AE, et al: Pediatric Psycho-Oncology, 2nd Edition. New York, Oxford University Press, 2015b

Zeltzer L, Krane EJ: Pain, in Pediatric Psycho-Oncology, 2nd Edition. Edited by Wiener LS, Pao M, Kazak AE, et al. New York, Oxford University Press, 2015, pp 91–104

14

Treatment Adherence

Treatment adherence, or treatment compliance, has been defined as the "extent to which a person's behavior…coincides with medical or health advice" (Haynes 1979, pp. 1–2). By contrast, nonadherence is defined as the "deviation from the prescribed medication regimen sufficient to influence adversely the regimen's intended effect" (Fine et al. 2009, p. 36). Nonadherence results in increased rates of medical morbidity and mortality. The failure to follow through on prescribed pediatric treatments such as medications, diet, and laboratory monitoring is a common reason for psychiatric consultation in the pediatric setting. Problems with treatment adherence frequently arise in adolescents who have chronic illnesses such as diabetes mellitus or in organ transplant recipients who may have complex medication regimens or stringent requirements for medical monitoring or dietary restrictions (Berquist et al. 2008; Connelly et al. 2015).

Epidemiology

Rates of treatment adherence vary between 4% and 60% depending on the pediatric condition, type of treatment, and the criteria used to define adherence (Killian et al. 2018). Reviews of relevant studies suggest that 33% of patients with acute physical conditions and 50%–55% of those with chronic ones fail to adhere to their treatment regimens (Shaw et al. 2003). A mean nonadherence rate of 30% was found in a systematic review of pediatric transplant recipients (Killian et al. 2018). Rates of adherence to medication are generally higher than those of adherence to other treatment measures such as dietary restrictions for diabetes or physical therapy for cystic fibrosis. Complexity of treatment regimen is associated with higher rates of nonadherence. Estimates of nonadherence are often based on patient report or provider estimates that likely underestimate the true rate of nonadherence (Connelly et al. 2015).

Consequences of Nonadherence

Nonadherence with pediatric treatment may result in adverse consequences that include pediatric, financial, and quality-of-life outcomes.

Pediatric Outcomes

Studies have shown a direct relationship between nonadherence and morbidity and mortality in several chronic illnesses, including asthma and diabetes. Pediatric kidney transplant recipients with medication nonadherence had more than twice the risk of biopsy-proven acute rejection, 1.6 times the risk of hospitalization, and 1.8 times the risk of graft loss (Connelly et al. 2015). Nonadherence in patients with infectious diseases, such as tuberculosis or HIV, is related to increased morbidity and to the emergence of drug-resistant infectious organisms. Nonadherence can also interfere with pediatric treatment decisions by leading physicians to misattribute treatment failures to ineffective treatment agents or by exposing patients to unnecessary diagnostic procedures.

Financial Outcomes

The increased morbidity associated with nonadherence has been related to higher health care costs due to unnecessary or extended hospital admissions. For example, a patient who loses a renal transplant may require hemodialysis, which imposes enormous costs on the health care system. Nonadherence can also burden family members who must miss work or incur childcare and transportation expenses. Persistently nonadherent patients have been shown to have approximately $33,000 higher medical costs after 3 years compared with patients with excellence adherence (Pinsky et al. 2009). Overall, poor adherence to treatment regimens is estimated to result in $100–$300 billion in health care in the United States annually (Aitken and Valkova 2013).

Quality-of-Life Outcomes

Nonadherence affects the quality of life of both the patient and family members (Connelly et al. 2015). The medical consequences of nonadherence can lead to decreased physical ability to participate in recreational and social activities. Children hospitalized for medical complications of nonadherence experience other negative consequences such as missing school, which frequently leads to lower academic performance.

Risk Factors

There has been fairly extensive research on the correlates of treatment adherence (Table 14–1). The results of these studies have been used to identify subjects at particular risk and to develop treatment interventions.

Patient Correlates

Several studies have established a relationship between treatment adherence and the presence of individual psychopathology, including depressive, anxiety, and posttraumatic stress disorders (Killian et al. 2018). Behavioral and emotional problems, feelings of pessimism, and denial of the illness have all been correlated with poor adherence in patients with renal disease and diabetes (Brownbridge and Fielding 1994). Adolescents, especially those with comorbid psychiatric illness, are at particular risk (Shaw et al. 2003). Patients with histories of child abuse and neglect have higher rates of nonadherence (Killian 2017). Patients who are less knowledgeable about their disease also have lower rates of adherence. A patient's past record of adherence is one of the strongest predictors of current and subsequent adherence.

Table 14–1.   Risk factors associated with treatment nonadherence in children and adolescents

Correlates	Risk factors
Patient	Past history of poor adherence
	Adolescence
	History of behavioral difficulties
	Past emotional difficulties
	Presence of denial regarding illness
	Lack of knowledge about disease/perceptions of disease severity
	Feelings of pessimism regarding illness
	Low self-esteem
	Internal locus of control
Family	Lack of parental supervision
	Single-parent family
	Parental conflict
	Parental psychopathology
	Child abuse and neglect
	Poor family support
	Low socioeconomic status
	Lack of family cohesion
	Poor pattern of family communication
Disease	Long duration of illness
	Few or no symptoms
Treatment	Complexity of the treatment regimen
	Unpleasant medication side effects
	Low level of perceived efficacy of treatment
	High financial costs

Family Correlates

Many studies have shown that adaptation to chronic physical illness is closely related to family demographics, including race, ethnicity, socioeconomic status, and financial stability (Killian et al. 2018). Single-parent families are at higher risk of poor adherence. Family support, expressiveness, harmony, cohesion, empathy, organization, and good conflict resolution skills are all positive aspects associated with successful adaptation. By contrast, parental depression and anxiety, parental stress, and parental substance abuse have been correlated with poor adherence. Additional family variables associated with nonadherence include the presence of family conflict, lack of parental supervision and support, and problematic communication styles.

Disease Correlates

Nonadherence is associated with diseases of long duration; adherence has been found to decline over time in patients with diabetes or arthritis and following renal transplantation. Adherence may decline more frequently in patients who are asymptomatic, such as successful organ transplant recipients. Perceptions of disease severity can influence adherence. Parental perceptions of higher disease severity are associated with higher rates of adherence, whereas patient perceptions of severity are negatively associated with adherence, possibly because of feelings of pessimism and hopelessness.

Treatment Correlates

Rates of adherence tend to be lower for illnesses with complex or difficult treatment regimens (Simons et al. 2010). Nonadherence is more likely for treatments that have unpleasant tastes or cosmetic side effects, a particular issue for adolescent patients. Rates of adherence are higher for treatments that have a high level of perceived efficacy and for those that benefit the patient immediately and measurably. In lower-income families, treatment cost can negatively affect adherence.

Developmental Influences

Data from studies on treatment adherence suggest that specific developmental factors play an important role. Numerous studies have shown that difficulties with treatment adherence increase markedly during adolescence (Killian et al. 2018). These findings may be understood by considering the developmental issues in adolescence that may directly interfere with an adolescent's ability to adapt to the diagnosis of a chronic illness. These issues include separation-individuation conflicts, difficulties with risk assessment, and peer group affiliations (Shaw 2001).

Separation-Individuation

The developmental task of separation-individuation is a core issue for adolescents that can result in parent-child conflict. Although there has been little empirical study of this issue in adolescents with chronic illness, clinical observations suggest that adolescents not infrequently act out conflicts with their parents through overt or covert refusal to adhere to medications and/or treatment. Some adolescents may decide to limit or avoid treatment in an effort to reduce feelings of dependency on their parents (Stein et al. 1999).

Separation-Individuation and Treatment Adherence

Chronic illness can interfere with the adolescent's separation from his or her parents if it creates physical limitations or the need for increased levels of parental involvement due to the demands of treatment. A struggle around the pediatric treatment may result in overt nonadherence and treatment refusal. Some adolescents may persistently maintain that they are fully adherent with their treatment despite clear medical evidence to the contrary. Lask (1994) classified these groups as either *refusers* or *deniers*.

Response by Caretakers

Parental reactions to the diagnosis of a serious physical illness in their child can enhance the potential for conflict around adherence. Parents who experience guilt related to their child's illness may compensate for these feelings by failing to set limits on their child's behavior. This type of parenting can indirectly encourage acting-out behaviors such as nonadherence. On the other hand, some parents of children with potentially life-threatening diseases, such as leukemia or asthma, respond with increased anxiety and hypervigilance. This anxiety may then foster overprotectiveness that clashes with an adolescent's need for autonomy.

Difficulties With Risk Assessment

Child and parent perceptions of the seriousness of the child's health condition as well as maternal perceptions of risks related to nonadherence are related to treatment adherence (Riekert and Drotar 2000). However, patients usually cannot accurately assess the risks of nonadherence. Adolescents may be particularly prone to misjudging the consequences of treatment nonadherence because of cognitive difficulties in assessing personal risk, lack of experience with the consequences of risk, ignorance, and denial (Brooks-Gunn 1993).

Cognitive Immaturity

Piaget's theory of cognitive development provides a model for understanding the developmental issues that contribute to poor treatment adherence (Inhelder and Piaget 1958). Young adolescents are likely to employ concrete operations in making treatment decisions and to perceive only a narrow range of solutions to difficulties related to their treatment. Adolescents tend to ignore long-term consequences and make premature decisions when faced with the need to conform to family or peer pressures.

Adolescent Omnipotence

Adolescents often feel invulnerable, and this feeling can contribute to a sense that they are immune to the potential negative consequences of high-risk behavior (Elkind 1967). This observation has led to speculation that poor adherence to pediatric treatment may be based on the patient's belief that he or she can get away with failing to adhere to the prescribed treatment.

Cognitive Limitations

Cognitive limitations related to the illness or treatment can interfere with the adolescent's ability to assess risk. Many chronic illnesses, such as renal and liver failure, directly affect cognitive and academic functioning. In addition, medications such as anticonvulsants and immunosuppressants used to treat many chronic pediatric conditions may impair cognitive functioning.

Peer Group Affiliation

The adolescent's desire for acceptance and conformity with his or her peers often conflicts with treatment adherence (Brooks-Gunn 1993). Chronic illness carries a stigma, and the pressures for conformity may result in resistance to treatment recommendations, particularly those that have cosmetic side effects (Friedman and Litt 1987). For example, corticosteroid medications used in asthma and juvenile rheumatoid arthritis as well as organ transplantation may result in significant changes in physical appearance (e.g., weight gain) that are troubling to adolescents. To reduce the stigma of their illness, some individuals avoid taking their medications in front of their peers or stop taking them altogether (Conrad 1985).

Psychiatric Factors Affecting Adherence

Nonadherence is common among adolescents, but there is a subset of physically ill adolescents who engage in severe risk-taking behaviors, including nonadherence, that indicate the presence of psychiatric comorbidity.

Depressive Disorders

Patients with depression may forget or ignore their pediatric treatment or, in severe cases, intentionally miss medications as an expression of their hopelessness or suicidality. Studies of patients receiving renal dialysis have demonstrated an association between poor treatment adherence and depressive symptoms as well as suicidal behavior (Brownbridge and Fielding 1994). Patients with terminal illnesses may consciously refuse treatment when they judge that the costs of treatment outweigh the benefits.

Posttraumatic Stress Disorder

There are a number of studies that have found symptoms of posttraumatic stress disorder as a consequence of physical trauma and physical illness (Green et al. 1997). There appears to be a direct relationship between symptoms of posttraumatic stress and nonadherence in pediatric liver transplant recipients (Shemesh et al. 2000). Patients who desire to avoid stimuli that remind them of their medical illness may avoid their medications or medical appointments.

Parent-Child Conflict

Family function plays a crucial role in the adaptation of children and adolescents to chronic illness (Lorenz and Wysocki 1991). Numerous studies have shown a direct relationship between family conflict and treatment adherence (Christiaanse et al. 1989). Other family correlates of adherence include parental coping, family support, family cohesion, efficacy of family communication, and parental supervision of the medical treatment (Beck et al. 1980; Hauser et al. 1990). Parental support is critical to ensuring adequate treatment adherence, and families with excessive levels of conflict are at particular risk for nonadherence.

Assessment of Treatment Adherence

To assess adherence, consultants must evaluate the different components of the treatment regimen. Common components include medications; diet; exercise; and monitoring, such as blood glucose or drug assays. Assessment of adherence in older children and adolescents is more complicated because of the parental supervisory role. For younger children whose parents are exclusively responsible for the treatment, the evaluation should focus on parental behavior. With adolescents, the situation is more complex because responsibility is shared between the patient and the parents (Smith and Shuchman 2005). Table 14–2 presents guidelines for the clinical assessment of treatment adherence.

Treatment Interventions

Studies on the efficacy of treatment interventions for adherence in children with chronic illnesses have been limited by several factors. It is difficult to obtain samples of adequate size and to standardize the definitions and measurement of adherence. Many studies have been single-sample studies that help to delineate intervention models but cannot be easily generalized to patients with different illness types or demographics (Shaw et al. 2001). There are few data on long-term outcome secondary to difficulties in recruitment and retention of study subjects.

When effective treatment interventions are being developed, it is critical to establish conceptual models of treatment adherence (Shaw and Palmer 2004). Research on the correlates of nonadherence is a useful first step that helps identify certain high-risk groups (e.g., adolescents). This research also suggests specific interventions, such as treatment aimed at reducing family conflict or improving family cohesion and communication. Conceptual mod-

Table 14–2.   Clinical assessment of treatment adherence in children and adolescents

Treatment regimen

Describe the frequency and timing of each component of the prescribed treatment regimen:

1. Medications

2. Outpatient appointments

3. Laboratory tests

4. Monitoring (e.g., blood glucose)

5. Diet (e.g., diabetes diet, fluid restrictions)

6. Exercise

Patient's understanding of illness and treatment

Describe the patient's understanding of the illness and treatment regimen, including the following:

1. Understanding of illness

2. Understanding of treatment regimen

3. Understanding of consequences of nonadherence

Treatment protocol

Describe the system used by the patient and family for taking the prescribed treatment:

1. Where are medications kept?

2. Who is responsible for remembering the treatment?

3. What is the degree of family supervision of the treatment?

   • Direct observation of treatment

   • Parent dispenses or administers treatment

   • Calls to remind patient

   • Absence of supervision

Table 14–2. Clinical assessment of treatment adherence in children and adolescents *(continued)*

Treatment protocol *(continued)*

4. What aids are used to facilitate treatment?

   • Medication dispensers or pillboxes

   • Pagers or alarm clocks

   • Telephone calls

   • Signs posted around house

5. What are the patient's responses to missed treatment?

   • No response

   • Additional make-up treatment

   • Checks blood sugar and adjusts next insulin dose

Pattern of adherence

Describe the pattern of missed treatments, including the following:

1. Frequency of missed treatment (e.g., once a day, once a week)

2. Days, times, and places of most frequently missed treatments (e.g., school days, weekends, mornings, evenings, home, school)

3. Circumstances associated with missed treatments (e.g., with one parent and not the other, in separated families, while one parent is away or out of town, when one parent is working longer hours, school vacations, sleepovers)

4. Patient's level of distress associated with missed treatments

Major reasons for nonadherence

1. Forgetfulness

2. Reluctance to take treatment

   • Taste

   • Difficulty swallowing

   • Side effects (e.g., cosmetic, nausea, low energy)

   • Embarrassment, teasing, social stigma

   • Lack of confidence in efficacy or lack of trust in doctor

   • Hopelessness about disease

Table 14–2. Clinical assessment of treatment adherence in children and adolescents *(continued)*

Major reasons for nonadherence (*continued*)

3. Treatment too complicated or difficult

4. Lack of resources

    • Cost of medications

    • Transportation difficulties

5. Anger and acting out in relation to the medical team

6. Lack of awareness or belief in possibility of negative medical consequences

7. Lack of supervision

    • Working parents

    • Parental resistance to providing supervision

8. Family psychopathology

    • Parental conflict

    • Parental disorganization

    • Poor communication

    • Parental psychiatric illness (e.g., depression, substance abuse)

9. Psychiatric illness

    • Depression

    • Attention-deficit/hyperactivity disorder

    • Posttraumatic stress symptoms

    • Oppositional defiant disorder

    • Cognitive deficits

els help to identify factors such as psychiatric comorbidity that may reduce the efficacy of treatment interventions.

The family should be the primary focus of interventions designed to improve adherence to therapeutic regimens in pediatric populations (Rapoff 1999). This conclusion is particularly important when parents have the primary responsibility for ensuring treatment adherence because of the child's age. Multicomponent interventions including education, parental involvement, self-monitoring, reinforcement, and problem-solving have been most successful in promoting adherence to chronic regimens (Fredericks and Dore-Stites 2010; Graves et al. 2010). Treatment approaches based on the major etiological factors related to nonadherence are given in Table 14–3.

Educational Interventions

Written and verbal educational interventions should be part of the routine care provided when patients are first diagnosed or when there is a simple goal, such as helping adolescents take on increased responsibility. Consultants must assess the knowledge of the patient and family regarding the illness and its treatment before initiating any adherence-enhancing program. It is important to review with the family the common principles of adolescent development and how they relate to treatment adherence. This assessment should emphasize the family's role in supporting their child's treatment by providing adequate supervision and should help the family anticipate difficulties that may interfere with adherence. The family should also receive guidance on how to respond to nonadherence. Families often react in an overly strong and punitive manner and withdraw privileges rather than increasing levels of supervision until such time that the adolescent demonstrates greater ability to take responsibility for the treatment.

Organizational Interventions

Simplification of the Medical Regimen

It is always important to simplify the treatment regimen wherever possible. Patients with chronic illnesses may be seen by several specialists, each of whom may be prescribing medications without awareness of the total burden of the treatment on the individual.

Memory Aids

Helpful strategies to remind patients about their treatments include the use of pagers, alarm clocks, and telephone calls or text messages from parents or pediatric clinics (Fredericks and Dore-Stites 2010). Other strategies include using pillboxes, storing medications in highly visible places, and posting reminders around the house.

Table 14–3. Treatment approaches for pediatric treatment adherence

Primary reason for nonadherence	Treatment modality
Forgetfulness	Increased parental supervision
	Memory aids (e.g., pillboxes, pagers, telephone reminders)
Inadequate awareness of consequences of nonadherence	Reeducation of patient and family regarding medical issues
Lack of appropriate parental supervision of treatment • Lack of awareness of need for parental supervision • Logistical issues (e.g., working parents)	Education of the family regarding adolescent developmental need for supervision Establishment of effective system for supervision of treatment
Adolescent developmental issues • Cognitive immaturity • Acting out of separation conflicts • Adolescent omnipotence or denial • Peer group issues	Education of the family Increased parental supervision Behavioral interventions (e.g., incentives, behavior modification programs) Possible referral for individual and/or family therapy in refractory cases
Family psychopathology • Parental conflict • Parental disorganization • Poor communication • Parental psychiatric illness (e.g., depression, substance abuse)	Family therapy Possible referral of parent for individual psychiatric treatment
Psychiatric illness • Depression • Attention-deficit/hyperactivity disorder • Posttraumatic stress symptoms	Individual psychotherapy Family therapy Possible use of psychiatric medications

Enhanced Supervision

The first step in treating nonadherence is to increase the level of supervision. This increase may involve parental observation or administration of treatments, more frequent clinic visits, or laboratory monitoring.

Behavioral Interventions

Data support the conclusion that interventions that integrate behavioral approaches including the use of incentives are more effective than programs based on educational and organizational approaches alone (Rapoff 1999). To implement these strategies, families need to understand the importance of reinforcing desired behaviors by providing incentives rather than focusing on negative behaviors. Specific behavioral plans with appropriate incentives and an effective system of monitoring and rewards should be tailored for each patient. For younger children, the program may involve a sticker chart tied to age-appropriate incentives. For adolescents, adherence may be tracked using signatures on a chart with a similar system of short- and longer-term incentives.

Psychotherapy Interventions

In situations in which psychiatric comorbidity has been identified, the patient and family may be referred for psychotherapy. Treatment may involve both individual and family therapy, with the goals of helping the family develop insight into the issues affecting adherence behaviors and promoting a sense of greater personal responsibility. Referrals for family therapy are specifically indicated for families who are unable to provide adequate supervision despite clear education about its importance. Family therapy may also be indicated when significant family conflict leaves the parents unable to coordinate their treatment efforts and motivates the child to act out family conflicts in the form of nonadherent behavior. Treatment intervention studies have targeted family variables, such as parent-adolescent conflict, in an effort to improve treatment adherence (Wysocki et al. 2000).

References

Aitken M, Valkova S: Avoidable costs in U.S. health care: the $200 billion opportunity from using medicines more responsibly. Parsippany, NJ, IMS Institute for Healthcare Informatics. June 2013. Available at: http://offers.premierinc.com/rs/381-NBB-525/images/Avoidable_Costs_in%20_US_Healthcare-IHII_AvoidableCosts_2013%5B1%5D.pdf. Accessed March 26, 2019.

Beck DE, Fennell RS, Yost RL, et al: Evaluation of an educational program on compliance with medication regimens in pediatric patients with renal transplants. J Pediatr 96(6):1094–1097, 1980 6989973

Berquist RK, Berquist WE, Esquivel CO, et al: Non-adherence to post-transplant care: prevalence, risk factors and outcomes in adolescent liver transplant recipients. Pediatr Transplant 12(2):194–200, 2008 18307668

Brooks-Gunn J: Why Do Adolescents Have Difficulties Adhering to Health Regimes? Hillsdale, NJ, Lawrence Erlbaum, 1993

Brownbridge G, Fielding DM: Psychosocial adjustment and adherence to dialysis treatment regimes. Pediatr Nephrol 8(6):744–749, 1994 7696117

Christiaanse ME, Lavigne JV, Lerner CV: Psychosocial aspects of compliance in children and adolescents with asthma. J Dev Behav Pediatr 10(2):75–80, 1989 2708540

Connelly J, Pilch N, Oliver M, et al: Prediction of medication non-adherence and associated outcomes in pediatric kidney transplant recipients. Pediatr Transplant 19(5):555–562, 2015 25917112

Conrad P: The meaning of medications: another look at compliance. Soc Sci Med 20(1):29–37, 1985 3975668

Elkind D: Egocentrism in adolescence. Child Dev 38(4):1025–1034, 1967 5583052

Fine RN, Becker Y, De Geest S, et al: Nonadherence consensus conference summary report. Am J Transplant 9(1):35–41, 2009 19133930

Fredericks EM, Dore-Stites D: Adherence to immunosuppressants: how can it be improved in adolescent organ transplant recipients? Curr Opin Organ Transplant 15(5):614–620, 2010 20651598

Friedman IM, Litt IF: Adolescents' compliance with therapeutic regimens. Psychological and social aspects and intervention. J Adolesc Health Care 8(1):52–67, 1987 3546226

Graves MM, Roberts MC, Rapoff M, et al: The efficacy of adherence interventions for chronically ill children: a meta-analytic review. J Pediatr Psychol 35(4):368–382, 2010 19710248

Green BL, Epstein SA, Krupnick JL, et al: Trauma and medical illness: assessing trauma-related disorders in the medical settings, in Assessing Psychological Trauma and PTSD. Edited by Wilson JP, Keane TM. New York, Guilford, 1997, pp 160–191

Hauser ST, Jacobson AM, Lavori P, et al: Adherence among children and adolescents with insulin-dependent diabetes mellitus over a four-year longitudinal follow-up: II. Immediate and long-term linkages with the family milieu. J Pediatr Psychol 15(4):527–542, 1990 2258799

Haynes RB: Introduction, in Compliance in Health Care. Edited by Haynes RB, Taylor DW, Sackett DL. Baltimore, MD, Johns Hopkins University Press, 1979, pp 1–18

Inhelder B, Piaget J: The Growth of Logical Thinking From Childhood to Adolescence. New York, Basic Books, 1958

Killian MO: Psychosocial predictors of medication adherence in pediatric heart and lung organ transplantation. Pediatr Transplant 21(4): 2017 DOI: 10.1111/petr.12899 28198130

Killian MO, Schuman DL, Mayersohn GS, et al: Psychosocial predictors of medication non-adherence in pediatric organ transplantation: a systematic review. Pediatr Transplant 22(4):e13188, 2018 29637674

Lask B: Non-adherence to treatment in cystic fibrosis. J R Soc Med 87(suppl 21):25–27, 1994 8201583

Lorenz RA, Wysocki T: From research to practice: the family and childhood diabetes. Diabetes Spectr 4:261–292, 1991

Pinsky BW, Takemoto SK, Lentine KL, et al: Transplant outcomes and economic costs associated with patient noncompliance to immunosuppression. Am J Transplant 9(11):2597–2606, 2009 19843035

Rapoff MA: Adherence to Pediatric Medical Regimens. New York, Kluwer Academic/Plenum, 1999

Riekert KA, Drotar D: Adherence to medical treatment in pediatric chronic illness: critical issues and answered questions, in Promoting Adherence to Medical Treatment in Chronic Childhood Illness: Concepts, Methods, and Interventions. Edited by Drotar D. Mahwah, NJ, Lawrence Erlbaum Associates, 2000, pp 1–32

Shaw RJ: Treatment adherence in adolescents: development and psychopathology. Clin Child Psychol Psychiatry 6:137–150, 2001

Shaw RJ, Palmer L: Consultation in the medical setting: a model to enhance treatment adherence, in The Stanford University School of Medicine Handbook of Psychiatric Treatment of Children and Adolescents: Treatment from a Developmental Perspective. Edited by Steiner H, Chang K, Lock J, et al. San Francisco, CA, Josey-Bass, 2004, pp 917–941

Shaw RJ, Palmer L, Hyte H, et al: Case study: treatment adherence in a 13-year-old deaf adolescent male. Clin Child Psychol Psychiatry 6:551–562, 2001

Shaw RJ, Palmer L, Blasey C, et al: A typology of non-adherence in pediatric renal transplant recipients. Pediatr Transplant 7(6):489–493, 2003 14870900

Shemesh E, Lurie S, Stuber ML, et al: A pilot study of posttraumatic stress and non-adherence in pediatric liver transplant recipients. Pediatrics 105(2):E29, 2000 10654989

Simons LE, McCormick ML, Devine K, et al: Medication barriers predict adolescent transplant recipients' adherence and clinical outcomes at 18-month follow-up. J Pediatr Psychol 35(9):1038–1048, 2010 20410021

Smith BA, Shuchman M: Problem of nonadherence in chronically ill adolescents: strategies for assessment and intervention. Curr Opin Pediatr 17(5):613–618, 2005 16160536

Stein MT, Shafer MA, Elliott GR, et al: An adolescent who abruptly stops his medication for attention-deficit hyperactivity disorder. J Dev Behav Pediatr 20(2):106–110, 1999 10219689

Wysocki T, Harris MA, Greco P, et al: Randomized, controlled trial of behavior therapy for families of adolescents with insulin-dependent diabetes mellitus. J Pediatr Psychol 25(1):23–33, 2000 10826241

PART III

Treatment and Intervention

15

Psychotherapy in the Pediatric Setting

The psychological reaction to any physical illness or disability can be viewed as a transitional process that begins with shock and disbelief and proceeds through feelings of anguish (sadness) and protest (anger) toward the gradual assimilation of illness information and adjustment to the implications of the disease. Tailored to the patient's individual developmental level, psychotherapy in the pediatric setting can help patients understand the meaning of and responses to their illnesses. Treatment can be targeted at assisting children or adolescents at various points along this grieving process by enhancing the use of adaptive coping mechanisms that promote the continued psychological development and adaptation to their illnesses.

In a multilevel meta-analysis of nearly 500 randomized trials over the past 50 years, the mean posttreatment effect size for psychotherapy was 0.46, with a 63% probability that youth receiving psychotherapy fare better than those in a control condition (Weisz et al. 2017). Effects varied across the problem targeted, with greater effect sizes for anxiety (0.61) and behavioral or conduct problems (0.46) compared with depression (0.22). In sum, psychotherapy is moderately effective in reducing psychiatric symptomatology and/or achieving illness remission. Although the studies generally excluded youth with physical illnesses, these findings nevertheless do lend support to the potential effectiveness of psychotherapy in the pediatric setting.

Models of Psychotherapy

Psychotherapy can provide a time and place where patients can effectively vent feelings of fear, anger, or sadness. Common elements of the interaction include support, reassurance, suggestion, explanation, and introspective exploration of the causes of a patient's feelings of demoralization (Goldberg and Green 1985). A number of different models of psychotherapy may be applicable in the inpatient setting, including supportive psychotherapy, psychodynamic psychotherapy, narrative psychotherapy, cognitive-behavioral therapy, coping skills training, medical hypnosis, mindfulness-based interventions, and group therapy.

Supportive Psychotherapy

Supportive psychotherapy aims to minimize levels of emotional distress through ego support, enhancement of coping mechanisms, and protection of self-esteem (Green 2015). In the pediatric setting, support may be brief (i.e., during a single visit) or more prolonged and ongoing. The treatment is focused on the here and now, providing the patient symptomatic relief by dissipating the powerful emotions that may have emerged in the context of the illness. The consultant is active and helpful in ways that work to contain anxiety and allow the patient to function (Green 2015). The goal is not to help uncover unconscious motivations and conflicts but to provide education, encouragement, and support. Reassurance and explanation are provided by pointing out the patient's strengths and by removing misconceptions about the illness or its treatment. The consultant aims to support and strengthen existing defenses to better facilitate patients' response to physical illnesses.

Psychodynamic Psychotherapy

Psychodynamic psychotherapy attempts to promote psychological maturation by exploring the turmoil of emotional upheaval caused by the illness.

The therapeutic task is to help patients acknowledge and put into perspective painful feelings of loss that are brought up in the context of their lives (Green 2015; Kernberg et al. 2012). Patients are made aware of previously unrecognized emotions that are blocked from consciousness by their defense mechanisms. It is hoped that by recognizing the intensity of these feelings, patients come to achieve some resolution of their personal conflicts. In addition, Schwab et al. (2013) described a psychodynamic approach to the evaluation of physically ill children that incorporates a focus on the traumatic reactions of their parents. Psychodynamic psychotherapy depends to a significant degree on the patient's ability to tolerate the anxiety that goes along with exploratory work. However, there may be limitations on the applicability of this type of therapy in the inpatient setting for several reasons: 1) acutely ill pediatric patients usually have a diminished capacity of self-expression or self-examination because of the direct effects of their illness; 2) younger patients may not be at a cognitive level to participate in this type of approach; 3) patients may already be overwhelmed emotionally by the constraints of their illness such that they cannot tolerate any additional anxiety that might be generated in an insight-oriented approach; and 4) the brief time available to intervene in a pediatric setting does not readily lend itself to this more reflective and emotion-generating treatment.

Narrative Therapy

Narrative therapy emphasizes the construction of meaning as a central concept and goal. In this approach, consultants allow patients to tell their stories, which in the pediatric setting are generally the stories of their physical illness. Consultants help patients make meaning of their stories and thereby increase self-understanding and understanding of others. Studies have shown positive emotional and physical effects in patients who have the opportunity to narrate their stories in a manner that improves their emotional regulation by facilitating attention and habituation to uncomfortable emotional experiences (Smith et al. 2015; Suedfeld and Pennebaker 1997; Travagin et al. 2015). When patients feel a sense of control over their emotions, they are better able to integrate difficult experiences and experience distress (Schwartz and Drotar 2004).

Cognitive-Behavioral Therapy

Cognitive-behavioral therapy (CBT) is problem-oriented treatment that seeks to identify and change maladaptive beliefs about the self, world, and future and to modify behavior. In physically ill youth, this therapy is based on the premise that patients can develop cognitive distortions that have an adverse impact on their illness and its treatment (Table 15–1). For example, an erroneous belief that important pediatric information is being withheld could lead to the belief that the prognosis is hopeless, which undermines the patient's willingness to cooperate with treatment. CBT can be used to address patients' specific emotional responses that result in distress about their illnesses or interfere with their treatment. It can be applied to counterbalance negative cognitions about physical symptoms and irrational thoughts of being physically ill as well as to treat disabling comorbid mood or anxiety symptoms.

CBT is also useful to address distress at the time of initial diagnosis, anxiety and pain during treatment, adherence to medical treatment, and skills to help with school reintegration (Pao and Bosk 2011). A randomized controlled trial suggested improvement in depression severity, global functioning, quality of life, and disease activity for both CBT and supportive psychotherapy in youth with comorbid inflammatory bowel disease and depressive disorders (Szigethy et al. 2014). In a systematic review, CBT was noted to have positive effects on symptoms of depression and anxiety in children with chronic physical illnesses (Bennett et al. 2015), and a Cochrane database review found that CBT can improve a child's medical symptoms (Eccleston et al. 2012).

Coping Skills Training and Medical Hypnosis

Coping skill techniques such as distraction, relaxation, and guided imagery as well as medical hypnosis are described in Chapter 18, "Preparation for Procedures." These techniques have applicability beyond preparing for procedures in that they can help patients manage disabling anxiety and distress they may experience in the ups and downs of complex physical illness and its treatment.

Mindfulness-Based Interventions

Mindfulness-based interventions are based on the premise of increasing personal awareness on the part of the patient with the goal of improving physical comfort and emotional distress as well as teaching acceptance-based positive

Table 15–1.   Common cognitive distortions in pediatric physical illnesses

Belief that

- Nothing will change the outcome of my illness

- Minor physical symptoms herald the return of my illness

- My illness is a punishment for bad behavior

- I will not be able to resume school or social activities

Fear about

- Inevitable progression of my illness

- Inevitability of pain

- Becoming a burden to my family

- Friends not wanting to associate with me

- Medical information being withheld

coping skills (Ahola Kohut et al. 2017). These approaches have been shown to be helpful in improving adaptation in pediatric patients (Zoogman et al. 2014). Mindfulness-based interventions have been offered in a group format to adolescents with chronic physical illness with the goal of reducing pain, fatigue, anxiety, and depression (Ahola Kohut et al. 2017). A systematic review of use of mobile apps and text messaging for physical and mental health interventions found promising and emerging efficacy as mobile health interventions (Rathbone and Prescott 2017). In this context, there are multiple web-based applications that can be downloaded to computers and/or mobile devices for use by children and their parents in the pediatric setting.

Group Therapy

Group therapy has been found to be useful in physically ill patients who have shared diagnoses or illness-related issues (Gore-Felton and Spiegel 2000; O'Dowd and Gomez 2001). Table 15–2 outlines the functions that group therapy may serve in physically ill patients. The targets of group interventions are attitude and behavior changes that will result in better self-care and, as a result, improved overall health. The heightened social support and reduced feelings of isolation afforded by a peer group with a similar illness or experience are the foundation of group therapy.

Educational groups disseminate information as well as provide a forum in which patients do not feel as if they are the only ones with their illness. These groups can be used to educate and introduce preventive health care (e.g., to adolescents with high-risk sexual behaviors) (Gore-Felton and Spiegel 2000). There are few data on the efficacy of these interventions, but their popularity would seem to support their value to participants, although similar cognitive-behavior-oriented groups more typically use problem-focused skills to help build patient coping skills. Groups for physically ill children must have activities that are developmentally appropriate (e.g., young children may have art projects, storytelling, or therapeutic play as opposed to conventional verbal techniques). Adolescents may be particularly receptive to group therapy with peers who have similar medical diagnoses.

Selection of a Psychotherapeutic Strategy

Factors that may influence the choice of psychotherapy approach include the level of personal functioning along with stability of interpersonal functioning. The assessment should take into account a patient's level of emotional development, intellectual capacity, and ability to assume responsibility. Patients who are more flexible or have a variety of coping responses with more apparent resilience in their functioning are more likely to tolerate psychodynamic treatment. Patients who have a greater tendency to use denial, avoidance, or distortion or who have trouble relating to others are more likely to respond to more supportive or concrete behavioral approaches. Consultants should strike a balance between the different models of psychotherapy, targeting the pragmatic integration of the diverse approaches into an effective treatment approach. Youth with chronic physical illnesses may be at different phases of their treatment, and thus different therapy models may be more effective. For instance, treatment at diagnosis may require a more supportive approach, with a transition to more psychodynamic goals as the illness progresses and as patients are more able to tolerate exploration of their illnesses. Supportive treatment may be especially necessary to prevent maladaptive emotional responses during acute exacerbations of an illness or at times of relapse.

Table 15–2. Functions of group therapy for physically ill patients

Social support

- Establishment of a new social network with common underlying medical issues

- Decreased feelings of stigma and difference

- Emotional expression

- Facilitation of the expression of common emotions of sadness, anger, and fear

- Discussion of issues of loss

- Increased understanding of illness

Education about illness and treatment

- Detoxification of death

  - Facilitation of discussion of issues related to dying

  - Exploration of fears associated with the process of dying

- Reordering of life priorities

- Accomplishing important life projects

Source. Adapted from Gore-Felton and Spiegel 2000.

Therapeutic Use of Play

In childhood, play is a major means of communication and a way that children express their feelings, memories, and reactions to stress, including medically traumatic experiences (Nabors et al. 2013). The direct and indirect (reactive) effects of a physical illness can interfere with the ability to play, and restoration of the ability to play may indicate improvement in the illness or response to psychotherapy. Play can provide a medium in which the experience of the illness can be more easily understood and mastered. Children with chronic illnesses and their siblings can experience a sense of mastery and benefit from expressing their feelings in unstructured pediatric play (Nabors et al. 2013). Play materials, including stuffed animals or dolls, art materials, and medical supplies, are needed. Real medical objects may be introduced to help desensitize the child and provide a sense of mastery.

Several play therapy techniques for physically ill children have been described (Sourkes and Wolf 2009). The consultant can make lists of things that the child does not like about being sick (e.g., medical procedures, nausea, hair loss, hospitalization). In letter writing, the patient and the consultant jointly write a letter to a parent, a friend, a physician, or even a stuffed animal. The child and the consultant may also elect to write an illustrated book about the illness and hospitalization. Even during play, the consultant may make use of a technique called the *therapist monologue* (Sourkes and Wolf 2009). In this technique, the consultant articulates hypothesized feelings or fears that the child may experience. These emotions are introduced to the child in general terms such as "some children feel…" without the expectation that the child respond to the comments. Nonverbal art techniques may be useful in helping gain access to and understanding of a patient's inner world. Techniques such as a feelings mandala project and feelings pie project (see Chapter 3, "Assessment in Pediatric Consultation-Liaison Psychiatry") can prove useful in facilitating the expression of emotional responses and cognitive misunderstandings. The kinetic family drawing technique, in which the child is asked to draw the change in the family following the diagnosis of his or her illness, is a similar approach for facilitating dialogue.

Selected Psychotherapy Issues in Pediatric Illness

There are several important issues to consider in psychotherapy with the physically ill children and adolescents.

Setting

Individual therapy in the hospital may occur at the patient's bedside or in a hospital conference room or hallway, often without the degree of privacy that is expected in the outpatient setting. Patients may be wearing hospital gowns or be attached to intravenous lines. Consultants have little or no control over the patient's schedule. It is not unusual for the consultant and patient to be interrupted numerous times at the bedside. The length of the session may be unpredictable, sometimes as short as only a few minutes. Despite these impediments, it is common for a solid therapeutic alliance or relationship to develop rapidly. This has been attributed to the fact that hospitalized patients are in a more vulnerable emotional state, with relatively fewer defense mechanisms and coping strategies (O'Dowd and Gomez 2001).

Duration

Lengths of hospital stays have decreased dramatically over the past several years, with the result being that consultants generally have time-limited involvement with most patients. This is best reflected in frequent use of brief supportive therapy techniques by consultants aimed at building and supporting coping strategies. Brief treatment approaches, however, are well suited to youngsters who are dealing with the trauma of pediatric illness as well as the attendant feelings of loss and grief. Patients who are dealing with the stress of a life-threatening illness may be more open to psychotherapy because illness may prompt patients to reevaluate their life circumstances (O'Dowd and Gomez 2001). However, consultants will generally find that hospitalized patients are not interested in exploring deep-seated psychological issues but may be open to exploring the current issues related to their physical illness.

Consistency

Fluctuations in a patient's health may significantly limit the consistency of treatment. Youngsters receiving stressful and intense treatment regimens may be unable to participate in therapy either while in the hospital or as an outpatient. They may also be reluctant to give up what available free time they have for something that is seen as dispensable. Children and adolescents in the terminal phases of their illness similarly have difficulties keeping appointments. In addition, patients often prefer to minimize or ignore their emotional reactions during periods of relatively good health and become more engaged in catching up on missed school and peer activities. Consultants require flexibility (e.g., changes in appointment times at short notice) and creativity (e.g., home visits) to maintain treatment consistency.

Illness as a Grieving Process

The bereavement model has been used to help conceptualize the process of adaptation to physical illness and to guide treatment intervention. In healthy grieving, emphasis is placed on the need to discover and accept both what has been lost and what "is still left behind" (Schneider 1984). In addition, this model emphasizes what is possible that would not have been possible if the loss of health had not occurred. The acceptance of illness is a process, and numerous events (e.g., relapse, developmental transitions) may trigger the grieving process. Ongoing losses in a chronic illness can complicate this process and extend the time needed to grieve.

Physical illness may involve loss in a number of areas: independence, sense of control, privacy, body image, relationships, roles inside and outside the family, self-confidence, self-esteem, productivity, self-fulfillment, future plans, fantasies of immortality, unhindered movement, familiar daily routines, uninterrupted sleep, ways of expressing sexuality, and pain-free existence (Lewis 1998). Many of the assumptions of the child's daily life, including their sense of the future, can be shattered by the diagnosis of an illness. Children and adolescents may experience overwhelming threats and fears, including threats to self-integrity and self-esteem, regressive fear of strangers on whom the patient must rely, separation anxiety, fears of loss of love and approval, fear of loss of control of bodily functions, and/or fear of pain and humiliation as well as guilt and fear of retaliation, reflecting the unconscious belief that illness may be a punishment for past behavior (Lipsitt 1996; Strain and Grossman 1975). Emotional adjustment is also shaped by the developmental capacity of children to understand their illness (Table 15–3).

As noted at the beginning of this chapter, emotional responses to physical illness can be viewed as a process that begins with shock or denial and proceeds through feelings of anguish and protest toward the assimilation of illness information and adjustment.

Denial

Denial is generally the first response to an illness as well as a common reaction in patients who have difficulty accepting distressing feelings or emotions. Denial serves an adaptive function in helping a patient at least temporarily ignore or minimize the overwhelming impact of stress that might otherwise threaten his or her psychological integrity. Denial is common during periods of illness quiescence when patients do not face the direct effects of their illness (e.g., pain). Denial becomes problematic when its use prevents acceptance of the realities of the illness. For example, denial may interfere with the acceptance of the diagnosis, delay the search for medical treatment, and interfere with treat-

Table 15–3. Children's conceptions of illness

Preoperational stage of cognitive development (<7 years)

- Belief in the power of magical thinking

- Limited ability to understand functions of organs

- Inability to understand processes and mechanisms of illness

- Tendency to define illness as occurring only when they are told they are ill

- Belief that illnesses are caused by concrete actions

- Belief that illness can be avoided by obeying a rigid set of rules

- Inability to explain why or how these rules prevent illness

- Expectation that recovery from illness occurs either automatically or by rigid adherence to rules

Concrete operational thinking stage of cognitive development (8–10 years)

- Beginning ability to explain complex mechanisms of physical causality

- Immature understanding of the mechanisms of illness

- Belief that outside factors both cause and cure illness

- Belief that illness is caused primarily by germs or contagion

- Inability to explain the mechanism by which germs cause illness

- Expectation that recovery from illness occurs by "taking care of themselves" and allowing medicines to act on the illness

- Limited understanding of how the body heals itself

- Tendency to be more passive about health care

Formal operational stage of cognitive development (10–12 years)

- Ability to think hypothetically and to fill gaps in knowledge with generalizations from prior experience

- More sophisticated notion of concepts of illness

- Greater ability to understand physiological functions of the body

- Understanding that there are many interrelated causes of illness

Table 15–3.   Children's conceptions of illness *(continued)*

Formal operational stage of cognitive development (10–12 years) *(continued)*

- Understanding that illnesses are caused and cured as a result of the complex interaction between host and agent factors

- Understanding that the body's response is critical if treatment is to be effective

- No longer holding the belief that the mere existence of things or events is sufficient to cause, treat, or prevent disease

- Ability to see how diverse factors actively interact to affect health

- Very limited ability to understand concepts of prevention

Source.   Adapted from Bibace and Walsh 1981; Perrin 1984.

ment adherence. Denial has the potential to affect the child's motivation for psychotherapy and make psychotherapeutic work difficult or even impossible.

Anxiety

Anxiety may accompany an illness, particularly when the prognosis is uncertain or unresolved (see Chapter 8, "Anxiety Symptoms and Trauma/Stress Reactions"). Depending on their developmental level, patients may have fears of being abandoned or physically harmed in addition to fear about venipuncture and procedures (Nabors et al. 2013). Fear of dying is not unusual for school-age children and adolescents in the midst of illness flares. Anxiety can interfere with a child's willingness or ability to disclose symptoms, resulting in treatment delays. In contrast, anxiety can also lead children to overinterpret physical symptoms, potentially leading to unnecessary medical investigations.

Anger

Anger is routine, although patients are generally more apt to use the word frustration when asked to name their feelings. Patients develop strong feelings of frustration, resentment, and hostility in the context of the losses (e.g., being with peers, being physically active) engendered by their illnesses. Children's unstructured medical play often reveals feelings of anger directed at doctors and caregivers (Nabors et al. 2013). Patient anger can be directed internally, toward family members, at the pediatric team, or toward all three. Children may judge family members or their peers as being insensitive or unsupportive or even blame ancestors for illnesses that are thought to have a genetic component. The pediatric team may be blamed for a wide range of problems, including poor communication, insensitivity, lack of time with the patient, medication side effects, school absences, or adverse outcomes. Wherever the anger is directed, it is often shown by means of oppositional behaviors, including disobedience, self-defeating behaviors, refusal to cooperate with procedures, or nonadherence with treatment.

Depression

Sadness commonly accompanies pediatric illnesses. As with anger, the intensity of this feeling ranges from an expected normal response to a change in one's life to clinical depression. It can be difficult to tease out the symptoms of reactive sadness from those of the direct physical effects of an illness (e.g., malaise) in physically ill youngsters (see "Chapter 7, Depressive Symptoms and Disorders"). Nevertheless, pediatric patients can manifest their sadness through both their mood and their behavior. They may be less active than expected, whether in the hospital or at home. They may become more focused on somatic concerns and be unwilling or unable to participate in daily activities.

Although most patients will emerge from this cycle of emotions and reestablish a healthy emotional equilibrium, an abnormal response occurs when the child is unable to effectively grieve the losses caused by the illness. Patients may be unable to recognize, experience, or put into perspective the feelings precipitated by the illness. Often, they may deny all emotions or may experience a specific mood to the relative exclusion of others, thus preventing emotional resolution regarding the loss of health. There may also be pathological grief manifestations that include excessive mood disturbances or behavioral problems.

Anticipatory Bereavement

The death of the child marks a tragic and dramatic intrusion into the normal order of the family life cycle. Children are supposed to outlive their parents, not the other way around. Decisions related to treatment during the terminal phase of an illness can be excruciating for parents who, on one hand, do not wish for their child to suffer but, on the other hand, cannot tolerate thoughts of ending treatment. Psychotherapy with the dying child is differentiated from routine psychotherapy by the simple fact that the patient is confronting the concrete reality of death and loss rather than unrealistic fears and fantasies. Patients are generally aware that death is approaching, with the only unknown being its time of occurrence. Nevertheless, awareness of death is a fluid rather than static state (Sourkes and Wolf 2009; Strada and Sourkes 2015). Children tend to "dose" themselves regarding the degree to which they can discuss their illness (e.g., one minute crying and the next minute playing a game). The level of awareness may fluctuate depending on their medical status. Therapy provides the opportunity for the expression of grief and integration of life experiences. It provides an opportunity for discussion of quality-of-life issues as well as facilitating the child's expression of his or her own wishes for what is left of his or her life.

Children and adolescents can derive great comfort from the safety of a therapeutic relationship in which there is the opportunity to discuss their awareness of impending death. The consultant bears witness to the child's extraordinary situation and responds within the context of that reality (Lindemann 1990). A shared knowledge of the fine line that separates living from dying, whether implicit or explicit, becomes the containment of the psychotherapy (Sourkes 1992).

The development of anticipatory bereavement suggests a patient's greater recognition of his or her poor prognosis. The grief related to the impending loss of important relationships becomes manifest in an increased sensitivity to separation without specific references to death or in the form of direct and explicit discussion about death (Sourkes 1992). There may be themes of presence and absence or disappearance and return. Patients can project their concerns onto significant adults as well as show concern about the emotional well-being of their parents or loved ones after their death. There may be fears about being replaced and resentment of healthy siblings. As death draws near, children often turn inward and withdraw from the external world. Normal responses at this time can include quietness, retreat from physical contact, and irritability. It is common for the patient to withdraw from the therapeutic relationship. In the terminal phase, consultants may get to see the child only in the presence of the parents. This may, however, be a time when important disclosures are made by the child.

Countertransference Issues for Consultants

In work with physically ill patients, consultants must possess a high threshold for witnessing and tolerating pain, particularly pain involving separation and loss (Sourkes 1992). Consultants are in the position of witnessing the patient's experience of his or her illness. This requires an ability to contain and process intense emotional feelings in order to allow the child to have access to his or her own feelings and reactions. This is all the more salient because children and adolescents often try to protect their parents by not disclosing the full extent of their own awareness of their illness and may not have another place to share their painful feelings.

Working with children can elicit issues from the consultant's own childhood. It is important to be aware of these reactions, particularly if the individual consultant has his or her own history of childhood loss. Consultants may also have feelings of guilt about their own health or that of loved ones in relation to the patient's illness. Guilt about being healthy may develop unexpectedly and intrude on the therapeutic process, causing consultants to withdraw instead of focusing on the patient's feelings of anger and isolation. It is common for consultants to develop a heightened appreciation for their own health and that of their families.

There is the potential for consultants to overidentify with the patient or the family. This is particularly true when an endearing patient and family are facing severe debilitating or chronic illness. This reaction may be intensified if the consultant is also a parent. Consultants must be alert to rescue fantasies that result in a failure to maintain appropriate therapeutic boundaries. It is possible for the therapist to develop competitive or angry feelings directed toward the parents. Parents similarly may harbor feelings of resentment about the special relationship that can develop between a child and the consultant at this critical time in the child's life.

Awareness of these issues is important for the therapeutic relationship. Children who become aware of negative feelings between the consultant and their parents may withdraw from the therapeutic relationship. A strong working partnership between consultants and parents diminishes this threat and facilitates the therapeutic work. The consultant's role as a therapist is to enhance the parents' understanding of their child's experience so that they can provide effective support to the child. Children may also be helped by the knowledge that the consultant can provide support to their parents.

Sourkes (1992) outlined a number of key aspects of therapeutic work with dying children and their potential implications for the countertransference; these are discussed in the following subsections.

Tolerance for Physical Pain

Consultants must be prepared to witness firsthand the realities of the child's illness. They must be able to tolerate the physical aspects of the child's treatment, including disfigurement or extreme pain. Consultants will often have to endure feelings of profound helplessness involved in watching suffering and yet still feel that they have something useful to offer. Adolescents in particular may heighten these doubts by making explicit accusations, directed toward the consultant, expressing their anger about the injustice of their illness. The consultant's credibility with the patient is based partially on his or her ability to tolerate the physical and emotional aspects of the patient's illness. Any unprocessed feelings of anxiety or discomfort have the potential of intruding into the therapeutic work.

Disclosure of Personal Information

Consultants must be prepared to disclose more personal information than may be typical in other types of treatment. Psychotherapy with a patient who has a life-threatening illness makes demands on the consultant to involve himself or herself to an extraordinary degree. As anxiety, anger, and sadness emerge, consultants may need to join the patient in expressing and exploring these emotions in a way that is linked to the patient's experience. For example, consultants may need to acknowledge that they also would be frightened or angry if faced with similar circumstances. The ability to share these emotions allows the patient to feel less alone and can strengthen the patient's sense of safety.

Consistency and Continuity

Consultants must recognize the importance of their presence in the patient's life as one of the key consistent and reliable figures. Although important in any form of psychotherapy, continuity is an absolute prerequisite in working with physically ill children. The work requires an ongoing availability and accessibility to the patient that is more pronounced than in routine psychotherapy. Consultants must accept the potential need for increased contact and be sure to plan carefully with regard to vacations and absences. Failure to acknowledge and confront these issues may result in countertransference feelings of irritation and resentment as well as feelings of guilt in relation to the patient's needs. There is the potential that consultants may withdraw at critical times from the patient (e.g., close to the time of the child's death).

Processing of Personal Losses

Consultants needs to develop ways to process and mourn the losses involved in the work. Without an outlet for these feelings, the consultant is at risk of harboring his or her own feelings of unresolved grief that may affect work with subsequent patients. Consultants should have access to ongoing support and consultation from peers and supervisors and engage in ongoing, honest appraisals of their capacity for repeated cycles of attachment and loss. Consultants may develop their own personal rituals regarding the death of their patients that can be helpful to facilitate further engagement in their work.

References

Ahola Kohut S, Stinson J, Davies-Chalmers C, et al: Mindfulness-based interventions in clinical samples of adolescents with chronic illness: a systematic review. J Altern Complement Med 23(8):581–589, 2017 28355082

Bennett S, Shafran R, Coughtrey A, et al: Psychological interventions for mental health disorders in children with chronic physical illness: a systematic review. Arch Dis Child 100(4):308–316, 2015 25784736

Bibace R, Walsh ME: Children's conceptions of health, illness, and bodily functions, in New Directions in Child Development. Edited by Bibace R, Walsh ME. San Francisco, CA, Jossey-Bass, 1981, pp 31–65

Eccleston C, Palermo TM, Fisher E, et al: Psychological interventions for parents of children and adolescents with chronic illness. Cochrane Database Syst Rev 15(8):CD009660, 2012 22895990

Goldberg RL, Green S: Medical psychotherapy. Am Fam Physician 31(1):173–178, 1985 3966306

Gore-Felton C, Spiegel D: Group psychotherapy for medically ill patients, in Psychiatric Care of the Medical Patient, 2nd Edition. Edited by Stoudemire A, Fogel BS, Greenberg DB. New York, Oxford University Press, 2000, pp 41–49

16

Family Interventions

Consultants are routinely called on to intervene with families of physically ill children and adolescents for issues such as 1) difficulties with emotional adjustment in family members, 2) family conflict related to the issues of parenting and responsibility for the pediatric treatment, and/or 3) conflict between the family and the pediatric team. Chronic physical illness commonly leads to alterations in the structure and functioning of the family system. From a family systems perspective, rules that have traditionally governed patterns of family interaction and the definition of roles within the family may be challenged by the demands of the illness. The quality of the marital relationship may be altered if one parent takes on a primary role in the management of the child's illness, with the potential for exclusion of the less involved parent. Similarly, an overly close relationship between the ill child and one of the parents has the potential to interfere with important developmental tasks, such as the need for increased autonomy in the adolescent. Successful families maintain their integrity in the face of chronic illness provided they are able to demonstrate the flexibility to make necessary changes to facilitate effective child-rearing in affected and healthy children and can support the goals of all family members.

Medical family therapy describes the biopsychosocial treatment of individuals affected by a child's physical illness (McDaniel et al. 1992). It emphasizes the collaboration between physicians, health care professionals, and family therapists. Medical family therapy provides a conceptual way to understand and promote the relationship among individuals involved in the treatment of the physically ill child. Its goals are 1) to provide a framework for working with chronic illness, 2) to recognize the impact of illness on the family, 3) to promote collaboration with health care professionals, and 4) to promote active involvement of the patient and family members in the management of the illness (Sholevar and Sahar 2003). This approach starts with a focus on the patient and often uses psychoeducational techniques to explain biopsychosocial concepts related to the illness and the developmental issues of the family.

Significant benefits from family system–based interventions in chronic pediatric illness have been demonstrated, including reduced levels of anxiety and conflict and improved school attendance (Distelberg et al. 2016). The paradigm of family-based integrated care has been adopted as a model for intervening in families of children with complex physical illness in a medical-psychiatric partial hospitalization program (Rickerby et al. 2017). In this model, mental health clinicians focus on the family beliefs regarding the physical illness and the relationships between family members. Cognitive-behavioral family-based therapy has been shown to be effective in the management of pediatric patients with chronic pain (Sieberg and Manganella 2015). These techniques have also been adapted specifically to address symptoms of trauma, anxiety, and depression in parents of physically ill children (Shaw et al. 2013, 2014).

Illness Course

The conceptualization of an illness life cycle involves the unfolding of an expected basic sequence (onset, course, outcome, and incapacitation) that evolves over time, with the illness impacting and being impacted by individual and family adaptation (Figure 16–1) (Newby 1996; Rolland 1987).

Physical illnesses in childhood can be classified as either acute or chronic onset. An acute-onset illness (e.g., meningitis) requires more rapid mobilization of family crisis-management skills, whereas a chronic-onset illness (e.g., rheumatoid arthritis) allows for a more protracted period of adjustment. Ill-

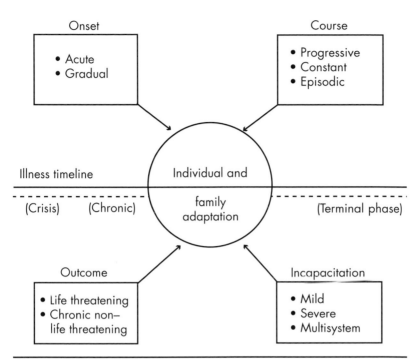

Figure 16–1.   Illness life cycle and the family.
Source.   Reprinted from Newby NM: "Chronic Illness and the Family Life-Cycle."
Journal of Advanced Nursing 23(4):786–791, 1996. Copyright © 1996, Blackwell Science, Ltd. Used with permission.

nesses may be characterized as being progressive, constant, or relapsing/episodic in terms of their chronological course. Progressive diseases (e.g., cystic fibrosis) are continuous and generally symptomatic, with a progression in illness severity. Disability increases in a stepwise or progressive fashion, with minimal periods of relief from the demands of the illness. In a constant-course illness (e.g., head injury) there is a period of stabilization after the initial diagnosis. Recurrence can occur, but in general there are stable and predictable changes to which the family must adapt. Relapsing/episodic illnesses (e.g., ulcerative colitis) are characterized by periods of stability, during which there is an absence of symptoms, alternating with flare-ups and exacerbations. Another critical variable is the extent to which the illness is likely to shorten the child's life. Illnesses may be progressive and terminal in nature or of minor severity. Prognosis can be defined in terms of the degree of incapacitation as a result of impairments in cognition, physical mobility, or disfigurement.

Finally, it is helpful to determine the phase at which the family is located in terms of the longitudinal course of the child's illness. Crisis, chronic, and terminal phases of an illness all require different responses on the part of family members (Rolland 1987). Periods of transition from one phase to another often require family members to reevaluate their circumstances and make changes to accommodate the new demands of the illness. Issues that are not resolved in one phase have the potential to create difficulties in subsequent stages. For example, parents who are unable to agree on career or work changes that are needed during the crisis phase may experience significant conflict or feelings of resentment that interfere with later adjustment.

Family Life Cycle

The family has been conceptualized as having its own life cycle, with characteristic developmental stages that include the single adult, the new couple, the family with young children, the family with adolescent children, the family launching young adult children, and the family in later life (Carter and McGoldrick 2005). Much as in theories of individual development, families are thought to have different developmental tasks associated with each stage of the family life cycle that include adjustments in the structure and nature of relationships to allow for the entry and exit of family members from the immediate family system. Specific hypotheses have been developed to conceptualize the specific psychological issues facing the family at each stage of development (Table 16–1).

Physical illness occurring in a child or adolescent at any one of these stages may interfere with the accomplishment of important developmental tasks. The resultant flow of stress through a family can be differentiated into *vertical stressors*, which are related to historical issues in the family of origin, and *horizontal stressors*, which are associated with developmental life cycle transitions and external factors such as physical illness (Figure 16–2; Carter and McGoldrick 2005). For instance, illness in an adolescent may result in the need for increased caretaking and supervision by parents at a time when the adolescent has normal developmental needs for greater autonomy and independence. The outcome may be a power struggle and oppositional behavior that is expressed

Table 16–1.   Illness and the family life cycle

Family life cycle stage	Psychological issues	Potential adverse impact of physical illness
Family with young children	Focus on the developmental issues of the child Develop confidence in parenting skills Preserve the intimacy of the couple Establish the role of extended family members	Parental difficulties in setting appropriate limits, with consequent tendency to foster oppositional behavior in the child Disagreement about parenting issues Negative impact on the marital relationship Intrusion of extended family in caretaking role
Family with adolescent children	Support increased autonomy of the adolescent while maintaining appropriate levels of supervision Gradual transition to a greater level of adolescent responsibility for the medical treatment	Illness interferes with appropriate adolescent needs for greater autonomy Increased feelings of insecurity in the adolescent and failure of individuation Acting out and oppositionality by the adolescent in response to constraints of medical illness Nonadherence with treatment
Family preparing for children to leave home	Support efforts of the young adult to leave home Young adult develops romantic and social relationships outside the family	Illness may limit or restrict academic and vocational plans of the young adult Interference with romantic and sexual relationships Ongoing financial dependency of the young adult on parents

Source.   Reprinted from Carter B, McGoldrick M: "Overview: The Expanded Family Life Cycle," in *The Expanded Family Life Cycle: Individual, Family, and Social Perspectives,* 3rd Edition. Edited by Carter B, McGoldrick M. Boston, MA, Allyn & Bacon, 2005, p, 2. Copyright © 2005, Pearson Education. Used with permission.

in the form of treatment nonadherence. Similarly, the arrival of grandparents in the home to provide help may be more problematic for the family with a new infant at a time when the parents have yet to figure out their new parental roles.

The concept of centripetal and centrifugal forces has been used to explain how physical illness may interfere with family development (Rolland 1987). Family systems commonly oscillate between periods of family closeness (centripetal period) and periods of family disengagement (centrifugal period). During a centripetal period (e.g., childrearing), external boundaries around the family are tightened, whereas personal boundaries between members are relaxed to facilitate the focus on child-rearing responsibilities. By contrast, in the transition to a centrifugal period (e.g., young adult children leaving home), the family structure shifts to support a loosening of the relationship between the child and the parents and a greater connection to the outside world.

Physical illness exerts a centripetal force on the family system. The demands of the pediatric treatment as well as the need to adjust to changes in the child's level of functioning may result in an inward family focus. Extended family members may be temporarily drawn back into the nuclear family to provide emotional and logistical support. Difficulties arise when the centripetal influence of the illness occurs at a time when the family is at a centrifugal stage of development. Developmental transitions that involve children leaving home may be prevented by the greater dependency that occurs in the context of the illness. Parents may also have to relinquish interests outside the family to focus on caretaking for a sick child.

Factors Affecting Family Adjustment

More than 50% of families with a physically ill child manage to establish a healthy level of functioning, although individual family members may be prone to symptoms of anxiety, depression, anger, and somatic complaints (Jacobs 2000). This positive response occurs across the wide range of illness factors as well as at different stages of the family life cycle. To more fully understand family adjustment to a child's physical illness, the following factors must be considered: illness factors, family belief system, and family structure.

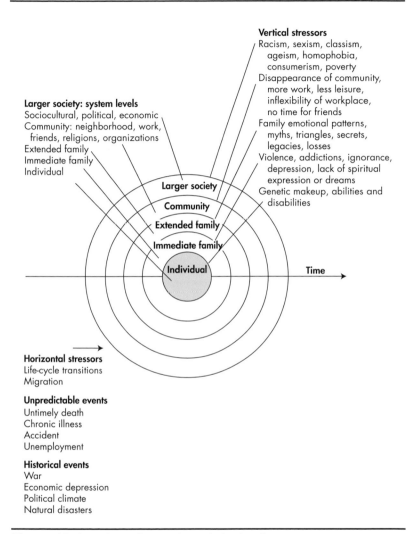

Figure 16–2.   Flow of stress through the family.

Source.   Reprinted from Carter B, McGoldrick M: "Overview: The Expanded Family Life Cycle," in *The Expanded Family Life Cycle: Individual, Family, and Social Perspectives,* 3rd Edition. Edited by Carter B, McGoldrick M. Boston, MA, Allyn & Bacon, 2005, p. 6. Copyright © 2005, Pearson Education. Used with permission.

Illness Factors

Degree of Predictability

The degree to which family members can anticipate acute exacerbations of the illness may affect their ability to make short- and long-term plans. The ability to plan for meaningful events (e.g., school attendance) for both ill and healthy siblings and even smaller daily routines (e.g., carpooling) is critical to the quality of family functioning. Unpredictability can create a cycle of anxiety and anger, particularly in families that have a history of early trauma or loss.

Degree of Disability

The extent of the child's physical disability has important implications for the way roles are allocated in the family. It may be necessary to engage additional childcare on a long-term basis in order for work and family routines to continue. Mothers remain more likely to give up employment or career aspirations to care for ill children, and the loss of income may affect the family's financial resources.

Stigma

Disorders with significant social stigma, such as AIDS, bring up some unique issues. Family members may be reluctant to share information about the child's illness with friends, family members, or professional colleagues. There may be a reluctance to have friends or friends of healthy siblings visit the home. This tendency toward collective shame may isolate family members from crucial sources of social support.

Degree of Monitoring

The degree of supervision and monitoring required for specific illnesses, such as in diabetes or cystic fibrosis, may have a significant impact on the autonomy of individual family members. Adolescents are particularly prone to resist these efforts and may fail to adhere to their treatment. Increased demands for adult supervision may also have an adverse impact on the parents' ability to work and participate in non-illness-related family events.

Prognosis

An uncertain prognosis can leave the family struggling with fears of relapse or death and can be a major source of stress in the family (Jacobs 2000). Illnesses

with a poor prognosis (e.g., acute myelogenous leukemia) are often characterized by the experience of anticipatory grief in family members as they imagine
the child's death. There is the potential for feelings of isolation of family members in families that are not able to discuss these concerns.

Family Belief System

Family behavior cannot be understood in isolation from the family's history.
Family coping patterns are transmitted across generations as family myths, ta-
boos, expectations, and belief systems. Stressors occurring as a result of the diagnosis of a pediatric illness may be intensified because of long-held family
beliefs and prior experiences of illness and loss. Family members may have
particular assumptions about illness and its prognosis as well as traditions and
expectations regarding caretaking behaviors during times of illness (Shaw and
Halliday 1992). Generally, family beliefs are related to illness permanence,
commitment, and connectedness. Family beliefs assist the family in preserving
a sense of competence and mastery during a time of crisis. For example, some
families may see illness as a test of the family strength and as a challenge to be
worked through to strengthen the family. There is often a polarity between family members' belief in their ability to master issues versus a fatalistic position in
which they believe they have no control over the outcome. The family's place
on this continuum often determines how well the family is able to adapt.

Family Structure

Family adaptation is influenced by unique family characteristics that shape
and influence children's behavior. The structural family approach has long
conceptualized the family as comprising different subsystems that are separated
from each other by boundaries and levels of authority (Table 16–2; Minuchin
1974). Healthy families have a wide range and flexibility in the way that their
subsystems interact with one another, but under conditions of stress they may
develop more rigid interactional patterns. Childhood physical illness stresses
the family structure and can result in family members having to negotiate new
patterns of interaction. Boundary regulation, enmeshment, overprotectiveness,
role allocation, hierarchy, rigidity, and communication problems are classic
concepts that have been used to characterize family behaviors in response to a
physical illness (Minuchin et al. 1978).

Table 16–2.   Family structure and physical illness

Concept	Definition	Relationship with physical illness
Boundary regulation	Management of space and privacy among individuals in the family, between generations, and between the family and the outside world	Boundaries are vulnerable to disruption in chronic illness. Individual family members may feel they have no right to private time when a sick family member needs emotional support. There is a potential for coalitions between one of the parents and the sick child or between one parent and a healthy sibling.
Enmeshment	Situation in which there is a high degree of involvement and lack of appropriate boundaries between family members	Boundaries with the outside world may become more rigid, particularly if the illness carries a social stigma. There is a potential for increased risk of enmeshment between the child and parent due to the child's increased need for emotional support. There is a potential for exclusion of the less involved parent and unaffected siblings. There is a potential for interference with the child's developmental needs for autonomy and privacy.
Overprotectiveness	Overly high degree of concern that family members show toward each other	Overprotectiveness is a common consequence of chronic illness. Excessive parental protective and nurturing responses may accompany even minor signs of emotional distress in the child. Parents may excuse their child from normal responsibilities or fail to set appropriate limits, fostering maladaptive patterns of behavior (e.g., nonadherence with treatment).

Table 16–2. Family structure and physical illness *(continued)*

Concept	Definition	Relationship with physical illness
Role allocation	Assignment of roles within the family structure	The ill child may assume a position of centrality within the family. Healthy siblings may be asked to take on caretaking roles or responsibilities that are not appropriate for their age. There may be a potential pressure on one of the parents to take on a full-time caretaking role while the other parent attempts to find new ways to increase the family's income.
Family hierarchy	Level of authority that exists in the family (healthy families are defined by having parents at the top of the hierarchy, with appropriate delegation of responsibilities to siblings and extended family members)	Families with a strict generational hierarchy may have difficulty in allowing healthy siblings to assume appropriate caretaking roles for an ill child. There is potential for inversion of the traditional power hierarchy, with the child using the physical illness to take on an unhealthy position of emotional dominance.
Rigidity	The family's generally appropriate tendency to maintain the status quo	The threat to a family's stability caused by a physical illness may lead the family to persist with rigid patterns of behavior. Attempts to maintain pre-illness routines that are no longer realistic may increase family stress. Families with rigid boundaries may have difficulties in mobilizing social support and allowing the entry of extended family members, pediatric staff, and outside agencies.

Table 16–2. Family structure and physical illness *(continued)*

Concept	Definition	Relationship with physical illness
Communication problems	Lack of transmitting information within the family	There is a potential for the gradual restriction of affect among family members. There is a potential to minimize discussion of important issues because of fears that tension may trigger episodes of the illness. There may be fears that strong emotional expression may worsen the patient's prognosis.

Source.   Adapted from Minuchin 1974.

Impact of Illness on Family Functioning

A family's emotional, cognitive, and behavioral responses are set in motion when a child develops a physical illness. The family experiences the vulnerability of their child along with their inability to control and protect the child from the illness. Successful adaptation requires that the family develop a good understanding of the illness and recognize potential complications and treatments. The family must continue to acknowledge their child's skills and abilities while at the same time accommodating changes in the child's health and ability. Parents must maintain discipline and encourage active contributions from their child and his or her siblings. Three developmental phases—crisis, chronic, and terminal— are helpful in understanding the impact of the illness on family functioning (Rolland 1987).

Crisis Phase

The crisis phase is the period immediately before and after the diagnosis of a physical illness. Pediatric activities are directed toward controlling the symptoms and progression of the illness. This phase is characterized by shock and bewilderment, which are the first feelings of grief regarding the potential loss of the healthy child (Sholevar and Sahar 2003). This is a time when there may be an oscillation between denial of the illness and acceptance of permanent change. The patient's (and family's) concerns and worries about a new diagnosis of a serious illness, such as cancer, can be summarized by the *five Ds*: distance, dependence, disability, disfigurement, and death (Rowland 1989).

The crisis phase represents an existential crisis during which a family may search for meaning in an effort to obtain a sense of mastery. During this time, families may turn to religious and spiritual support. Families may respond to their need for meaning in different ways, including resignation (assuming a passive role in the search for meaning by resigning oneself to circumstances), reconciliation (a more active approach in which the patient or family may believe there is a reason for the illness of which they are not aware but are able to accept), and remonstration (in which there is a continued search for meaning throughout the course of the illness) (Taylor 1995). Table 16–3 outlines family coping tasks during the crisis phase. Anxiety levels are generally high, which can make it difficult for family members to integrate new pediatric information. Additional tasks may include learning how to live with pain and disability as well as adapting to the pediatric setting.

Table 16–3.   Family coping tasks during the crisis phase of the illness

Obtain and retain information about the disease.

Explain the illness to healthy siblings and family members.

Mobilize support from friends and extended family.

Manage the emotional reactions to the illness (e.g., anxiety, depression).

Temporarily reallocate family resources.

Source.   Adapted from Jacobs 2000.

The new illness generally necessitates that other family problems be temporarily placed on hold. If these issues have previously been problematic or difficult to negotiate, the centrality of the illness may serve the role of helping the family avoid having to deal with them. This is common in parents who have unresolved marital issues. Illness may be used to regulate marital distance or parental conflict. Parenting can become an adversarial process if the illness polarizes or fragments the family such that opposing sides are taken regarding issues related to the illness.

Chronic Phase

The chronic phase unfolds after the initial adjustment to a physical illness. In many ways, this is a maintenance period characterized by the hope of minimizing the risk of relapse through appropriate pediatric care. Social support and rehabilitation are important in this phase to reduce disability and maximize functioning. Illnesses can have stable, progressive, and episodic courses of varying time length. In the treatment of cancer, for example, families enter a phase in which they hope for long-term remission but remain aware of the potential for recurrence. As fears about recurrence lessen, patients may be defined as long-term survivors. If the illness is fatal, the chronic phase becomes a period of living in limbo.

Children and their families may have delayed emotional reactions to their illness. It is not unusual for an ill child to be at a different phase in his or her reaction to the illness after treatment ends than other family members are, with family members wanting to move on and to restore a sense of normalcy that may not be possible for the child. Families may experience a sense of abandonment by the pediatric team due to the reduction in frequency of medical appointments. Common concerns in the chronic phase include fears of recurrence, body image concerns, school and academic difficulties, peer problems, and/or awareness of longer-term illness complications. Family members may mourn the loss of past and future opportunities for their child and/or maintain crisis patterns of behavior from the crisis phase that have the potential to reinforce the child's sick role. The term *illness-maintaining behaviors* has been used to describe patterns of poor treatment adherence, excessive dependency on the sick role, behavioral problems, and depression (Frey 1984).

Families with adaptive coping mechanisms during the chronic phase are able to contain the impact of the illness and prevent it from dominating family life. Their goals should be one of restoring a sense of normalcy and reestablishing important family routines that accommodate the demands of the child's illness. It is important wherever possible for the family to accept the permanent changes brought about by the illness and to positively redefine the developmental trajectory of both the child and the family.

Terminal Phase

In the terminal phase, the inevitability of death becomes apparent and dominates family life. The major task is for family members to process their emotional feelings and make preparations for the loss of their child. This is the phase in which anticipatory bereavement and preparation for death occur. It is a time for the family to review their child's life, address family conflicts, communicate important messages, and prepare to say goodbye. Adjustments in the family's daily routine become necessary as the child's health deteriorates. The most common problem that arises is disagreement between parents when their respective treatment goals are different from each other's or from those of the child. In some circumstances, families may attempt to push for or seek out increasingly aggressive or unrealistic treatment options.

Reactions of Siblings

In a meta-analysis, siblings of children with chronic health conditions were found to be especially vulnerable to internalizing problems and negative self-attributes, with older siblings and siblings of children with life-threatening or highly intrusive illnesses more at risk (Vermaes et al. 2012). Siblings have been reported to have a variety of reactions, such as envy; worry about health issues; anger, loneliness, and isolation; feelings of guilt; and school difficulties, including missing school more often because of somatic complaints (Williams et al. 2009). Siblings who have poor relationships with their parents or who are in the middle of an important developmental transition appear to have a decreased ability to tolerate the stresses related to the diagnosis of an illness in a family member (Stewart et al. 1992). Despite these problematic reactions, there are studies that have shown positive effects on siblings, such as greater feelings of closeness and sensitivity to the feelings of others (Nabors et al. 2013).

Families generally have limited emotional and financial resources, and their priorities may need to be reordered following the diagnosis of a physical illness. These changes have the potential to interfere with the goals and routines of healthy siblings. Parents, for example, may have to struggle with how to distribute the available resources and balance the good of one child against that of the other. Siblings are vulnerable to the absence of their parents, who are pulled into caretaking responsibilities for the ill child. Siblings may be put into situations of early responsibility at the expense of their own developmental needs. Parents do experience feelings of guilt or may believe that they have failed their children in fundamental ways by burdening them with additional stress. Siblings are often aware of these concerns and may further suppress their reactions in an effort to avoid further burdening their parents.

Siblings may have confusion about the illness (Table 16–4). Although siblings may overhear snippets of information from conversations between parents and with physicians, they are often not given adequate explanations about the illness. As a result, siblings can arrive at theories of illness based on their own fears and immature perceptions and can develop inappropriate feelings of responsibility or concerns about their own health. Siblings may struggle with conflicting emotions regarding their ill sibling. There can be strong feelings of resentment and complaints about unfairness regarding special treatment or privileges afforded the ill child. Siblings may be called on to explain and defend the ill sibling and to protect him or her from being rejected or teased. Siblings may feel embarrassed or ashamed about the illness and the way it reflects on their family. Normal sibling rivalry may become associated with feelings of guilt in siblings who do not feel justified in having negative thoughts.

Table 16–4.   Questions siblings have regarding their physically ill brother or sister

Questions about causation or prognosis

• What caused my brother's/sister's illness/disability?

• Will it get worse?

• Will she/he ever get well?

• Will she/he die?

• Will I catch what my brother/sister has?

• Has my own health been bought at the cost of my brother's/sister's health?

• Is my brother/sister somehow defective or less of a person?

• Why didn't my parents stop this from happening?

• How can I explain this to other people?

Questions about their own health

• Am I ill/handicapped too?

• How many of my brother's/sister's characteristics do I share?

• Will the same thing happen to me sometime or am I safe?

Questions about unfairness

• Why did this happen to our family?

• What did we do to deserve this?

• Why should I have to live with this when my friends don't?

• Why are there different rules for my brother/sister than for me?

• Am I not as important as my brother/sister?

Questions about feelings

• Do I have the right to be angry at someone who is ill/helpless?

• How come all the money (time, love, etc.) goes to my brother/sister?

• Doesn't anyone know that what I need is important, too?

• How can I help my brother/sister and still get other kids to like me?

• Do I have to love him/her when he/she makes me so unhappy?

• Whom do my parents love most?

Table 16–4. Questions siblings have regarding their physically ill brother or sister *(continued)*

Questions about the future of their brother or sister

- Why do I hear a lot about ill/handicapped children but never hear about them as grown-ups?
- What happens to ill or handicapped children when they grow up?
- Do ill/handicapped children grow up at all?

Questions about their own future

- Will I be able to have my own children?
- Do I carry a defective gene that I will pass on to other generations?
- Will I have a defective child?
- Will some accident or disease strike my life unexpectedly when I'm a grown-up as it did with my parents?
- Will this brother/sister compromise what I want to do with my own grown-up life?

Questions about responsibility

- How much do I owe my brother/sister?
- How much responsibility can I leave to others?
- Where does ultimate responsibility lie for my brother/sister?
- Will I be responsible for my brother/sister when he/she grows up?
- Do my parents expect me to take charge when they no longer can?
- Will I be able to do a good job in caring for my brother/sister?
- Will I find a spouse who will want to share this job?
- How much of what I need and want am I supposed to give up so my brother/sister can be happy, included, and well?
- Do I have to achieve twice as much to make up for what my brother/sister lacks?
- Am I responsible for the care of my parents? Am I responsible for supporting and comforting them?

Source. Adapted from Siemon M: "Siblings of the Chronically Ill or Disabled Child," in *Nursing Clinics of North America* 19(2):302, 1984. Copyright © 1984, Elsevier, Inc. Used with permission from Elsevier.

Working Relationship With the Pediatric Team

Although strong working relationships develop between the family and the pediatric team, the impact of these relationships on the course of the illness is often underestimated. Interactions between the family and the pediatric team directly influence the family's experience of their child's illness (see Chapter 2, "Coping and Adaptation in Physically Ill Children"). The large number of health care providers generally involved in giving complex pediatric care increases the opportunities for breakdowns in communication and conflict around care. Some families welcome the entry of outside caretakers, whereas others are more apprehensive and may want to limit access of medical providers to their children. Problems can arise when parents and the pediatric team are in conflict over the treatment plan. Pediatric team members may even experience pressures to join in a coalition with one parent against the other regarding treatment planning decisions.

As an example, providers and family members must be able to work through the grieving process in a terminal illness to prepare for the death of the child. Family members may avoid dealing with these feelings by failing to integrate information from the pediatric team, by maintaining unrealistic expectations of the team, and by taking out their feelings of anger on the team members. Physicians in turn may experience feelings of failure, sadness, and anger related to their inability to cure the child and may withdraw emotionally at critical points during the child's treatment.

An intervention model for the early recognition and prevention of breakdowns in the working relationship between the family and the pediatric team has been described (DeMaso and Bujoreanu 2013). In this model, three types of family involvements in medical decision making are described: collaborative partnership, deferential partnership, and problematic partnership.

The *collaborative partnership*, which constitutes the majority of working relationships, is characterized by honesty, respect, and compassion with a sense of working together. Families who, for cultural, religious, or personal reasons, adopt a more passive and deferential stance with respect to the medical team characterize the *deferential partnership*. This type of relationship can bring up potential challenges in a health care system where joint decision-making and open discussion about treatment options are valued. The third type of working relationship, the *problematic partnership*, which is based on work by Affleck and

Tennen (1991), accounts for approximately 20% of families and is the one that is most likely to lead to the involvement of consultants. Examples include families who engage in threatening or intimidating behavior with the team, have a tendency to blame the staff for adverse outcomes, use foul language and make offensive comments, or demonstrate entitled parental attitudes. These families often interfere with the provision of good quality patient care and engender reactions on the part of the team that include anger, avoidance, and sometimes deviations from the appropriate standard of care. In the following subsections, we describe a pragmatic approach developed by DeMaso and Bujoreanu (2013) for responding to these problematic partnerships.

Step 1: Prevention

Timely and consistent communication by all members of the treatment team with the family about their child's care is the first step in helping prevent threats to the partnership. This should occur in the context of providing emotional and social support along with appropriate boundaries and setting of limits. This is often best accomplished by frequent multidisciplinary meetings and involvement of the family in family-centered rounds.

Step 2: Recognition

The pediatric team should be aware of any of the early warning signs for the development of a problematic working relationship. Issues should be actively and directly addressed and not ignored with the hope that they will resolve by themselves. Members of the pediatric team should also recognize the ways in which their own attitudes and behaviors may contribute to poor communication. The responsible pediatric team physician should have an active role in the patient's care rather than delegating responsibilities to consultants and ancillary services. Interpreter services should be used whenever necessary. It also is important not to deviate from the standard of care in the case of VIP families and to be aware of how staff burnout or the fear of lawsuits may influence interactions with the family.

Step 3: Resolution

Once the problematic aspects of working relationships are identified, direct and open communication between the responsible physician and pediatric team and the parents can settle most difficulties. If not already involved, the social worker can be called on to help facilitate these discussions. Psychiatric consultation should be requested when there are concerns about mental health, substance abuse issues, or safety concerns regarding the parents. A multidisciplinary treatment team meeting should be held early to identify the potential concerns and to decide on the appropriate response. Subsequent firm and supportive limit setting regarding unacceptable parent behaviors best addresses the situation and is particularly necessary in the context of threatening, demeaning, or intimidating behavior directed toward pediatric team members. Involvement of legal services and patient relations may also be necessary.

Family Intervention Guidelines

Consultants aim to facilitate a system of support for the physically ill child or adolescent through the promotion of collaboration between the patient, the family, and the pediatric team. In this context, consultants can help the family acknowledge the extent of the illness, manage their emotional reactions, and adjust to the demands of the illness and its treatment. These goals are often achieved by helping empower parents to participate in the management of the illness, encouraging the involvement of less-involved parents, advocating for consensus regarding parenting tasks, supporting cooperation among siblings, and/or addressing individual concerns of the child.

Assessment Phase

Effective consultation to any family requires an ability to understand the challenges brought about by the illness. The previous discussions regarding illness factors, the family life cycle, factors affecting family adjustment, illness impact on family functioning, sibling reactions, and relationship with the pediatric team provide consultants with a theoretical foundation for their assessment (see Chapter 2, "Coping and Adaptation in Physically Ill Children"). It is important to have an understanding of any prior psychiatric consultations and intervention efforts so that consultants can understand what has worked and what has not worked well in the past.

Assessing the Family's Reaction to the Referral

Direct consultation for family members is common when the working relationship between the family and the pediatric team is showing signs of tension. It is important for consultants to demonstrate empathy for and understanding of the pediatric team referral concerns. Consultants should be alert for any systems issues involving the pediatric team, including feelings of anger or blame on the part of either the family or the pediatric team. In the initial contact with family members, it is important to assess their attitudes toward both the referral and the physician making the referral. Referrals prompted by a breakdown in the working relationship between the family and the pediatric team generally have some elements of poor communication, lack of trust, and/or frustration related to failures in making a diagnosis or in implementing effective treatment interventions.

Engaging the Family

Rather than focusing on chronic family issues, it is much more helpful to focus on the current problems that are directly related to the illness. Even if the difficulties in managing the illness are reflective of more long-standing problems, the family's focus at the time of referral is usually on the illness. An intervention that results in a successful experience in managing the illness will reinforce confidence in the consultant. The objective can be conceptualized as maintaining a successful balance between managing the illness and maintaining family priorities. The following assessment methods may be useful in engaging the family.

- The *family circle method* consists of asking family members to draw a circle and place their family members and other important people inside the circle. This technique helps assess closeness between individual family members as well as particular coalitions or subgroups.
- The *family genogram* is a diagram that can be helpful in assessing family genetic relationships, relationship issues, and the family's past experience of medical issues. The family genogram can also be used to note important life events in the family.
- The *family timeline* is a chronological description of the important life events within the immediate and extended family.

Providing Education and Normalizing Reactions to the Illness

Although it is the task of the pediatric team to educate the patient and family about the illness, it is important for consultants to evaluate the family's understanding of illness—what did they hear? It is not unusual, given the shock and numbness that accompany a new physical illness diagnosis, for parents to have difficulty integrating complex medical concepts and treatments. Consultants can take an active role in educating the family about developmental issues that may interfere with the child's ability to understand his or her illness and to take responsibility for treatment. The family may need guidance about the need to talk openly with their child about the illness as well as the importance of encouraging and answering questions in a direct yet age-appropriate manner. Normalization of the illness experience is an important therapeutic intervention. Families generally respond well to information that validates their own experience of and reactions to their child's illness. The family may need permission to place normal plans and activities on hold or encouragement to solicit and utilize support from extended family and outside agencies.

Identifying Major Family Concerns

The initial assessment should include an itemization of the major concerns of the family. For example, the concerns of mothers of children facing pediatric heart disease and depressive illnesses have been categorized into concerns regarding medical prognosis, quality of life, psychosocial functioning, effects on family, and financial issues (Snell et al. 2010; Van Horn et al. 2001). Consultants can assist by asking family members about their concerns and having them comment on the relevance of these issues to their own family (Table 16–5). An awareness of specific family concerns can help improve clinical care by enabling consultants to anticipate and address concerns in a proactive way. The results may also inform the development of supportive mental health interventions for families dealing with a major illness. For instance, parents can be supported in providing siblings with information that validates their concerns (Lane and Mason 2014).

Treatment Phase

After the assessment, consultants move into the treatment or intervention phase. This may range from support and education within the role of consultant to a more defined role as a family therapist. Consultants should involve the social work service if not already doing so, given the important role consultants play in working with the family in the hospital setting. The following

Table 16–5.   Common family concerns regarding
                    illness diagnosis

How to discuss implications of the illness with the affected child

How to discuss the illness with healthy siblings

Emotional impact of the illness on the child

Emotional impact of the illness on healthy siblings

How to manage involvement of extended family members and friends

Educational impact of illness on the affected child

How to delegate and manage treatment responsibilities

Conflict or disagreement between parents regarding the medical treatment plan

Increased risk of marital conflict

Impact of illness on parents' work schedule and career goals

How to manage limit setting and expectations of responsibilities for the affected child

Tendency of children to protect their parents due to their concerns about the burden of the illness

subsections detail these intervention principles, which are critical to employ when working with families facing pediatric illness.

Delegating Responsibility for Treatment

Consultants can assist the family in delegating responsibility for different components of a child's treatment. It is common to find that one family member takes on a disproportionate share of responsibility, with the most common dynamic in two-parent families being maternal overload and paternal distance. Common interventions include involving peripheral family members, delegating limited responsibilities to other family members, and giving increased self-care responsibility to the child. Lack of communication between parents regarding these issues may result in significant tension or marital conflict. Single-parent families struggle with not having someone with whom to share treatment responsibilities, and creative efforts are required to increase social support.

Establishing Appropriate Parental Authority

Parents are often reluctant to set limits or to discipline the ill child, particularly during the early phases of the illness. The natural tendency to overcompensate early in an illness, if not corrected, may result in behavior problems and feelings of vulnerability in the child as well as anger and resentment among siblings. Consultants can empower parents to resume their practice of setting age-appropriate limits, which is beneficial for all children in the family. Parents are encouraged to be consistent in their expectations of responsible behavior in both healthy and affected children.

Processing the Impact of the Illness on Family Life

Life-threatening illness introduces issues of uncertainty and potential loss into the family system. To some degree, the impact depends on the nature of the specific illness, its timing in the family life cycle, and family coping mechanisms. In addition to its effect on physical health, chronic illness may result in significant changes in a child's role and lifestyle. Role reversals, for example, may result in the delegation of responsibilities to healthy siblings and reduced responsibilities for the ill child. There can be a progressive organization of family life around the ill child to the detriment of the developmental needs of the family. The first step in the treatment is recognition by the family of the profound and pervasive consequences of the disability. All family members should be given an opportunity to openly discuss the impact of the illness on their respective lives.

Intervening With Siblings

There are several ways to help meet the needs of siblings, including education about the illness, encouragement to express feelings, and opportunities for experiences separate from their sibling's illness (Siemon 1984). Cognitive-behavioral and psychoeducational group interventions have been found to be helpful in improving family relationships and enhancing self-esteem and coping in siblings (Bellin and Kovacs 2006). If group intervention is used, siblings are best divided by age groups into 5–10 years and 11 years and older (Lane and Mason 2014). Open and clear communication about the illness is strongly encouraged because efforts to protect healthy siblings from this information can lead to increased feelings of loneliness and anxiety. Siblings appreciate being involved in decision making and responsibilities that are appropriate for their developmental age. Although it is impossible to completely shield siblings from the impact of the illness, the family should strive to strike a balance such that no one individual in the family is overwhelmed by the demands of the illness. Siblings need to know that their parents can understand their feelings of embarrassment, anger, and confusion. Siblings who feel confident in their parents' resilience are more able to express their own thoughts and feelings and feel secure in their parents' ability to protect the ill child. Parents may need to anticipate questions and concerns and not assume the siblings will independently raise these issues. Table 16–6 lists some general approaches that may be helpful to siblings.

Reestablishing the Family Balance

Families generally respond well to interventions that help reestablish a balance so that the illness does not continue to consume family life. In the chronic phase of the illness, consultants can help the family gain perspective on the illness. Family members can be prompted to recall priorities and routines that were present before the illness. During the chronic phase, consultants can support a shift of attention away from the ill child. Narrative family therapy is useful in helping understand the family's definition of the illness and its impact (White and Epston 1990). Treatment techniques using this model include externalizing the problem and enlisting the family's ability to minimize the impact of the illness on the family's experience. Families may develop rigid or even incorrect narratives about the illness or specific family members that can be revised to allow for greater flexibility and appreciation of different future outcomes. Family therapy can help families take on a broader perspective and reduce the tendency to become overly focused on the illness. Consultants can help the family acknowledge constraints caused by the illness, normalize the family's emotional responses, increase family support, and reinforce the continuance of normal family rituals.

Consultants should be alert to dysfunctional family dynamics when there is resistance to establishing balance within the family. The resistance may lie in the need to resume normal family tasks that involve greater degrees of separation between family members and may also be present when the illness diverts attention away from problematic family conflicts. For instance, the ill child may have a central role in protecting the parents, including hiding legitimate physical and psychological needs.

Table 16–6. Assisting siblings with adjustment to a child's illness

Speak directly in an age-appropriate manner about the illness

Encourage questions about their sibling's illness

Have scheduled family meetings to discuss new information and check in on how individual family members are coping

Spend time alone with each sibling

Encourage attention to healthy siblings when people are focusing on the illness

Include siblings in decision-making

Anticipate behavior problems and regression in healthy siblings

Alert teachers to the stress of the illness at home

Facilitate participation of siblings in camps and social support groups

References

Affleck G, Tennen H: The effect of newborn intensive care on parents' psychological well-being. Child Health Care 20(1):6–14, 1991 10109769

Bellin MH, Kovacs P: Fostering resilience in siblings of youths with a chronic health condition: a review of the literature. Health Soc Work 31(3):209–216, 2006 16955659

Carter B, McGoldrick M: Overview: the expanded family life cycle, in The Expanded Family Life Cycle: Individual, Family, and Social Perspectives, 3rd Edition. Edited by Carter B, McGoldrick M. Boston, MA, Allyn & Bacon, 2005, pp 1–26

DeMaso DR, Bujoreanu IS: Enhancing working relationships between parents and surgeons. Semin Pediatr Surg 22(3):139–143, 2013 23870207

Distelberg BJ, Emerson ND, Gavaza P, et al: A cost-benefit analysis of a family systems intervention for managing pediatric chronic illness. J Marital Fam Ther 42(3):371–382, 2016 27282311

Frey J 3rd: A family/systems approach to illness-maintaining behaviors in chronically ill adolescents. Fam Process 23(2):251–260, 1984 6734795

Jacobs J: Family therapy in chronic medical illness, in Psychiatric Care of the Medical Patient, 2nd Edition. Edited by Stoudemire A, Fogel BS, Greenberg DB. New York, Oxford University Press, 2000, pp 31–39

Lane C, Mason J: Meeting the needs of siblings of children with life-limiting illnesses. Nurs Child Young People 26(3):16–20, 2014 24708334

McDaniel SH, Hepworth J, Doherty W: Medical Family Therapy. New York, Basic Books, 1992

Minuchin S: Families and Family Therapy. Cambridge, MA, Harvard University Press, 1974

Minuchin S, Rosman BL, Baker L: Psychosomatic Families: Anorexia Nervosa in Context. Cambridge, MA, Harvard University Press, 1978

Nabors L, Bartz J, Kichler J, et al: Play as a mechanism of working through medical trauma for children with medical illnesses and their siblings. Issues Compr Pediatr Nurs 36(3):212–224, 2013 23845098

Newby NM: Chronic illness and the family life-cycle. J Adv Nurs 23(4):786–791, 1996 8675898

Rickerby ML, DerMarderosian D, Nassau J, et al: Family Based Integrated Care (FBIC) in a partial hospital program for complex pediatric illness: fostering shifts in family illness beliefs and relationships. Child Adolesc Psychiatr Clin N Am 26(4):733–759, 2017 28916011

Rolland JS: Chronic illness and the life cycle: a conceptual framework. Fam Process 26(2):203–221, 1987 3595826

Rowland JH: Developmental stage and adaptation: adult model, in Handbook of Psychooncology: Psychological Care of the Patient With Cancer. Edited by Holland JC, Rolland JH. New York, Oxford University Press, 1989, pp 25–43

Shaw MC, Halliday PH: The family, crisis and chronic illness: an evolutionary model. J Adv Nurs 17(5):537–543, 1992 1602067

Shaw RJ, St John N, Lilo EA, et al: Prevention of traumatic stress in mothers with preterm infants: a randomized controlled trial. Pediatrics 132(4):e886–e894, 2013 23999956

Shaw RJ, St John N, Lilo E, et al: Prevention of traumatic stress in mothers of preterms: 6-month outcomes. Pediatrics 134(2):e481–e488, 2014 25049338

Sholevar GP, Sahar C: Medical family therapy, in Textbook of Family and Couples Therapy: Clinical Applications. Edited by Sholevar GP, Schwoeri, LD. Washington, DC, American Psychiatric Publishing, 2003, pp 747–767

Sieberg CB, Manganella J: Family beliefs and interventions in pediatric pain management. Child Adolesc Psychiatr Clin North Am 24(3):631–645, 2015 26092744

Siemon M: Siblings of the chronically ill or disabled child: meeting their needs. Nurs Clin North Am 19(2):295–307, 1984 6233538

Snell C, Marcus NE, Skitt KS, et al: Illness-related concerns in caregivers of psychiatrically hospitalized children with depression. Residential Treatment for Children and Youth 27(2):115–126, 2010

Stewart DA, Stein A, Forrest GC, et al: Psychosocial adjustment in siblings of children with chronic life-threatening illness: a research note. J Child Psychol Psychiatry 33(4):779–784, 1992 1601948

Taylor EJ: Whys and wherefores: adult patient perspectives of the meaning of cancer. Semin Oncol Nurs 11(1):32–40, 1995 7740221

Van Horn M, DeMaso DR, Gonzalez-Heydrich J, et al: Illness-related concerns of mothers of children with congenital heart disease. J Am Acad Child Adolesc Psychiatry 40(7):847–854, 2001 11437024

Vermaes IP, van Susante AM, van Bakel HJ: Psychological functioning of siblings in families of children with chronic health conditions: a meta-analysis. J Pediatr Psychol 37(2):166–184, 2012 21994420

White M, Epston D: Narrative Means to Therapeutic Ends. New York, WW Norton, 1990

Williams PD, Ridder EL, Setter RK, et al: Pediatric chronic illness (cancer, cystic fibrosis) effects on well siblings: parents' voices. Issues Compr Pediatr Nurs 32(2):94–113, 2009 21992093

17

Psychopharmacological Approaches and Considerations

Psychiatric consultants are often called on to make recommendations about the use of psychotropic medications, including assistance in interpreting medication side effects and potential drug interactions. There may be requests for medication evaluations for distressed parents and family members. Effective pharmacological interventions can help patients relieve emotional and behavioral distress related to their illness or treatment as well as support the pediatric team in its care of patients.

A target symptom approach works well in the pediatric setting. Although medication use considerations by physicians frequently center on the presence or absence of a psychiatric disorder, medications target specific clinical symptoms as opposed to specific diagnostic entities. In the pediatric setting, these target symptoms generally fall into one or more of the following categories: agitation, anxiety, delirium, depression, fatigue, insomnia, pain, psychosis, or

441

withdrawal. Table 17–1 is an outline of medications that consultants can consider for these target symptom categories when formulating recommendations.

Pharmacokinetics

Pharmacokinetics describes the absorption, distribution, metabolism, and elimination of medications (Robinson and Owen 2005).

Absorption

Medications can be administered by several routes, including oral, intravenous, intramuscular, subcutaneous, rectal, transdermal, or sublingual. *Drug bioavailability* is the rate and extent to which a drug's active ingredients are absorbed and made available for therapeutic action. The rate of absorption is influenced by drug formulation, drug interactions, and gastric motility, which all become important factors when rapid onset of action is required.

The extent of drug absorption is more relevant in the chronic administration of medications. Properties that affect absorption include the surface area, mucosal integrity/function, gastric pH, and local blood flow. In general, gastric absorption is increased when the stomach is empty, although gastrointestinal side effects are often increased when medications are taken without food. Drugs given orally that are absorbed through the gastrointestinal tract may be altered by first-pass hepatic metabolism. Sublingual and topical administration of drugs minimizes the first-pass effect, and rectal administration reduces the effect by 50%. Intravenous drug delivery offers 100% bioavailability and generally results in a more rapid therapeutic effect.

Distribution

Serum pH, blood flow, protein binding, fat solubility, and the degree of ionization influence the distribution of a medication. With the exception of lithium, methylphenidate, and venlafaxine, most psychoactive drugs are 80%–95% bound to proteins, either albumin or α_1 glycoprotein. In general, only the unbound or free drug is pharmacologically active. Drugs such as the selective serotonin reuptake inhibitors (SSRIs) tend to bind to albumin, whereas other drugs, such as the tricyclic antidepressants (TCAs), amphetamines, and benzodiazepines, bind to globulins. Decreases in protein binding increase the availability of the drugs for therapeutic action and may increase the incidence

Table 17–1. Target symptom approach in pediatric consultation-liaison psychiatry

Target symptom	Medication considerations
Acute agitation	Antipsychotic agent
	Benzodiazepine
	Diphenhydramine (younger children)
	Valproic acid
Anxiety	Antidepressant
	Benzodiazepine (only situational anxiety)
	Buspirone
	Gabapentin
	Clonidine
Delirium	Antipsychotic agent
Depression	Selective reuptake inhibitor
	Norepinephrine selective reuptake inhibitor
	Psychostimulant
Fatigue	Psychostimulant
	Modafinil
Insomnia	Diphenhydramine
	Benzodiazepine
	Trazodone
	Hypnotics (e.g., zolpidem or zaleplon)
	Amitriptyline
	Mirtazapine
	Gabapentin
	Ziprasidone

Table 17–1.   Target symptom approach in pediatric consultation-liaison psychiatry *(continued)*

Target symptom	Medication considerations
Pain	Tricyclic antidepressant
	Norepinephrine selective reuptake inhibitor (e.g., duloxetine or venlafaxine)
	Analgesic
	Gabapentin
Psychosis	Antipsychotic agent
Withdrawal	Benzodiazepine
	Buprenorphine
	Methadone
	Clonidine

of medication side effects. Drugs with a narrow therapeutic range, such as divalproex sodium, may be more susceptible to alterations in protein binding.

Albumin binding is decreased in many illnesses, including cirrhosis, pneumonia, malnutrition, acute pancreatitis, renal failure, and nephrotic syndrome. In patients with these conditions, albumin-bound drugs with a low therapeutic index may increase in concentration, causing toxicity. In other diseases, such as hypothyroidism, albumin binding may be increased. Plasma concentrations of α_1 glycoprotein may increase in patients with Crohn's disease, renal failure, rheumatoid arthritis, surgery, and trauma. In general, if protein binding is affected by disease, it may be necessary to make adjustments to medication dosages.

Metabolism

Drugs are primarily metabolized in the liver and gastrointestinal tract and then excreted through the kidney. Water-soluble drugs are readily excreted by the kidneys, but fat-soluble drugs tend to accumulate until they are converted into water-soluble compounds or metabolized by the liver into inactive compounds. Drugs are absorbed from the gastrointestinal system, pass through the liver prior to entering the systemic circulation, and undergo first-pass metabolism in the liver and intestinal wall. Hepatic metabolism may be either phase I or phase II metabolism.

Phase I metabolism, which involves oxidation (via the cytochrome P450 [CYP450] mono-oxygenase system), reduction, or hydrolysis, prepares the drug for excretion or further metabolism by the phase II pathways. Phase II metabolism consists of conjugation of the drug or its metabolites with hydrophilic compounds in pathways such as glucuronidation, acetylation, and sulfation. This produces a form of the drug that is more readily excreted. First-pass metabolism can result in significant changes in the activity of a medication and may explain why there is often a big difference in potency when medications are given parenterally rather than orally.

Hepatic metabolism may be limited by both the hepatic blood flow that delivers the drug to the hepatic metabolizing enzymes and the intrinsic capacity of the enzymes involved in metabolism. Hepatic blood flow may be altered in patients with liver disease because of portosystemic shunting and may be increased in those with chronic respiratory illness, acute viral hepatitis, or diarrhea and in patients taking certain medications (e.g., clonidine). In practice, however, only severe cirrhosis has clinically significant effects on hepatic blood flow. Hepatic metabolism is also affected by enzyme inhibition or induction caused by specific medications, whereas hepatic diseases, such as acute viral hepatitis, may limit phase I metabolism. Liver disease does not generally have clinically significant effects on glucuronide conjugation reactions because of its large reserve of enzymes.

Elimination

Drugs and metabolites may be excreted through the kidneys as well as into the bile, feces, sweat, saliva, or tears. Lithium, gabapentin, amantadine, and topiramate are primarily excreted through the kidneys without hepatic metabolism. The half-life is a measure of the amount of time needed to excrete half of the drug from the plasma and determines the frequency of administration that is required to achieve a steady-state drug concentration. The half-life of highly protein-bound psychoactive drugs is greatly increased. Although the kidney is primarily involved in drug elimination, renal disease may also affect absorption, distribution, and metabolism of drugs.

Drug-Drug Interactions

Drug-drug interactions are a common cause of patient morbidity (Owen and Crouse 2017). They may be pharmacokinetic or pharmacodynamic. Pharmacokinetic interactions involve changes in the absorption, distribution, metabolism, or excretion that influence drug concentration. Pharmacodynamic interactions involve alterations in the pharmacological response to a drug and can occur directly or by alterations in drug receptor site binding.

Cytochrome P450 System

The CYP450 system is a family of mostly hepatic enzymes that perform oxidative phase I metabolism. CYP450 enzymes exist in a number of body tissues, including the gastrointestinal tract, liver, and brain. The hepatic CYP450 system is responsible for most metabolic drug interactions. The major CYP450 enzyme families that are active in humans are CYP1, CYP2, and CYP3. These families are further divided into subfamilies that include CYP1A2, 2C9, 2C19, 2D6, 2E1, and 3A4. Substrates are those agents that are metabolized by the cytochrome enzyme.

An inhibitor may decrease or block enzyme activity required for drug metabolism and cause an elevated concentration of the circulating drug with potential to increase therapeutic or toxic effects. An inducer increases the activity of the metabolic enzyme and results in a decreased concentration in the amount of circulating drug and increased concentration of metabolites. This may lead to decreased therapeutic effect or to increased toxicity due to toxic metabolites. Knowledge of whether a drug has an inhibitory or inductive effect on a specific enzyme may help predict potential drug interactions.

Uridine Glucuronosyltransferases

Phase II metabolism usually follows phase I metabolism and generally plays a minor metabolic role. There are some medications, such as lamotrigine, morphine, and lorazepam, that are primarily metabolized by phase II metabolism. Phase II reactions are conjugation reactions in which water-soluble molecules bind with the drug to make it more easily excreted.

The most common phase II enzymes are the uridine glucuronosyltransferases (UGTs). The UGTs are further classified into 1A and 2B. These enzyme systems also have substrates, inhibitors, and inducers (e.g., glucuronidation of lorazepam is competitively inhibited by the nonsteroidal anti-inflammatory drugs).

P-Glycoproteins

P-glycoproteins participate in the transport of substances out of the body into the gastrointestinal tract, bile, and urine. They are involved in blocking gastrointestinal absorption and are part of the first-pass effect, functioning as "gatekeepers" for CYP3A4 metabolism. The P-glycoprotein transporter does not affect drug metabolism but rather influences drug bioavailability by removing P-glycoprotein substrates and returning them into the gut lumen. P-glycoprotein inhibitors antagonize this process and precipitate retention of P-glycoprotein substrates. For example, omeprazole, which is an inhibitor of the P-glycoprotein transporter system, may lead to increased serum concentrations of carbamazepine, a substrate for this system.

Identifying Drug Interactions

Most pharmacokinetic drug–drug interactions involve the effect of a drug on the CYP450-mediated metabolism of another agent. For these interactions to have clinical importance, the drug needs to have a narrow therapeutic index and only one primary P450 enzyme involved in its metabolism. Agents that interact with different CYP450 enzyme subfamilies do not influence the primary drug's metabolism.

The addition of an interacting drug to a medication regimen in which one drug is at a steady-state concentration may have important effects. If the new drug is an inhibitor of a P450 enzyme, substrate drug concentrations and the potential for toxicity will rise. By contrast, the addition of a drug that is an enzyme inducer will increase elimination of the substrate drug and lower its therapeutic effect. Similarly, withdrawal of an interacting drug from the drug regimen may have important results. Withdrawal of a drug that inhibits metabolism will result in increased metabolism of the substrate drug and lowered therapeutic effect. These changes may require alterations in the dosages of the primary substrate drug to maintain clinical efficacy and minimize potential toxic side effects. If a new, important substrate drug is introduced to a drug regimen that already contains an interacting drug, alterations to the dosage may also need to be made to obtain the desired therapeutic action. Monitoring of drug levels wherever possible helps facilitate safe clinical practice.

Drug interactions that affect renal elimination are important only if the drug is excreted primarily through the kidney. Changes in urine pH may modify elimination of specific drugs. For example, drugs such as antacids that alkalinize the urine may reduce the excretion of drugs such as amphetamine and TCAs.

Psychotropic Medication Use in Specific Physical Illnesses

Hepatic Disease

Hepatic disease may affect drug distribution because of changes in hepatic blood flow, effects on protein binding, and changes in volume of distribution due to peritoneal ascites (Beliles 2000b). The primary effects are reduced availability of medications for drug metabolism and the potential for increased serum drug levels. In acute hepatitis, there is generally no need to modify drug dosage because drug metabolism is only minimally altered and the change is transient. In chronic hepatitis and cirrhosis, however, there is destruction of hepatocytes, and drug dosages may need to be modified. Mild elevations in liver transaminases (i.e., alanine transaminase and aspartate transferase) are common and usually benign and require investigation only if elevated two to three times above baseline. By contrast, elevations in bilirubin or alkaline phosphatase suggest involvement of the biliary tract and may require further evaluation.

Liver cirrhosis may distort liver architecture and alter hepatic blood flow. In severe disease, portosystemic shunting may affect 60% or more of portal vein flow that diverts circulating drugs away from the liver, resulting in decreased drug extraction and first-pass metabolism. By contrast, hepatic blood flow may be increased in viral hepatitis and in patients with chronic respiratory problems. Medications with high baseline rates of clearance by the liver (e.g., haloperidol, paroxetine, sertraline, nefazodone, venlafaxine, TCAs, midazolam) are significantly affected by alterations in hepatic blood flow.

Albumin and α_1 glycoproteins that are produced in the liver may be reduced in patients with infectious and inflammatory hepatic disease, whereas surgery, trauma, and cirrhosis may result in elevated protein levels. Elevated serum bilirubin levels are found in acute viral hepatitis and primary biliary cirrhosis. Bilirubin has a strong affinity for albumin binding sites and may displace medications (e.g., divalproex sodium, phenytoin). In steady-state situations, changes in protein binding may result in elevated, unbound, active forms of a drug in the presence of normal serum total drug concentrations. Because it is often difficult to predict changes in drug protein binding, it is important to pay close attention to the clinical and toxic effects of psychotropic medications and not rely exclusively on serum drug concentrations.

In general, for patients with hepatic disease, it is necessary to use lower dosages of medications (Table 17–2). Initial dosing of medications should be reduced in patients with hepatic disease, and titration should proceed more slowly. For drugs that have significant hepatic metabolism, intravenous administration may be preferred. In general, parenteral administration of drugs avoids first-pass metabolic effects, and the dosing and action of drugs are similar to those in patients with normal hepatic function.

Gastrointestinal Disease

Gastrointestinal disease primarily affects drug absorption (Beliles 2000b). Examples of conditions that affect absorption include diseases affecting gastrointestinal motility, surgical alteration of the gastrointestinal tract (e.g., bypass surgery, G-tube and J-tube placement), short bowel syndrome, and celiac disease. Any conditions that divert blood away from the gastrointestinal tract (e.g., congestive heart failure, shock) may also affect absorption. Administration of antacid medications may similarly reduce gastric absorption.

Gastric motility may be affected by a number of pediatric conditions and by specific medications. For example, gastric motility is delayed in patients with diabetes mellitus, gastritis, and pyloric stenosis. Anticholinergic medications delay gastric motility. A number of medications are given to increase gastrointestinal motility, including metoclopramide, cisapride, and propantheline. In general, slowed gastrointestinal motility results in better absorption of poorly soluble drugs and vice versa. Enteric-coated preparations of medications are likely to have increased rates of drug absorption in patients with reduced gastric acidity. Orally administered drugs may be poorly absorbed in patients with malabsorption syndromes. If absorption is an issue, liquid formulations of drugs and alternative routes of administration such as sublingual, intramuscular, and intravenous may be preferred. Gastrointestinal disease affecting the large intestines generally has little effect because most medications are absorbed more proximally.

Table 17–2.   Medication use in hepatic disease

Medication class	Impact of hepatic disease on drug dosing	Potential drug effect on liver function
Antidepressants	Antidepressants that are metabolized by phase I hepatic oxidative metabolism require an approximately 50% dose reduction.	Tricyclic antidepressants may exacerbate hepatic encephalopathy by anticholinergic action.
	Doses of bupropion should not exceed 75 mg/day in patients with cirrhosis.	Minor elevations in transaminases are common and usually benign.
	Trazodone requires dose reduction because of prolonged clearance of trazodone in patients with hepatic disease.	Sertraline's short half-life and less potent inhibition of CYP2D6 make it the preferred SSRI in hepatic disease.
Antipsychotics	Atypical antipsychotics that are metabolized by phase I hepatic oxidative metabolism require dose reduction.	Chlorpromazine is associated with intrahepatic cholestasis and obstructive hepatic disease.
		Low-potency drugs may precipitate hepatic encephalopathy in patients with cirrhosis.
		Discontinue clozapine in patients with marked transaminase elevations or jaundice.

Table 17–2. Medication use in hepatic disease *(continued)*

Medication class	Impact of hepatic disease on drug dosing	Potential drug effect on liver function
Anxiolytics/hypnotics	Benzodiazepine half-lives are increased in hepatic disease.	Avoid use of benzodiazepines in patients at risk of hepatic encephalopathy.
	Lorazepam, oxazepam, and temazepam require no dose adjustment in hepatic disease because they are metabolized by phase II hepatic oxidative metabolism.	
	Zaleplon and zolpidem require dose reduction.	
Mood stabilizers	Carbamazepine, divalproex, lamotrigine, and topiramate require dose reduction and close monitoring.	Depakote is associated with hepatic failure in 1 in 40,000 cases.
	No dose adjustment is required for lamotrigine, gabapentin, or lithium.	Carbamazepine use is associated with hepatitis.
		Carbamazepine and valproic acid are contraindicated in patients with preexisting hepatic disease.
ADHD medication	Atomoxetine requires 25%–50% reduction in dose.	

Note.   CYP=cytochrome P450; SSRI=selective serotonin reuptake inhibitor.
Source.   Adapted from Beliles 2000a; Jacobson 2002; Robinson and Owen 2005.

Many psychotropic medications have the potential to cause gastrointestinal side effects. Medications with anticholinergic side effects can slow gastrointestinal motility, affect absorption, and cause constipation. By contrast, SSRIs increase gastric motility and may cause diarrhea. SSRIs also have a potential to increase the risk of gastrointestinal bleeding, especially when coadministered with nonsteroidal anti-inflammatory drugs. Using extended- or controlled-release preparations of medications may reduce gastrointestinal side effects, particularly in cases in which gastric distress is related to rapid increases in plasma drug concentrations.

Renal Disease

Renal insufficiency results in a functional loss of nephrons. This is generally a transient and reversible phenomenon in acute renal failure, but in chronic renal failure it may be permanent and lead to the need for dialysis. Pharmacodynamic effects of renal failure include increased receptor sensitivity, and pharmacokinetic effects include delayed drug clearance (Beliles 2000b). Renal insufficiency may result in decreased absorption of drugs from the small intestine due to the gastric-alkalinizing effects of increased ammonia levels that develop in the presence of excess urea. Renal insufficiency may increase the volume of distribution of water-soluble or protein-bound drugs, with a consequent reduction in plasma levels at normal drug dosages. Plasma protein binding of drugs may be reduced in nephrotic syndrome as a result of decreases in albumin concentration. Displacement of highly protein-bound drugs may result in increased availability of these drugs for renal filtration and excretion. Renal insufficiency may also be associated with decreased first-pass metabolism and influence hepatic clearance due to CYP2D6 inhibition. Renal excretion or clearance is reduced in renal failure and is significant for drugs that are cleared primarily by renal excretion. Renal blood flow may be altered by changes in glomerular vasculature, severe dehydration, and conditions affecting other organ syndromes (e.g., cirrhosis).

In general, initial dosages of medications should be reduced or dosing intervals lengthened in patients with renal failure (Table 17–3). The *rule of two-thirds* is that dosages of medications should be reduced by one-third of the normal dosage in patients with renal insufficiency. However, most psychotropic medications, with the exception of lithium and gabapentin, do not require significant adjustments to dosing in patients with renal failure. It is important to carefully monitor serum concentrations in patients with renal insufficiency, particularly for medications with a narrow therapeutic index. Lithium may be given to renal transplant recipients; however, cyclosporine may elevate serum lithium levels by decreasing lithium excretion, necessitating a dosage adjustment. Patients with renal failure and those on dialysis appear to be more sensitive to the side effects of the TCAs, possibly because of the accumulation of hydroxylated tricyclic metabolites. However, SSRIs have generally supplanted the use of TCAs in the treatment of depression in patients with renal insufficiency.

Hemodialysis

Special consideration should be given to patients on hemodialysis. During hemodialysis, there may be an initial lowering of the plasma drug concentration followed by a rebound after dialysis as the drug redistributes from the periphery to the circulation. Drugs that are highly protein bound (this includes most of the psychotropic agents with the exception of lithium, divalproex sodium, venlafaxine, gabapentin, and topiramate) are generally not significantly cleared by dialysis. Drugs such as lithium and gabapentin are completely removed by dialysis, and the common practice is to administer these medications after dialysis. Drugs with a narrow therapeutic index should be avoided wherever possible in patients who are on dialysis. In addition, patients on dialysis often have significant fluid shifts and are at risk of dehydration. Neuroleptic malignant syndrome may be more likely in these situations (see Chapter 6, "Neurocognitive Disturbances"). Another common issue is that of orthostatic hypertension, which occurs particularly following dialysis.

Cardiac Disease

Cardiac disease may influence the pharmacokinetics of medications. For example, congestive heart failure may result in decreased perfusion of drug absorption sites both in the gastrointestinal tract and in skeletal muscle, affecting drugs given both orally and by intramuscular injection (Beliles 2000b). Sympathetic activity may redistribute blood flow to the brain and heart, reducing perfusion of the liver, kidney, and other organs, with the potential to affect drug distribution. Local edema may also reduce epithelial permeability and increase drug absorption. Cardiac patients are commonly treated with anticoagulant medications (e.g., warfarin) that are highly protein bound. In these situations,

Table 17–3. Medication use in renal disease

Medication class	Impact of renal disease on drug dosing	Potential drug effect on renal function
Antidepressants	SSRIs and TCAs require no dose adjustment except in severe renal insufficiency.	Patients with renal insufficiency are more susceptible to TCA side effects especially sedation and anticholinergic effects.
	Venlafaxine requires 25%–75% reduction in dose because of reduced renal clearance.	
Antipsychotics	Risperidone requires dose reduction.	Antipsychotic agents are generally safe.
Anxiolytics/hypnotics	Benzodiazepines, especially chlordiazepoxide, require dose reduction because of increased half-life in renal insufficiency.	Barbiturate use should be avoided due to the risk of excessive sedation.
	Lorazepam and oxazepam are preferred because of the absence of active metabolites.	
Mood stabilizers	Lithium, topiramate, and gabapentin require 50%–75% reduction in dose.	Lithium is contraindicated in acute renal failure but is considered safe in chronic renal failure with a dose adjustment.
	Divalproex sodium requires no dose adjustment.	Lithium requires dose reduction in patients on hemodialysis
		Lithium should be given after dialysis.

Note.   SSRI=selective serotonin reuptake inhibitor; TCA=tricyclic antidepressant.
Source.   Adapted from Beliles 2000a; Jacobson 2002; Robinson and Owen 2005.

it may be necessary to reduce the dosage of highly protein-bound psychotropic agents to reduce the potential risk of elevated levels of anticoagulants.

Potential cardiovascular side effects of psychotropic medications include orthostatic hypotension, conduction disturbances, and arrhythmias (Table 17–4). Orthostatic hypotension is one of the most common cardiovascular side effects that complicate the use of TCAs. The risk is increased in patients who have impaired left ventricular function. If TCAs are used in patients with cardiac disease, nortriptyline is thought to be less likely to result in orthostatic hypotension. Trazodone may result in orthostatic hypotension and exacerbate myocardial instability. As a result, SSRIs and bupropion are preferred as antidepressant agents in patients with cardiac disease.

There is the potential for increased cardiac morbidity and mortality, particularly in patients with preexisting cardiac conduction problems such as atrioventricular block. Intravenous haloperidol has been associated with the development of arrhythmias, including QT_c prolongation and torsades de pointes, and may depress cardiovascular function (Beliles 2000a). Both TCAs and lithium may exacerbate congestive cardiac failure. Some of the calcium channel–blocking agents, such as diltiazem and verapamil, may slow atrioventricular conduction and may theoretically interact with the TCAs. Patients with Wolff-Parkinson-White syndrome who have a short PR interval (less than 0.27 seconds) and widened QRS interval associated with paroxysmal tachycardia are at high risk of life-threatening ventricular tachycardia that may be exacerbated by the use of TCAs.

Quinidine-like effects of the TCAs and antipsychotic agents may lead to prolongation of the QT_c interval with increased risk of ventricular tachycardia and ventricular fibrillation, particularly in patients with congenital heart disease. Patients with a baseline QT_c interval of greater than 440 msec should be considered at particular risk. The range of normal QT_c values in children is 400 msec ± 25–30 msec. A QT_c value that exceeds two standard deviations (> 450–460 msec) is considered too long and may be associated with increased mortality (Labellarte et al. 2003). An increase in the QT_c of greater than 60 msec from baseline is also associated with increased mortality. It is important to keep in mind that computer readouts of the electrocardiogram are not reliable, particularly in situations of tachycardia or bradycardia. Situations that should prompt cardiology consultation include QT_c duration longer than 480 msec, QT_c prolongation longer than 60 msec over baseline, prolonged QT_c dura-

Table 17–4.   Medication use in cardiac disease

Medication class	Potential drug effect on cardiac function
Tricyclic antidepressants	Increased cardiac morbidity and mortality due to arrhythmias
	Side effects in healthy individuals limited to orthostatic hypotension.
	Nortriptyline the preferred TCA because of its lower likelihood of hypotension
	Potential for delayed cardiac conduction, increased heart rate, and heart block
	Prolonged PR interval, QRS duration, and QTc interval
	Potential torsades de pointes in patients with preexisting conduction disturbances
	Potential for ventricular tachycardia or fibrillation in patients with Wolff-Parkinson-White syndrome
Selective serotonin reuptake inhibitors	Isolated reports of bradycardia and atrial fibrillation with fluoxetine
	Citalopram and escitalopram not recommended in cardiac disease with prolonged conduction times
Antipsychotics	Orthostatic hypotension associated with use of clozapine, quetiapine, and low-potency antipsychotics
	Risk of prolonged QTc interval with use of pimozide, thioridazine, mesoridazine, droperidol, risperidone, ziprasidone, and high-dose intravenous haloperidol
Anxiolytics/ hypnotics	Benzodiazepines and buspirone thought to be free from cardiovascular effects
Mood stabilizers	Possible sinus node dysfunction or first-degree atrioventricular block with use of lithium
	Carbamazepine associated with atrioventricular conduction disturbances
	Lamotrigine associated with QT interval prolongation
	Divalproex sodium thought safe

Table 17–4.   Medication use in cardiac disease *(continued)*

Medication class	Potential drug effect on cardiac function
Psychostimulants	FDA warning to avoid using psychostimulants with structural and other serious cardiac disorders
	Although methylphenidate and amphetamines may be safe in low doses, consultation with a cardiologist is recommended.

Note.   FDA=U.S. Food and Drug Administration; TCA=tricyclic antidepressant.
Source.   Adapted from Beliles 2000a; Robinson and Owen 2005.

tion that continues after the medication has been discontinued, or the presence of cardiovascular symptoms.

Respiratory Disease

The benzodiazepines are the psychiatric medications of most concern in patients with pulmonary disease due to the risk of respiratory depression (see Table 17–5). There is particular concern in patients who retain carbon dioxide. Both buspirone and trazodone have been recommended as alternative medications for the treatment of anxiety and insomnia.

Medication Selection and Target Symptoms

Psychotropic medications are selected to address target symptoms that cause significant subjective distress or functional impairment (Klykylo 2014). Target symptoms are often specific dimensions of a psychiatric diagnosis (e.g., sad mood as a symptom of depression). Target symptoms may also be a common shared dimension of multiple psychiatric disorders. For example, sleep disturbance can be a symptom common to depressive disorders, bipolar disorder, delirium, moderate to severe substance use disorders, adjustment disorders, or sleep disorders. Target symptoms may cause clinically significant distress or impairment in functioning even when full categorical criteria for a psychiatric disorder are not met. A target symptom approach to prescribing should take into account differential diagnosis, possible symptom etiologies, and existing evidence of both clinical safety and effectiveness pertaining to the symptoms

Table 17–5.   Medication use in respiratory disease

Medication class	Potential drug effect on respiratory function
Antidepressants	Selective serotonin reuptake inhibitors generally do not cause problems
	Patients needs to be monitored for anticholinergic side effects.
	Monoamine oxidase inhibitors may interact with sympathomimetic medications used in asthma treatment.
Antipsychotics	Patient needs to be monitored for anticholinergic side effects.
	Laryngeal dystonia can occur and may affect respiratory status.
	Clozapine has been associated with respiratory arrest and depression as well as allergic asthma.
Anxiolytics/hypnotics	Respiratory depression and failure are possible with benzodiazepines.
	Baseline blood gas analysis should be considered prior to use of benzodiazepines.
	Oxazepam, lorazepam, and temazepam have fewer respiratory depressant effects.
	Buspirone, zolpidem, and zaleplon are thought to be safe.

Source.   Adapted from Beliles 2000a; Jacobson 2002; Robinson and Owen 2005.

being treated. In the rest of this chapter, we focus on several common target symptoms facing psychiatric consultants: acute agitation, anxiety, depression, fatigue, and insomnia.

Acute Agitation

Acute agitation encompasses a psychological state (feelings of inner tension or arousal) and a motor state (pacing, hand-wringing, fidgeting) that occurs commonly in the pediatric hospital setting—for example, in states of acute intoxication, sedative withdrawal, delirium, or other neurocognitive disorders as well as in the context of emergency room evaluation, or in patients with depressive, bipolar, or psychotic disorders (DeMaso and Walter 2019). In these situations, rapid control of agitation is needed to prevent harm or injury to both the patient and staff. Principles of the management of acute agitation include targeting treatments toward the etiology and root causes of the aggression and adopting a multimodal approach that includes nonpharmacological management (Gerson et al. 2019). Etiologies to be considered include delirium, substance intoxication/withdrawal, catatonia, and comorbid psychiatric illness (anxiety, trauma, mania, psychosis, and behavioral disorders), each of which may suggest specific pharmacological agents (Table 17–6). Individuals with autism spectrum disorder and developmental delays are particularly prone to acute agitation in the emergency department and inpatient setting, and history from family members can help identify precipitants and possible intervention strategies (Gerson et al. 2019).

Unfortunately, the literature on the psychopharmacological treatment of acutely agitated children seen in emergency department settings remains sparse (Hilt and Woodward 2008). When we extrapolate from adult studies, it is clear that the two most common categories of psychiatric medications used are the antipsychotics and benzodiazepines, either alone or in combination. Some data suggest that a combination of medications, most commonly haloperidol with lorazepam, is more effective than one alone (Battaglia et al. 1997). Medication choice may also be influenced by whether or not the patient is willing and able to take oral medications.

The management of acute agitation associated with delirium is described in Chapter 5 ("Delirium"). Medication guidelines for agitation derived from causes other than delirium are presented in Table 17–7 and 17–8. The management assumes that psychosocial crisis management techniques to control the behavior have either been unsuccessful or are simultaneously being implemented (Pappadopulos et al. 2003).

Benzodiazepines

Although benzodiazepines differ in potency, speed of onset of action, and route of administration, there are no data to support the use of one specific benzodiazepine over another in terms of therapeutic efficacy. Available in oral, intramuscular, and intravenous formulations, lorazepam is the most frequently

Table 17–6.   Selected medications for agitation, aggression, irritability, and psychosis

Generic (brand) Name	FDA-approved indication (pediatric age range in years)	Target symptoms	Daily starting dose	Daily therapeutic dosage range[a]	Selected medical monitoring and precautions
Second-generation antipsychotics					
Aripiprazole (Abilify) *Note:* available in liquid preparation	Bipolar (10–17) Schizophrenia (13–17) Irritability in autism (6–17) Tourette's disorder (6–17)	Mania Psychosis Irritability Aggression Agitation Vocal/motor tics	Bipolar and schizophrenia: 2 mg Autism: 2 mg Tourette's: 2 mg	Bipolar and schizophrenia: 10–30 mg Autism: 5–15 mg Tourette's: 5–20 mg	BMI, BP, P, fasting glucose and lipids, abnormal movements; compulsive behaviors; NMS; leukopenia/ neutropenia/ agranulocytosis; seizures

Table 17–6. Selected medications for agitation, aggression, irritability, and psychosis *(continued)*

Generic (brand) Name	FDA-approved indication (pediatric age range in years)	Target symptoms	Daily starting dose	Daily therapeutic dosage range[a]	Selected medical monitoring and precautions
Second-generation antipsychotics (continued)					
Olanzapine (Zyprexa) *Note:* available in liquid, dissolvable, and intramuscular preparations	Bipolar (13–17) Schizophrenia (13–17)	Mania Psychosis Agitation	2.5 mg	2.5–10 mg	BMI, BP, P, fasting glucose and lipids, abnormal movements; skin rash; NMS; leukopenia/ neutropenia/ agranulocytosis; seizures

Table 17–6.   Selected medications for agitation, aggression, irritability, and psychosis *(continued)*

Generic (brand) Name	FDA-approved indication (pediatric age range in years)	Target symptoms	Daily starting dose	Daily therapeutic dosage range[a]	Selected medical monitoring and precautions
Second-generation antipsychotics (continued)					
Quetiapine (Seroquel)	Bipolar (10–17) Schizophrenia (13–17)	Mania Psychosis Agitation	25 mg bid	Bipolar: 400–600 mg Schizophrenia: 400–800 mg	BMI, BP, P, fasting glucose and lipids, abnormal movements; ophthalmological exam; NMS; leukopenia/ neutropenia/ agranulocytosis; seizures; QT prolongation

Table 17–6. Selected medications for agitation, aggression, irritability, and psychosis *(continued)*

Generic (brand) Name	FDA-approved indication (pediatric age range in years)	Target symptoms	Daily starting dose	Daily therapeutic dosage range[a]	Selected medical monitoring and precautions
Second-generation antipsychotics (continued)					
Risperidone (Risperdal) *Note:* available in liquid and dissolvable preparations	Bipolar (10–17) Schizophrenia (13–17) Irritability in autism (5–17)	Mania Psychosis Irritability Aggression Agitation	Bipolar and schizophrenia: 0.5 mg Autism: <20 kg: 0.25 mg; ≥20 kg: 0.5 mg	Bipolar and schizophrenia: 1–6 mg Autism: 0.5–3 mg	BMI, BP, P, fasting glucose and lipids, prolactin, abnormal movements; NMS; leukopenia/ neutropenia/ agranulocytosis; seizures

Table 17–6. Selected medications for agitation, aggression, irritability, and psychosis (*continued*)

Generic (brand) Name	FDA-approved indication (pediatric age range in years)	Target symptoms	Daily starting dose	Daily therapeutic dosage range[a]	Selected medical monitoring and precautions
Second-generation antipsychotics (*continued*)					
Paliperidone (Invega) *Note:* Available in liquid and IM preparations	Schizophrenia (12–17)	Psychosis	3 mg	<51 kg: 3–6 mg ≥51 kg: 3–12 mg	BMI, BP, P, fasting glucose and lipids, prolactin, abnormal movements, QT prolongation; NMS; potential for GI obstruction; leukopenia/ neutropenia/ agranulocytosis; seizures

Table 17–6. Selected medications for agitation, aggression, irritability, and psychosis *(continued)*

Generic (brand) Name	FDA-approved indication (pediatric age range in years)	Target symptoms	Daily starting dose	Daily therapeutic dosage range[a]	Selected medical monitoring and precautions
Second-generation antipsychotics (continued)					
Lurasidone (Latuda)	Schizophrenia (13–17)	Psychosis	40 mg	40–80 mg	BMI, BP, P, fasting glucose and lipids, prolactin, abnormal movements; NMS; leukopenia/ neutropenia/ agranulocytosis; seizures
Asenapine (Saphris)	Bipolar (10–17)	Mania Psychosis	2.5 mg bid	5–20 mg	BMI, BP, P, fasting glucose and lipids, prolactin, abnormal movements; QT prolongation; NMS; leukopenia/ neutropenia/ agranulocytosis; seizures

Table 17–6.   Selected medications for agitation, aggression, irritability, and psychosis (*continued*)

Generic (brand) Name	FDA-approved indication (pediatric age range in years)	Target symptoms	Daily starting dose	Daily therapeutic dosage range[a]	Selected medical monitoring and precautions
First-generation antipsychotics					
Haloperiol (Haldol) *Note:* Available in liquid and intramuscular preparations	Psychosis Tourette's disorder Severe behavioral disorders Agitation (3–17)	Mania Psychosis Irritability Aggression Agitation Vocal/motor tics	0.05 mg/kg/day	0.05–0.15 mg/kg/ day	BP; P; abnormal movements; QT prolongation; NMS; encephalopathy when combined with lithium; leukopenia/ neutropenia/ agranulocytosis

Table 17–6.   Selected medications for agitation, aggression, irritability, and psychosis *(continued)*

Generic (brand) Name	FDA-approved indication (pediatric age range in years)	Target symptoms	Daily starting dose	Daily therapeutic dosage range[a]	Selected medical monitoring and precautions
Mood stabilizer					
Lithium carbonate *Note:* available in liquid preparation	Bipolar (12–17)	Mania	1,800 mg/day for acute mania Target level: 1.0–1.5 mEq/L	900–1,200 mg/day for long-term control Target level: 0.6–1.2 mEq/L	Serum level, CBC with differential, thyroid function, BUN/creatine, urinalysis, electrolytes, FBS; ECG; encephalopathy when combined with haloperidol

Note.   BMI=body mass index; BP=blood pressure; BUN=blood urea nitrogen; CBC=complete blood count; ECG=electrocardiogram; FBS=fasting blood sugar; GI=gastrointestinal; IM=intramuscular; NMS=neuroleptic malignant syndrome; P=pulse.
[a]Doses shown in table may exceed maximum recommended dose for some children.

Source.   DeMaso DR, Walter HJ: "Psychopharmacology," in *Nelson Textbook of Pediatrics*, 21st Edition. Edited by Kliegman RM, Stanton BF, St. Geme J, et al. Philadelphia, PA, Elsevier, 2019, pp. 189–196. Copyright © 2019, Elsevier, Inc. Used with permission.

Table 17–7. Medication management of acute moderate agitation in children and adolescents

Medication recommendations for moderate agitation

Moderate agitation consists of raising voice/yelling/screaming, being verbally aggressive, threatening posture (e.g., clenched fists), pacing, rocking, throwing small objects without aiming at others, and self-injuring that does not break skin (e.g., light scratching, hitting self lightly, or brief head banging). If patient refuses medications by mouth and there is concern for progression to serious harm to self or others, proceed to medication recommendations for severe agitation.

Parameter	Child (weighing 25–50 kg)	Adolescent (weighing > 50 kg)
Preferred agent(s)	Diphenhydramine or lorazepam	Diphenhydramine or lorazepam
Administration route	PO	PO
Initial dosing *(Prescribers to use discretion and order lower or higher doses as appropriate)*	Diphenhydramine 25 mg or lorazepam 0.5–1 mg	Diphenhydramine 50 mg or lorazepam 1–2 mg
Repeat dosing *(60 minutes after initial dose if ineffective)*	Diphenhydramine 25 mg or lorazepam 0.5–1 mg	Diphenhydramine 25 mg or lorazepam 1–2 mg
Subsequent frequency	Q4–6 hours *Not to exceed 100 mg of diphenhydramine or 2 mg of lorazepam in 24 hours*	Q4–6 hours *Not to exceed 150 mg of diphenhydramine or 4 mg of lorazepam in 24 hours*

Source. Boston Children's Hospital, Patient Care Manual, Pharmacy and Therapeutics, 2019.

used benzodiazepine for treatment of acute agitation. Intramuscular midazolam has been used to treat acute agitation, with reported superior results compared with both haloperidol and lorazepam, although midazolam's short duration of action limits its utility and there is the potential for paradoxical agitation following its withdrawal (Rund et al. 2006). Diazepam should not be administered intramuscularly because of erratic absorption and unpredictable drug levels. Limitations in the use of benzodiazepines with children may

Table 17–8. Medication management of acute severe agitation in children and adolescents

Medication recommendations for severe agitation

Severe agitation consists of imminent risk to self or others, e.g., attempting to seriously injure self (attempts to strangle or cut self, deep scratches, forceful or prolonged head banging), being combative, being assaultive, moving or throwing large objects, or destroying property.

Parameter	Child (weighing 25–50 kg)	Adolescent (weighing > 50 kg)
Preferred agent(s)	Olanzapine[a] (orally disintegrating tablet) or haloperidol[b] and diphenhydramine[c] or lorazepam	Olanzapine[a] (orally disintegrating tablet) or haloperidol[b] and diphenhydramine[c] and/or lorazepam
Administration route	PO or IM	PO or IM
Initial dosing	Olanzapine 2.5 mg or haloperidol 2 mg and diphenhydramine 25 mg or lorazepam 0.5–1 mg	Olanzapine 5 mg or haloperidol 5 mg and diphenhydramine 50 mg and/or lorazepam 1–2 mg
Repeat dosing (45 minutes after initial dose if ineffective)	Olanzapine 2.5 mg or haloperidol 2 mg and diphenhydramine 25 mg or lorazepam 0.5–1 mg	Olanzapine 5 mg or haloperidol 2.5 mg and diphenhydramine 25 mg and/or lorazepam 1–2 mg
Subsequent frequency	Q4hr	Q4hr
	Do not exceed:	*Do not exceed:*
	Olanzapine 10 mg in 24 hours	Olanzapine 15 mg in 24 hours
	Haloperidol 5 mg in 24 hours	Haloperidol 10 mg in 24 hours
	Diphenhydramine 100 mg in 24 hours	Diphenhydramine 150 mg in 24 hours
	Lorazepam 3 mg in 24 hours	Lorazepam 6 mg in 24 hours

[a]Do NOT use IM olanzapine within 4 hours of IM/IV lorazepam because of risk of cardiopulmonary depression.
[b]Use of haloperidol in combination with citalopram, escitalopram, or fluoxetine may increase risk of QTc prolongation, and thus haloperidol should only be used in such combinations if benefits outweigh risks.
[c]Use of diphenhydramine with haloperidol is preferred to use of haloperidol alone to avoid risk of acute dystonic reactions.
Source.   Boston Children's Hospital, Patient Care Manual, Pharmacy and Therapeutics, 2019.

occur as a result of excessive sedation and/or behavioral/emotional disinhibition, and this may limit their usefulness in this population. Following extended use of benzodiazepines (>2 weeks), gradual tapering of the dose by 10%–25% every 7 days is recommended (Cummings and Miller 2004).

Antipsychotic Agents

The Treatment Recommendations for the Use of Antipsychotics for Aggressive Youth (TRAAY) supported the use of antipsychotic agents in the treatment of acute aggression (Pappadopulos et al. 2003; Schur et al. 2003). While haloperidol remains one of the most commonly used agents, intramuscular and oral formulations of aripiprazole, olanzapine, and ziprasidone, and rapidly disintegrating formulations of aripiprazole, olanzapine, and risperidone, have all been shown to be comparable in efficacy to haloperidol with or without lorazepam for acute agitation in adults with schizophrenia or mania, leading to their use in agitation experienced by children and adolescents (Andrezina et al. 2006; Daniel et al. 2001; Wright et al. 2001). Although there is a literature base that supports haloperidol's safety and efficacy in intravenous use (Citrome 2002), and even one report of intranasal use (Miller et al. 2008), caution should be exercised with the off-label use of intravenous haloperidol, which does not have approval from the U.S. Food and Drug Administration (FDA) because of concerns about QTc prolongation, particularly in the context of patients who have underlying cardiac abnormalities, hypothyroidism, electrolyte imbalances, and familial long QT syndrome, and in those taking other QTc-prolonging medications (Levenson et al. 2017).

Current emergency department practices tend to favor risperidone or olanzapine for patients who are willing to take oral medications because of the more favorable side effect profile (Hilt and Woodward 2008). However, for patients requiring intramuscular administration, ziprasidone and olanzapine have become widely acceptable alternatives to the use of haloperidol. In one study, intramuscular ziprasidone was found to be significantly more effective than haloperidol in reducing symptoms of acute agitation (Brook et al. 2000). There are also data describing the use of intravenous ziprasidone in the treatment of acute delirium (Young and Lujan 2004). Tollefson et al. (1997) have also reported on the safe and effective use of intramuscular olanzapine. Droperidol, once a popular medication choice in the emergency department setting, is now rarely used following the FDA warning regarding cardiac toxicity.

Antihistamines

Diphenhydramine and hydroxyzine are frequently used to treat children with acute agitation and can be administered by oral, intramuscular, and intravenous routes. The main limitations include anticholinergic side effects, cardiac conduction abnormalities, and the potential to increase delirium (Cummings and Miller 2004).

Mood Stabilizers

There are preliminary data supporting the use of intravenous valproic acid in combination with antipsychotics or benzodiazepines to help reduce agitation and aggressive behavior in pediatric patients (Battaglia et al. 2018). However, the delay in its onset of action and potential hepatic side effects limit its efficacy (Cummings and Miller 2004).

Anxiety Symptoms

Symptoms of anxiety in physically ill patients are significantly elevated compared with the general pediatric population. Commonly encountered diagnoses include separation anxiety disorder, generalized anxiety disorder, social anxiety disorder, and panic disorder as well as specific phobias related to the medical treatment environment (see Chapter 8, "Anxiety Symptoms and Trauma/ Stress Reactions"). Selected medications for anxiety symptoms are presented in Table 17–9.

Antidepressants

These medications target the presynaptic and postsynaptic receptors affecting the release and reuptake of brain neurotransmitters, including norepinephrine, serotonin, and dopamine (DeMaso and Walter 2019). There is strong evidence for their effectiveness in the treatment of anxiety disorders with a large effect–sized number needed to treat (NNT; an estimate of the number of patients need to be treated in order to impact one person) of only 3 (95% confidence interval [CI], 2–5) (Correll et al. 2011). Although there are some studies supporting the use of non-SSRI antidepressants (Rynn et al. 2015; Strawn et al. 2015), and duloxetine has received FDA approval for anxiety for youth ages 7–17 years, these medications lack rigorous evidence to support their use, rendering them generally a second-line treatment option, with SSRIs being the first-line treatment for anxiety. The applicability of these findings to

Table 17–9.   Selected medications for depression and anxiety

Name	FDA-approved indications (pediatric age range in years)	Target symptoms	Daily starting dose	Daily therapuetic dosage range[a]	Selected medical monitoring and precautions
Selective serotonin reuptake inhibitors					
Citalopram (Celexa)	None	Depression Anxiety Obsessions/ compulsions	10 mg	10–40 mg	Suicidal ideation; QT prolongation at doses >40 mg; abnormal bleeding; mania; serotonin syndrome; DS
Escitalopram (Lexapro)	Depression (12–17)	Depression Anxiety Obsessions/ compulsions	5 mg	5–20 mg	Suicidal ideation; abnormal bleeding; mania; serotonin syndrome; DS
Fluoxetine (Prozac)	Depression (8–17) OCD (7–17)	Depression Anxiety Obsessions/ compulsions	10 mg (ages 6–12) 20 mg (ages 13–17)	Depression: 10–20 mg Anxiety, OCD: 10–60 mg	Suicidal ideation; abnormal bleeding; mania; serotonin syndrome

Table 17–9. Selected medications for depression and anxiety *(continued)*

Name	FDA-approved indications (pediatric age range in years)	Target symptoms	Daily starting dose	Daily therapuetic dosage range[a]	Selected medical monitoring and precautions
Selective serotonin reuptake inhibitors (continued)					
Sertraline (Zoloft)	OCD (6–17)	Depression Anxiety Obsessions/ compulsions	25 mg (ages 6–12) 50 mg (ages 13–17)	12.5–200 mg	Suicidal ideation; abnormal bleeding; mania; serotonin syndrome; DS
Atypical antidepressants					
Bupropion (Wellbutrin XL)	None	Depression	150 mg	150–300 mg	Suicidal ideation; neuropsychiatric reaction, seizures (>300 mg/day), BP; mania; contraindicated in patients with seizure and eating disorders

Table 17–9. Selected medications for depression and anxiety *(continued)*

Name	FDA-approved indications (pediatric age range in years)	Target symptoms	Daily starting dose	Daily therapeutic dosage range[a]	Selected medical monitoring and precautions
Atypical antidepressants *(continued)*					
Duloxetine (Cymbalta)	Anxiety (7–17)	Depression Anxiety	30 mg	30–60 mg	Suicidal ideation; BP; pulse; liver damage; severe skin reactions; abnormal bleeding; mania; serotonin syndrome; DS
Mirtazapine (Remeron)	None	Depression	7.5 mg	7.5–45 mg	Suicidal ideation; weight; somnolence; agranulocytosis; QT prolongation; mania; serotonin syndrome; DS
Venlafaxine (Effexor XR)	None	Depression Anxiety	37.5 mg	37.5–225 mg	Suicidal ideation; BP; abnormal bleeding; mania; serotonin syndrome; DS

Table 17–9. Selected medications for depression and anxiety *(continued)*

Name	FDA-approved indications (pediatric age range in years)	Target symptoms	Daily starting dose	Daily theraputic dosage range[a]	Selected medical monitoring and precautions
Tricyclic antidepressants					
Amitriptyline (Elavil)	None	Depression	10 mg	10–200 mg	Suicidal ideation; BP; pulse; ECG; blood level; mania; seizures; serotonin syndrome; DS
Anxiolytic agents (situational use)					
Lorazepam (Ativan)	None	Anxiety	0.5 mg	0.5–2 mg	Respiratory depression; sedation; physical and psychological dependence; paradoxical reactions

Table 17–9.   Selected medications for depression and anxiety *(continued)*

Name	FDA-approved indications (pediatric age range in years)	Target symptoms	Daily starting dose	Daily therapuetic dosage range[a]	Selected medical monitoring and precautions
Anxiolytic agents (situational use) *(continued)*					
Clonazepam (Klonopin)	None	Panic	0.5 mg	0.5–1 mg	Respiratory depression; sedation; physical and psychological dependence; paradoxical reactions; suicidal ideation
Hydroxyzine (Atarax, Vistaril)	Anxiety	Anxiety	50 mg	50 mg (age <6 years) 50–100 mg (age ≥ 6 years)	QT prolongation

Note.   BP = blood pressure; DS = discontinuation syndrome; ECG = electrocardiogram; OCD = obsessive-compulsive disorder.

[a]Doses shown in table may exceed maximum recommended dose for some children.

Source.   Reprinted from DeMaso DR, Walter HJ: "Psychopharmacology," in *Nelson Textbook of Pediatrics*, 21st Edition. Edited by Kliegman RM, Stanton BF, St. Geme J, et al. Philadelphia, PA, Elsevier, 2019, pp. 189–196. Copyright © 2019, Elsevier, Inc. Used with permission.

youth with physical illnesses, given their lack of participation in nearly all medication studies, is a limitation.

Benzodiazepines

These medications have been used for the short-term relief of situational or acute anxiety, including in specific situations where there are concomitant physical symptoms, such as nausea or muscle spasms. Their efficacy as chronic (taken more than 4 months) anxiolytic medications is poorer, and their chronic use carries a significant risk of physical and psychological dependence (De-Maso and Walter 2019). Common reported side effects of benzodiazepines include sedation, disinhibition, and behavioral dyscontrol.

Propranolol

There is insufficient evidence to support the use of propranolol in the treatment of children with anxiety disorders (Patel et al. 2018). However, there may be some benefits in specific situations, for example, for performance anxiety. Blood pressure and heart rate should be monitored as well as a baseline electrocardiogram.

Buspirone

Buspirone is an azapirone anxiolytic with a primary indication for chronic generalized anxiety. It has little potential for abuse or physical dependency and is considered an agent of choice when risk for substance abuse accompanies a need to treat anxiety. The anxiolytic effects of buspirone can take weeks to be felt, thus requiring adjunctive treatments when acute anxiety must be addressed. Buspirone metabolism and clearance are decreased in hepatic and renal disease.

Depressive Symptoms

Numerous studies have shown increased rates of depression in physically ill children and adolescents, including patients with inflammatory bowel disease, cancer, and asthma (Apter et al. 2003; Mrazek 2003; Szigethy et al. 2004). First-line treatment for depression nearly always begins with psychotherapy, such as cognitive-behavioral therapy or interpersonal psychotherapy. However, for youth who present with moderate/severe depressive symptoms or with depression that is unresponsive to psychotherapy, an antidepressant should be considered.

Antidepressants

There is weaker evidence for the effectiveness of antidepressants in depressive disorders in comparison with anxiety disorders, with a small effect–sized NNT of 10 (95% CI, 7–15) (Correll et al. 2011). However, more recently a broad and important role for antidepressant medications in pediatric internalizing conditions has been postulated on the basis of findings from National Institute of Mental Health–funded depression trials combined with the demonstrated efficacy of serotonin reuptake inhibitors for anxiety disorders (Walkup 2017). Fluoxetine (ages 8–17 years) and escitalopram (ages 12–17 years) have FDA approval for use in pediatric depression. Although there are studies supporting the use of non-SSRI antidepressants (Bridge et al. 2005; Daviss et al. 2001), as with anxiety disorders, these medications lack rigorous evidence and are generally considered a second-line option. Again, as with anxiety disorders, the applicability of these findings to youth with physical illnesses has not been fully studied.

Studies have shown no greater efficacy for TCAs compared with placebo, and these agents are not currently recommended, particularly because of their unfavorable side effect profile and risk of lethality following overdose. However, clinical indications for their use at lower doses exist for specified situations (e.g., enuresis, migraine prophylaxis).

Medication algorithms for childhood major depression have been developed to guide treatment, including the Texas Children's Medication Algorithm Project (Hughes et al. 2007). In the case of the physically ill child, there may be specific circumstances that influence the choice of a therapeutic agent. The choice of a specific antidepressant may be guided by consideration of its side effects, half-life, and potential drug interactions. For patients who are taking multiple medications for their physical illness, for whom drug interactions are a concern, escitalopram may have benefits over other SSRIs. For example, in children with chronic pain syndromes, venlafaxine may have dual benefits in terms of its demonstrated antidepressant and analgesic actions (Kiayias et al. 2000). For patients with low energy or attentional issues, bupropion may have additional benefits.

Psychostimulants

Historically, psychostimulants have been recognized to have euphoric and alerting properties that suggest their usefulness in treating depressive symptoms. A

Cochrane database review of randomized controlled trials on the use of psychostimulants, including dexamphetamine, methylphenidate, methylamphetamine, pemoline, and modafinil, found some evidence for the short-term treatment of depressive symptoms and fatigue (Candy et al. 2008). The authors concluded that there might be clinical situations, including the physically ill child, in which psychostimulants could play an adjunction role in a patient's care. A recent systematic review found similar improvement in the treatment of major depressive episodes while calling for more study of the use as adjunctive or monotherapy in adults (McIntyre et al. 2017).

Fatigue

Fatigue and depressive symptoms have considerable overlap and often coexist in patients with cancer and other physical diseases. Cancer-related fatigue is well known and is often accompanied by insomnia, pain, and depression, which arise as a direct result of the cancer and/or as a side effect of its treatment (Wang and Woodruff 2015). The prevalence of cancer-related fatigue ranges from 4% to 91%, depending on the specific cancer population studied and the methods of assessment (Breitbart and Alici-Evcimen 2007). These findings have led many researchers to examine the role of psychotropic medications to treat fatigue. Most of the research, however, has been based on work with adult patients, and results of studies listed must be interpreted cautiously before extrapolating treatment guidelines for pediatric patients.

Psychostimulants

In the pediatric setting, these medications are commonly used as agents to help treat symptoms of fatigue and depression in physically ill patients. A Cochrane database review concluded that the findings were significant enough to support the use of methylphenidate to treat cancer-related fatigue in adult patients (Minton et al. 2008). An updated meta-analysis of five placebo-controlled trials similarly confirmed that psychostimulants consistently showed a small but favorable improvement in cancer-related fatigue (Minton et al. 2011). Although there are fewer data on other diseases, a randomized controlled study of adults with HIV disease found that psychostimulants improved quality of life and reduced fatigue (Breitbart et al. 2001). There have been other studies involving cancer-related fatigue, with less positive findings regarding the impact of psychostimulants (Auret et al. 2009; Carroll et al. 2007). The importance of considering potential side effects of psychostimulants, including irritability, anorexia, insomnia, labile mood, nausea, and tachycardia, when making treatment decisions was stressed.

There has been interest in the use of modafinil in the management of fatigue in physically ill adults with breast and brain cancer (Carroll et al. 2007). One Phase III trial reported that modafinil significantly benefited patients undergoing chemotherapy with severe baseline fatigue who had severe fatigue at baseline (Jean-Pierre et al. 2010), whereas no reduction in fatigue was observed in a 4-week, randomized multicenter trial in a cohort of adult patients with advanced lung cancer (Spathis et al. 2014).

Antidepressants

In the Cochrane database review noted above in the discussion of psychostimulants, no data were found to support the use of antidepressants for fatigue (Breitbart and Alici-Evcimen 2007; Minton et al. 2008). However, a double-blind, placebo-controlled study of paroxetine showed some benefits for cancer-related fatigue (Roscoe et al. 2005), and bupropion was shown to have some benefits because of its ability to increase neurotransmission (Moss et al. 2006).

Insomnia

Inability to sleep is a common complaint and referral question in youth with physical illnesses. A chart review of 9,440 pediatric inpatients found that 6% of all hospitalized children were prescribed medications for sleep, with antihistamines the most frequently prescribed medication (36.6%), followed by benzodiazepines (19.4%) and hypnotic agents (2.2%). While nonpharmacological sleep hygiene measures are the first-line treatment approach, medications can be considered when these approaches have been ineffective and pain is managed adequately. However, there are few studies to guide consultants in the use of pharmacological approaches to sleep disturbance in the context of physical illness, and this has led to a number of agents being used to treat insomnia, including antihistamines, benzodiazepines, nonbenzodiazepine hypnotics, melatonin, and trazodone, among others (Economou et al. 2018; Meltzer et al. 2007).

Diphenhydramine

Various studies have been done to evaluate the usefulness of diphenhydramine, an antihistaminergic drug, in sleep disorders of both adults and children. In general, data suggest its usefulness in decreasing both sleep latency times and night time awakenings (Pelayo and Dubik 2008; Pelayo and Yuen 2012). However, at least one study of infants ages 6–15 months found no benefit for diphenhydramine over placebo (Merenstein et al. 2006), and there are some data suggesting that tolerance develops to habitual use (Pelayo and Yuen 2012).

Benzodiazepines

Benzodiazepines have been used extensively in adults with insomnia and appear to reduce sleep latency and slow-wave sleep (Economou et al. 2018; Pelayo et al. 2004). Despite their widespread use in inpatient pediatric settings, benzodiazepines are not recommended for children with insomnia, unless they are being used concomitantly for other primary psychiatric conditions or as part of treatment for other physical symptoms, such as nausea.

Nonbenzodiazepine Hypnotics

The nonbenzodiazepine sedatives zolpidem, eszopiclone, and zaleplon are used in the treatment of insomnia. These agents are rapidly absorbed and have short half-lives (Pelayo and Yuen 2012). Their use in children is considered "off label," and therefore no official dosing guidelines are available. These newer medications preserve the overall sleep architecture and do not typically have the insomnia rebound effects experienced with benzodiazepine hypnotics when they are abruptly stopped. A study of the use of zolpidem in a sample of 21 children found it to be well tolerated, although further efficacy studies are needed (Blumer et al. 2008). Eszopiclone has a longer half-life than zolpidem and zaleplon, a feature that theoretically may be helpful in children, because they typically sleep longer than adults. To date, there are no published studies in children (Pelayo and Yuen 2012).

Melatonin

Melatonin is a commonly used sleep medication that is thought to possess both a phase-setting effect and a direct hypnotic effect (Economou et al. 2018; Pelayo and Yuen 2012). In a case series of 15 neurologically impaired children with chronic sleep disturbances, including fragmented sleep and delayed sleep phase, a significant subjective improvement in sleep was reported (Touitou 2001). Two other pediatric studies also demonstrated beneficial effects of melatonin in terms of a reduction in initial insomnia and enhanced total sleep time (Van der Heijden et al. 2007; Weiss et al. 2006). Although melatonin has a safe pharmacokinetic profile with mild and few side effects, the National Sleep Foundation has warned against using melatonin in patients with immune disorders, in those with lymphoproliferative disorders, and in those taking corticosteroids or other immunosuppressants, given its ability to enhance immune function (Touitou 2001).

Trazodone

Trazodone is a 5-HT$_2$ receptor antagonist that blocks histamine receptors and with sedating properties that is very widely used for the treatment of insomnia (Owens et al. 2010). However, despite the fairly widespread use of this agent, the data on the effectiveness of trazodone in psychitrically healthy subjects are limited, and there is little evidence to suggest that trazodone improves sleep in patients without a mood disorder. Furthermore, no safety data exist on trazodone used at hypnotic doses, and there are reported associations with cardiac arrhythmias and priapism. Available data also suggest tolerance occurs to its hypnotic effects.

Mirtazapine

Mirtazapine is a tetracyclic antidepressant that appears to have utility in the treatment of insomnia. Kim et al. (2008) found that mirtazapine helped reduce symptoms of nausea, sleep disturbance, and pain and improved quality of life and symptoms of depression in adult cancer patients. To date, there have been no studies in pediatric patients. Mirtazapine may be a particularly effective treatment option in physically ill patients who have disease or treatment-related physical symptoms, including poor appetite and pruritus (Shaw et al. 2007).

Tricyclic Antidepressants

TCAs, in particular amitriptyline, are commonly used in the medical setting for the treatment of insomnia, particularly for patients with symptoms of neuropathic pain (Economou et al. 2018). Imipramine has similarly been used in these situations. TCAs suppress slow-wave sleep and are quite sedating, although their use can be complicated because of anticholinergic side effects, as well as the potential to prolong the QTc interval. Cardiac monitoring is advised.

Clonidine

Clonidine, a centrally acting α_2-adrenergic receptor agonist that works presynaptically to inhibit norepinephrine activity and decrease sympathetic outflow, also has sedative effects, which become advantageous in the setting of management of sleep (Blackmer and Feinstein 2016). Common side effects include hypertension, bradycardia, and anticholinergic effects; rapid discontinuation can lead to tachycardia, hypertension, and shortness of breath (Economou et al. 2018; Pelayo and Yuen 2012). Clonidine has been used at night to promote sleep in children with attention-deficit/hyperactivity disorder, which could prove helpful for youth with co-occurring physical illness. It may also be useful to treat posttraumatic stress disorder and nightmares. However, caution should be exercised in patients with cardiac issues or those taking CNS-depressant medications.

Ziprasidone

Ziprasidone has been studied in the context of adult patients with bipolar disorder and found to have beneficial effects on sleep induction, sleep continuity, and sleep architecture (Monti 2016; Monti et al. 2017). The sedating side effects of ziprasidone have resulted in its use in patients with insomnia, particularly in the context of delirium and bipolar disorder. However, the potential for long-term side effects with all of the antipsychotics make them unsuitable as a primary treatment for insomnia.

Gabapentin

Gabapentin, an α_2-δ voltage-gated calcium channel ligand that is widely used for the treatment of epilepsy, neuropathic pain, and restless legs syndrome, can enhance slow-wave sleep in both healthy individuals and epileptic patients and can improve slow-wave sleep and sleep efficiency and reduce nighttime awakening in patients with primary sleep disorders (Liu et al. 2017). In a meta-analysis, gabapentin was found to be helpful in the treatment of sleep disturbance in adult patients with medical illness when used at an average dosage of approximately 1,800 mg/day (Liu et al. 2017). A review of sleep disorders in children with neurodevelopmental disorders has also described efficacy of gabapentin for sleep difficulties (Blackmer and Feinstein 2016).

Conclusion

Because this chapter does not go into depth regarding any one medication, consultants wanting the most up-to-date information regarding specific medications are referred to one or both of the following sites: the U.S. National Library of Medicine's DailyMed (https://dailymed.nlm.nih.gov) and the FDA website (https://www.fda.gov).

Overall, there remains a paucity of information in the literature pertaining to the pharmacological treatment of children and adolescents with physical illnesses. Studies to date have essentially excluded youngsters with comorbid pediatric conditions. Clinical experience suggests that the target symptoms outlined in this chapter will respond to psychotherapy and psychotropic medications. Psychiatric consultants working in the pediatric setting require a solid understanding of pediatric psychopharmacology. Nonprescribing consultants should establish a consulting relationship with a child and adolescent psychiatrist familiar with the pediatric setting. As in all psychiatric practice, both patients and family members should be given full explanations of the indications for medication treatment as well as the potential risks and benefits. Informed consent should also always be obtained prior to initiation of a new medication.

References

Alexander M, Vaughan B, Urion D, et al: Adderall use in children and adolescents. Pediatric Views, 2005. Available at http://www.childrenshospital.org/views/june05/adderall.html. Accessed April 23, 2006.

Andrezina R, Marcus RN, Oren DA, et al: Intramuscular aripiprazole or haloperidol and transition to oral therapy in patients with agitation associated with schizophrenia: sub-analysis of a double-blind study. Curr Med Res Opin 22(11):2209–2219, 2006 17076982

Apter A, Farbstein I, Yaniv I: Psychiatric aspects of pediatric cancer. Child Adolesc Psychiatr Clin N Am 12(3):473–492, vii, 2003 12910819

Auret KA, Schug SA, Bremner AP, Bulsara M: A randomized, double-blind, placebo-controlled trial assessing the impact of dexamphetamine on fatigue in patients with advanced cancer. J Pain Symptom Manage 37(4):613–621, 2009 18790598

Battaglia C, Averna R, Labonia M, et al: Intravenous valproic acid add-on therapy in acute agitation adolescents with suspected substance abuse: a report of six cases. Clin Neuropharmacol 41(1):38–42, 2018 29303801

Battaglia J, Moss S, Rush J, et al: Haloperidol, lorazepam, or both for psychotic agitation? A multicenter, prospective, double-blind, emergency department study. Am J Emerg Med 15(4):335–340, 1997 9217519

Beliles KE: Alternative routes of administration of psychotropic medications, in Psychiatric Care of the Medical Patient, 2nd Edition. Edited by Stoudemire A, Fogel BS, Greenberg DB. New York, Oxford University Press, 2000a, pp 395–405

Beliles KE: Psychopharmacokinetics in the medically ill, in Psychiatric Care of the Medical Patient, 2nd Edition. Edited by Stoudemire A, Fogel BS, Greenberg DB. New York, Oxford University Press, 2000b, pp 272–394

Blackmer AB, Feinstein JA: Management of sleep disorders in children with neurodevelopmental disorders: a review. Pharmacotherapy 36(1):84–98, 2016 26799351

Blumer JL, Reed MD, Steinberg F, et al; NICHD PPRU Network: Potential pharmacokinetic basis for zolpidem dosing in children with sleep difficulties. Clin Pharmacol Ther 83(4):551–558, 2008 17957186

Breitbart W, Alici-Evcimen Y: Update on psychotropic medications for cancer-related fatigue. J Natl Compr Canc Netw 5(10):1081–1091, 2007 18053430

Breitbart W, Rosenfeld B, Kaim M, et al: A randomized, double-blind, placebo-controlled trial of psychostimulants for the treatment of fatigue in ambulatory patients with human immunodeficiency virus disease. Arch Intern Med 161(3):411–420, 2001 11176767

Bridge JA, Salary CB, Birmaher B, et al: The risks and benefits of antidepressant treatment for youth depression. Ann Med 37(6):404–412, 2005 16203613

Brook S, Lucey JV, Gunn KP; Ziprasidone I.M. Study Group: Intramuscular ziprasidone compared with intramuscular haloperidol in the treatment of acute psychosis. J Clin Psychiatry 61(12):933–941, 2000 11206599

Candy M, Jones L, Williams R, et al: Psychostimulants for depression. Cochrane Database Syst Rev 2(2):CD006722, 2008 18425966

Carroll JK, Kohli S, Mustian KM, et al: Pharmacologic treatment of cancer-related fatigue. Oncologist 12(Suppl 1):43–51, 2007 17573455

Citrome L: Atypical antipsychotics for acute agitation: new intramuscular options offer advantages. Postgrad Med 112(6):85–88, 94–96, 2002 12510449

Correll CU, Kratochvil CJ, March JS: Developments in pediatric psychopharmacology: focus on stimulants, antidepressants, and antipsychotics. J Clin Psychiatry 72(5):655–670, 2011 21658348

Cummings MR, Miller BD: Pharmacologic management of behavioral instability in medically ill pediatric patients. Curr Opin Pediatr 16(5):516–522, 2004 15367845

Daniel DG, Potkin SG, Reeves KR, et al: Intramuscular (IM) ziprasidone 20 mg is effective in reducing acute agitation associated with psychosis: a double-blind, randomized trial. Psychopharmacology (Berl) 155(2):128–134, 2001 11401000

Daviss WB, Bentivoglio P, Racusin R, et al: Bupropion sustained release in adolescents with comorbid attention-deficit/hyperactivity disorder and depression. J Am Acad Child Adolesc Psychiatry 40(3):307–314, 2001 11288772

DeMaso DR, Walter HJ: Psychopharmacology, in Nelson Textbook of Pediatrics, 21st Edition. Edited by Kliegman RM, Stanton BF, St. Geme J, et al. Philadelphia, PA, Elsevier, 2019, pp 189–196

Economou NT, Ferini-Strambi L, Steiropoulos P: Sleep-related drug therapy in special conditions: children. Sleep Med Clin 13(2):251–262, 2018 29759275

Gerson R, Malas N, Feuer V, et al: Best practices for evaluation and treatment of agitated children and adolescents (BETA) in the emergency department: consensus statement of the American Association for Emergency Psychiatry. West J Emer Med 20(2):409–418, 2019 30881565

Hilt RJ, Woodward TA: Agitation treatment for pediatric emergency patients. J Am Acad Child Adolesc Psychiatry 47(2):132–138, 2008 18216715

Hughes CW, Emslie GJ, Crismon ML, et al: Texas Children's Medication Algorithm Project: update from Texas Consensus Conference Panel on Medication Treatment of Childhood Major Depressive Disorder. J Am Acad Child Adolesc Psychiatry 46(6):667–686, 2007 17513980

Jacobson S: Psychopharmacology: prescribing for patients with hepatic or renal dysfunction. Psychiatric Times, November 2002, pp 65–69

Jean-Pierre P, Morrow GR, Roscoe JA, et al: A phase 3 randomized, placebo-controlled, double-blind, clinical trial of the effect of modafinil on cancer-related fatigue among 631 patients receiving chemotherapy: a University of Rochester Cancer Center Community Clinical Oncology Program Research base study. Cancer 116(14):3513–3520, 2010 20564068

Kiayias JA, Vlachou ED, Lakka-Papadodima E: Venlafaxine HCl in the treatment of painful peripheral diabetic neuropathy. Diabetes Care 23(5):699, 2000 10834432

Kim SW, Shin IS, Kim JM, et al: Effectiveness of mirtazapine for nausea and insomnia in cancer patients with depression. Psychiatry Clin Neurosci 62(1):75–83, 2008 18289144

Klykylo W: General principles of psychopharmacotherapy with children and adolescents, in Green's Child and Adolescent Clinical Psychopharmacology, 5th Edition. Edited by Klykylo WM, Bowers R, Weston C, et al. Philadelphia, PA, Wolters Kluwer/Lippincott Williams & Wilkins, 2014, pp 6–41

Labellarte MJ, Crosson JE, Riddle MA: The relevance of prolonged QTc measurement to pediatric psychopharmacology. J Am Acad Child Adolesc Psychiatry 42(6):642–650, 2003 12921471

Levenson JL, Ferrando SJ, Owen JA: Surgery and critical care, in Clinical Manual of Psychopharmacology in the Medically Ill, 2nd Edition. Edited by Evenson JL, Ferrando SJ. Arlington, VA, American Psychiatric Association Publishing, 2017, pp 565–596

Liu GJ, Karim MR, Xu LL, Wang SL, et al: Efficacy and tolerability of gabapentin in adults with sleep disturbance in medical illness: a systematic review and meta-analysis. Front Neurol 8:316, 2017 28769860

McIntyre RS, Lee Y, Zhou AJ, et al: The efficacy of psychostimulants in major depressive episodes: a systematic review and meta-analysis. J Clin Psychopharmacol 37(4):412–418, 2017 28590365

Meltzer LJ, Mindell JA, Owens JA, et al: Use of sleep medications in hospitalized pediatric patients. Pediatrics 119(6):1047–1055, 2007 17545369

Merenstein D, Diener-West M, Halbower AC, et al: The trial of infant response to diphenhydramine: the TIRED study—a randomized, controlled, patient-oriented trial. Arch Pediatr Adolesc Med 160(7):707–712, 2006 16818836

Miller JL, Ashford JW, Archer SM, et al: Comparison of intranasal administration of haloperidol with intravenous and intramuscular administration: a pilot pharmacokinetic study. Pharmacotherapy 28(7):875–882, 2008 18576902

Minton O, Stone P, Richardson A, et al: Drug therapy for the management of cancer related fatigue. Cochrane Database Syst Rev 1(1):CD006704, 2008 18254112

Minton O, Richardson A, Sharpe M, et al: Psychostimulants for the management of cancer-related fatigue: a systematic review and meta-analysis. J Pain Symptom Manage 41(4):761–767, 2011 21251796

Monti JM: The effect of second-generation antipsychotic drugs on sleep parameters in patients with unipolar or bipolar disorder. Sleep Med 23:89–96, 2016 27692282

Monti JM, Torterolo P, Pandi Perumal SR: The effects of second-generation antipsychotic drugs on sleep variables in healthy subjects and patients with schizophrenia. Sleep Med Rev 33:51–57, 2017 27321864

Moss EL, Simpson JS, Pelletier G, et al: An open-label study of the effects of bupropion SR on fatigue, depression and quality of life of mixed-site cancer patients and their partners. Psychooncology 15(3):259–267, 2006 16041840

Mrazek DA: Psychiatric symptoms in patients with asthma causality, comorbidity, or shared genetic etiology. Child Adolesc Psychiatr Clin N Am 12(3):459–471, 2003 12910818

Owen JA, Crouse EL: Pharmacokinetics, pharmacodynamics, and principles of drug-drug interactions, in Clinical Manual of Psychopharmacology in the Medically Ill. Edited by Evenson JL, Ferrando SJ. Arlington, VA, American Psychiatric Association Publishing, 2017, pp 3–44

Owens JA, Rosen CL, Mindell JA, et al: Use of pharmacotherapy for insomnia in child psychiatry practice: A national survey. Sleep Med 11(7):692–700, 2010 20621556

Pappadopulos E, Macintyre Ii JC, Crismon ML, et al: Treatment recommendations for the use of antipsychotics for aggressive youth (TRAAY). Part II. J Am Acad Child Adolesc Psychiatry 42(2):145–161, 2003 12544174

Patel DR, Feucht C, Brown K, et al: Pharmacological treatment of anxiety disorders in children and adolescents: a review for practitioners. Transl Pediatr 7(1):23–35, 2018 29441280

Pelayo R, Dubik M: Pediatric sleep pharmacology. Semin Pediatr Neurol 15(2):79–90, 2008 18555194

Pelayo R, Yuen K: Pediatric sleep pharmacology. Child Adolesc Psychiatr Clin N Am 21(4):861–883, 2012 23040905

Pelayo R, Chen W, Monzon S, et al: Pediatric sleep pharmacology: you want to give my kid sleeping pills? Pediatr Clin North Am 51(1):117–134, 2004 15008585

Robinson MJ, Owen JA: Psychopharmacology, in The American Psychiatric Press Textbook of Psychosomatic Medicine. Edited by Levenson JL. Washington, DC, American Psychiatric Publishing, 2005, pp 871–922

Roscoe JA, Morrow GR, Hickok JT, et al: Effect of paroxetine hydrochloride (Paxil) on fatigue and depression in breast cancer patients receiving chemotherapy. Breast Cancer Res Treat 89(3):243–249, 2005 15754122

Rund DA, Ewing JD, Mitzel K, et al: The use of intramuscular benzodiazepines and antipsychotic agents in the treatment of acute agitation or violence in the emergency department. J Emerg Med 31(3):317–324, 2006 16982374

Rynn MA, Walkup JT, Compton SN, et al: Child/adolescent anxiety multimodal study: evaluating safety. J Am Acad Child Adolesc Psychiatry 54(3):180–190, 2015 25721183

Schur SB, Sikich L, Findling RL, et al: Treatment recommendations for the use of antipsychotics for aggressive youth (TRAAY). Part I: a review. J Am Acad Child Adolesc Psychiatry 42(2):132–144, 2003 12544173

Shaw RJ, Dayal S, Good J, et al: Psychiatric medications for the treatment of pruritus. Psychosom Med 69(9):970–978, 2007 17991825

Spathis A, Fife K, Blackhall F, et al: Modafinil for the treatment of fatigue in lung cancer: results of a placebo-controlled, double-blind, randomized trial. J Clin Oncol 32(18):1882–1888, 2014 24778393

Strawn JR, Prakash A, Zhang Q, et al: A randomized, placebo-controlled study of duloxetine for the treatment of children and adolescents with generalized anxiety disorder. J Am Acad Child Adolesc Psychiatry 54(4):283–293, 2015 25791145

Szigethy E, Levy-Warren A, Whitton S, et al: Depressive symptoms and inflammatory bowel disease in children and adolescents: a cross-sectional study. J Pediatr Gastroenterol Nutr 39(4):395–403, 2004 15448431

Tollefson GD, Beasley CM Jr, Tran PV, et al: Olanzapine versus haloperidol in the treatment of schizophrenia and schizoaffective and schizophreniform disorders: results of an international collaborative trial. Am J Psychiatry 154(4):457–465, 1997 9090331

Touitou Y: Human aging and melatonin. Clinical relevance. Exp Gerontol 36(7):1083–1100, 2001 11404053

U.S. Food and Drug Administration: FDA public health advisory: suicidality in child and adolescents being treated with antidepressant medications, October 15, 2004. Available at http://www.fda.gov/cder/drug/antidepressants/SSRI-PHA200410.htm. Accessed March 27, 2019.

Van der Heijden KB, Smits MG, Van Someren EJ, et al: Effect of melatonin on sleep, behavior, and cognition in ADHD and chronic sleep-onset insomnia. J Am Acad Child Adolesc Psychiatry 46(2):233–241, 2007 17242627

Walkup JT: Antidepressant efficacy for depression in children and adolescents: industry- and NIMH-funded studies. Am J Psychiatry 174(5):430–437, 2017 28253735

Wang XS, Woodruff JF: Cancer-related and treatment-related fatigue. Gynecol Oncol 136(3):446–452, 2015 25458588

Weiss MD, Wasdell MB, Bomben MM, et al: Sleep hygiene and melatonin treatment for children and adolescents with ADHD and initial insomnia. J Am Acad Child Adolesc Psychiatry 45(5):512–519, 2006 16670647

Wright P, Birkett M, David SR, et al: Double-blind, placebo-controlled comparison of intramuscular olanzapine and intramuscular haloperidol in the treatment of acute agitation in schizophrenia. Am J Psychiatry 158(7):1149–1151, 2001 11431240

Young CC, Lujan E: Intravenous ziprasidone for treatment of delirium in the intensive care unit. Anesthesiology 101(3):794–795, 2004 15329607

18

Preparation for Procedures

Children and adolescents are exposed to the potential of having invasive pediatric procedures throughout their lifetime. For instance, healthy children receive an average of 28 immunizations during the first 6 years of life (Centers for Disease Control and Prevention 2018). Many youth are also exposed to more invasive, painful, and anxiety-provoking medical and surgical experiences well beyond that of an immunization or even a routine venipuncture. More than 27 million U.S. children younger than 15 years are seen annually in emergency departments, with more than 650,000 admitted to the hospital for a mean of 3 days (Rui and Kang 2015). Youth with disabling chronic physical illnesses are at greater risk for an increased number of pediatric procedures compared with their peers. In this context, the issue of preparation for pediatric procedures is critical for a large population of children and adolescents.

Effective Preparation for Procedures

Effective preparation for pediatric procedures has four primary components: 1) encouraging trusting relationships, 2) providing emotional support, 3) giving age-appropriate information, and 4) helping children develop coping strategies to use before and during procedures (Mednick 2010). Effective psychological interventions can help youngsters and their parents cope with challenging pediatric interventions by providing them with an increased sense of control and mastery, which in turn helps to minimize the pain resulting from these interventions as well as decrease the adverse emotions experienced prior to and during procedures (Mednick 2010).

Effective preparation has been shown to provide comfort to a child, reduce a child's level of distress both before and after hospitalization, and shorten the length of a procedure (Butler et al. 2005). Emotional factors, such as elevated levels of anxiety, distress, anger, and depressed mood, may increase pain perception and make subsequent medical procedures more stressful (Blount et al. 1991; Kain et al. 2006, 2007). Poor management of pain in early childhood may alter the neuronal circuits that process pain and result in accentuated behavioral response to pain in later childhood (Koller and Goldman 2012; Ruda et al. 2000). These findings suggest that childhood pediatric experiences can continue to have a significant impact on individuals throughout their lives, making the effective preparation for procedures an important opportunity to facilitate successful coping and adaptation well beyond childhood. In this chapter, we outline approaches for consultants to consider in order to reduce the distress children experience when undergoing stressful and invasive pediatric procedures.

Assessment of Adaptation and Coping

Prior to any intervention to reduce procedural distress, it is important for consultants to understand the *correlates of adjustment* in childhood physical illness, including coping style, temperament, developmental level, medical severity, medical distress, long-term adaptation, and family factors (see Chapter 2, "Coping and Adaptation in Physically Ill Children") as well as prior psychological techniques that may have been used to facilitate or improve the child's level of coping (Table 18–1).

During the assessment, consultants are well served to consider involving a child life specialist, if one is not already involved, given this specialty's expertise in preparing children and their families for pediatric procedures. Today, children's hospitals routinely include child life programs, as evidenced by the more than 400 programs in operation in North America (Committee on Hospital

Table 18–1.   Assessment of children's responses to prior medical procedures (parent report)

How well does your child understand the procedure protocol?

Has your child had prior painful or stressful procedures?

Did your child experience anxiety or distress during these procedures? Rate on a scale from 1 to 5.

What aspect of the procedure was most distressing to your child?

Did your child report any distressing images, nightmares, or memories after the procedure?

What techniques has your child used to reduce his or her level of anxiety? Indicate one or more of the following: breathing, deep muscle relaxation, being held, massage, distraction, guided imagery, hypnosis, behavior modification

Rate the effectiveness of each technique in reducing your child's level of anxiety.

What is the optimal timing for your child to be prepared for a procedure?

What behaviors indicate that your child is experiencing distress or pain?

Have you received any instruction on coping strategies to assist your child during the procedure?

What incentives would be helpful as a reward for your child after the procedure?

Care and Child Life Council 2014). To varying degrees, these programs are also provided in community hospitals with pediatric units, ambulatory clinics, emergency departments, hospice and palliative care programs, camps for children with chronic illness, rehabilitation settings, and some dental and physician offices. Preparing children and their families for hospitalization, clinic visits, surgeries, and diagnostic or therapeutic procedures is an important element of a child life program (Committee on Hospital Care and Child Life Council 2014).

Preparation Through Education

Effective preparation for procedures includes information content, modeling, exposure, and coping skill training. Fostering trust, reducing uncertainty, correcting misconceptions, enhancing the child's belief in his or her ability to cope with a procedure, and minimizing distress are the potential benefits in providing advance information about a procedure to a child (Jaaniste et al. 2007). Providing accurate, minimally threatening information regarding upcoming procedures promotes accurate expectations and allows a child to focus on specific concrete sensations and concerns as well as to implement adaptive coping strategies (Mednick 2010; Jaaniste et al. 2007).

Content of Information

Children should be given developmentally appropriate verbal explanation of what they will see, hear, feel, and smell during, before, and after a procedure. It is helpful to discuss what is likely to happen after the procedure to avoid any unpleasant surprises. The decision on how much information to give is influenced by a child's maturity, temperament, and desire and need for information, which is often signaled by the child's specific questions (Mednick 2010). Language used should be simple, unambiguous, and appropriate to the child's cognitive and developmental level. Content should be accurate but as non-threatening as possible. Children who are given information that turns out not to be true are more likely to develop a distrustful relationship with the pediatric team that may negatively affect future interactions. Children should be encouraged to ask questions so that their concerns can be elucidated and misconceptions corrected (Table 18–2).

Timing of Information

Careful consideration must be given to timing when information is provided. The ideal time to prepare a child for a pediatric procedure greatly depends on age and developmental maturity. Preparing older children for procedures about 1 week in advance allows them adequate time to process the information and to rehearse the new coping skills without the increasing anticipatory anxiety. Children younger than 6 years usually do best if prepared 1–2 days prior to the procedure (Mednick 2010). Adolescents generally do best when they are included from the beginning in the decision-making process regarding a planned pediatric intervention.

Parental Presence

It is important to include parents in the preparation process, especially for younger children (Mednick 2010). Children are usually sensitive to how their

Table 18–2.   Guidelines for teaching children about pediatric procedures

Provide information in a developmentally appropriate format.

Include in explanations what the child will hear, see, and smell, as well as sensations he or she will feel prior to, during, and after the procedure.

Keep language simple and nonthreatening, with no ambiguity.

Ask the child to repeat back what he or she learned and to ask questions in order to correct any misconceptions.

Use visual aids and actual medical equipment when available to enhance learning and memory.

Source.   Adapted from Mednick 2010.

parents are responding to situations and often look to their parents for signals on how they should react. Parents who display signs of anxiety tend to exacerbate their child's level of distress. Providing information and support to parents through involvement in preparation activities is likely to reduce parental anxiety, with positive indirect benefits for their children (Mednick 2010). While older children are often more independent, younger children frequently require more direct help from adults to understand information and utilize coping skills. In situations where parents remain excessively anxious following preparation interventions, parental presence may do more harm than good. In such a situation, the value of the presence of the parent should be carefully considered. It may be helpful to explore the option of including other supportive adult figures to improve the child's procedural experience.

Preparation Through Modeling

Modeling is based on social learning theory, which asserts that individuals learn by observing the behaviors of others and the outcomes of these behaviors (Bandura 1977). In modeling, the patient may be introduced to a peer who has already successfully gone through the same medical event and can demonstrate effective coping skills or may watch a video showing another child successfully completing the procedure with the help of appropriate coping strategies. The effectiveness of modeling appears to be enhanced when the model is of similar age and ethnicity to the patient (Melamed et al. 1976). Modeling is likely to be particularly useful with younger children because they are better able to absorb visible demonstrations of the information rather than spoken explanations (Jaaniste et al. 2007). Beneficial effects of preparation programs appear to last for at least a month, and children older than 7 years appear to benefit more than do younger children.

The use of simulation for procedure preparation analogous to current pediatric procedure simulation training for health care givers offers potential future approaches that can combine education, modeling, and medical play. This emerging future can be seen in the online self-cathing experience journal designed to increase understanding and acceptance of clean intermittent catheterization, available at http://experiencejournal.com/journals/self-cathing (Holland et al. 2015) or in the use of a virtual reality exposure tool for elective pediatric day surgery (Eijlers et al. 2017).

Preparation Through Exposure

Medical play is a vehicle for self-expression, allowing children to express their thoughts and feelings, assimilate reality, resolve internal conflicts, and achieve mastery (Mednick 2010). It allows them an opportunity to examine medical equipment that they may experience during the planned procedure, which serves to familiarize the child with the equipment and provide an opportunity to gain mastery over the feared objects (Mednick 2010). Exposure to the equipment helps to desensitize the child, with the result that there is a less fearful reaction at the time of the procedure. Medical play can also be used as a way to prepare children for procedures by using the equipment in role-plays with a doll and/or another person. This is a particularly useful activity with younger children, who learn best by doing.

Coping Skills Training

Coping skills that may be used during the procedure itself include distraction, breathing, progressive muscle relaxation, guided imagery, reinforcement, and medical hypnosis. These interventions have consistently been shown to reduce levels of distress and improve levels of cooperation in children and adolescents undergoing stressful procedures. The addition of training in the use of coping skills appears to have added benefits when compared with interventions that use only education or modeling (Mednick 2010).

General Principles

Whenever possible it is preferable to perform procedures in a treatment room rather than at the bedside in order to preserve the room or bed as a safety zone for the hospitalized child. Local anesthesia, including EMLA cream (lidocaine 2.5% and prilocaine 2.5%), can be used for needle procedures. For procedural pain that is known to be severe and stressful, the use of pharmacological agents is important to reduce pain to levels that are acceptable for the child. This may include the use of analgesic agents, including local anesthetics and nerve blocks, as well as anxiolytics or sedative medications to reduce anxiety. Although anxiolytics alone do not provide analgesia, their adjunctive use has been shown to reduce the child's level of distress not only during the procedure but also for subsequent procedures (Mednick 2010). In rare circumstances, general anesthesia can be considered for particularly distressing procedures and/or for children who appear to have overwhelming and disabling anxiety.

Parental presence is generally helpful. Because children seldom spontaneously engage in coping behaviors, repeated prompting by adults is often necessary (Mednick 2010). Parents can be directed to assist with nonprocedural talk, humor, distraction, and encouragement of learned coping skills. Efforts to give the child a feeling of being in control may be used, such as the choice of which arm will be used for the blood test, what type of bandage he or she will get, or which coping strategies the child will use.

Parents (and children) can be encouraged to repeat positive thoughts or statements during the procedure (Mednick 2010). Positive statements assist the child in feeling calmer and more relaxed, whereas negative messages may increase symptoms of anxiety and distress. Examples of positive statements to be repeated during a procedure could include the following: "This will be over soon," "I am [or you are] going to get through this," "I am relaxed and calm," "I am a very strong boy/girl," "This gets easier each time I do it," and "The pain is not as bad as I thought."

It is helpful to debrief the child after the procedure and to provide praise for any successful coping efforts, even if the overall experience was not positive. Giving a child a sense of success and accomplishment during the procedure may facilitate improved performance during subsequent procedures. It is helpful to discuss which parts of the intervention were successful and which were not so that the child can build on the experience to improve his or her coping skills. *Transformation* refers to the attempt to change a child's evaluation of the event from horrible or awful to simply irritating or unfortunate (Chen et al. 1999). The goal is to modify or change the frequency of unwanted thoughts and behaviors that result from pain. This approach can be useful for children older than 8 years who are able to self-initiate and maintain its use.

Distraction

Distraction involves a purposeful refocusing of attention from the threatening, anxiety-provoking aspects of a situation to less threatening thoughts, objects, sights, or sounds (Mednick 2010). Techniques are adapted according to the age and developmental level of the child. For infants, rocking or patting them or having them suck on a pacifier can help distract them. Toddlers respond well to blowing bubbles or party blowers or the imaginary blowing out of birthday candles. The use of pop-up books or singing can also be helpful. Young children like to hold stuffed animals or toys or be comforted by having their arm touched or stroked during the procedure.

With older children and adolescents, distraction techniques include listening to music through headphones, counting backward, playing video games, or watching movies during the procedure. Sometimes, attention can be focused on parts of the body that are not in pain. Older children may respond well to the explanation of how difficult it is to pay attention to more than one thing at a time (e.g., doing homework when the television is on in the same room). Similarly, children may relate to the experience of not noticing an injury sustained during a sports game until after the game is over. It is helpful to teach several distraction strategies so that the child has the option of trying out different techniques as needed. For those children who are extremely vigilant and prefer not to be distracted from the procedure, it may be more helpful to develop a plan in which the child's attention is specifically focused on what is happening and the child verbalizes changes in sensations as the procedure progresses.

Relaxation

Relaxation is a behavior that is generally incompatible with the experience of anxiety, distress, or pain (Mednick 2010). Commonly used relaxation strategies include breathing exercises, progressive muscle relaxation, and guided imagery. Whereas deep breathing and progressive muscle relaxation are intended to directly influence somatic reactions, imagery-based relaxation aims to induce somatic reactions indirectly by influencing cognitions (Mednick 2010). Although no technology-based interventions are specifically recommended in this text, consultants should be aware that there are easily downloaded apps that offer patients and families ready access to user-friendly programs that can facilitate the use of relaxation techniques. In addition, although primarily used in outpatient settings, biofeedback-assisted relaxation training may prove useful as a therapeutic tool for treating pain and anxiety in the inpatient hospital setting (McKenna et al. 2018).

Breathing

Some of the distraction techniques, such as blowing bubbles, party blowers, or pinwheels, use the benefits of breathing to help promote muscle relaxation. Even children as young as 4 years can be taught to take slow, deep breaths with an emphasis on breathing out slowly and fully.

Diaphragmatic Breathing

Older children and adolescents can be taught the technique of diaphragmatic breathing by watching their hands move up and down on their stomachs during breathing. One technique that can be used to help teach the principle of diaphragmatic breathing is as follows. The child is asked to lie down on the floor or on the bed. A small book is placed on the child's stomach near the belly button. The child is asked to imagine that the book is a boat sitting on the child's stomach. The child is told that breathing in fills the stomach with air and makes a wave that causes the boat to rise up. As the child breathes out, the air leaves the stomach and the wave falls.

Alternate Nostril Breathing

For alternate nostril breathing, the child is asked to sit in a comfortable position with the left hand on the left knee and the right index and middle fingers in the center of the eyebrows. The child closes the right nostril with the right thumb and breathes in through the left nostril, closes it with the ring finger, pauses, and then exhales through the right nostril. Then, with the right nostril open, the child inhales slowly, closes it with the thumb, pauses, and exhales though the left nostril. The child then inhales through the left nostril, pauses, and moves to the right. This pattern is repeated 5–10 times. The child then puts the right hand on the right knee and resumes normal breathing..

Progressive Muscle Relaxation

Progressive muscle relaxation is used to distract patients from their pain and to reduce the intensity of their pain experience (Abel and Rouleau 2000). Muscle relaxation results in a reduction of muscle tension and may reduce autonomic nervous system reactivity. In the tension-relaxation method, the child is taught to constrict the muscles for 5–10 seconds and then relax specific muscle groups (Table 18–3). It can be combined with suggestions of relaxation, heaviness, and warmth and images of relaxing situations. With serial sessions, the number of muscle groups is reduced until the child can attain a state of relaxation using a relaxation cue word.

In the suggestion method, the patient is given repeated suggestions of calmness, relaxation, heaviness, and warmth combined with pleasant imagery but without initially tensing the muscles. In the technique of differential relaxation, the child learns to relax one part of the body while maintaining tension in other parts. For example, in the treatment of migraine headaches, the patient learns to relax the jaw and shoulders but keeps tension in arms and trunks. Patients may be given the procedures in digital format or referred to relaxation apps to facilitate the use of the relaxation techniques at home.

Guided Imagery

Generally, children are easily able to focus their attention and become absorbed in their own world of fantasy or imaginary play. Younger children in particular are able to shift backward and forward between fantasy and reality while listening to an absorbing story that is being told to distract them from the procedure. Guided imagery with younger children generally involves the use of storytelling. Older children and adolescents may respond to more conventional scripts that contain pleasant or relaxing images. Some children prefer calm soothing images such as lying in bed or rocking in a chair or hammock. Others prefer more active images in which they participate as a character in a story. The ability to engage in this technique is facilitated if the child has a feeling of trust in the consultant.

Table 18–3. Progressive muscle relaxation exercise: sample script

Instructions

Have the patient sit (or lie) quietly in a comfortable position. With a calm and nonrushed approach, use the following script as a guideline for progressive muscle relaxation. This process of tensing and relaxing the muscles is repeated on the left side of the body and can also incorporate the muscles in the legs and in the face. The exercise should last 10–20 minutes. You may choose to record the session so that the patient can practice using the recording.

Suggested script

- Close your eyes as you take in a deep breath through your nose, filling your lungs completely, and then slowly breathe out. Take another deep breath in and feel the air filling up your chest, like a big balloon.

- Continue taking slow, deep breaths in three or four times through your mouth, noticing the feeling of the air as it flows gently and easily in and out of your body. Feel your body relaxing, with all the tension draining from your muscles, as you become softer and floppy like a big rag doll.

- Now focus your attention on your right hand. Squeeze your hand tightly together, as tightly as you can, noticing the feeling of your fingernails pushing into the palm of your hand. Hold your hand tightly clenched as we count slowly...1...2...3...4...5.... Notice how your hand feels slightly warm and tense as you squeeze tightly. Notice how different it feels from your other hand.

- Quickly relax your hand and notice the feeling of the blood rushing back into your hand, with a slight warm feeling, as your hand relaxes and sinks down on to the bed. Now bend your right arm at the elbow, tightening the muscles in your arm. Squeeze tightly as we count slowly...1...2...3...4...5.... Now release your arm and allow it to become relaxed and floppy. Notice the difference in sensations between your right arm and left arm.

- Now push your arm down into the bed and against the side of your body, squeezing very tightly as we count again slowly...1...2...3...4...5.... Release the muscles and allow the arm to sink back down into the bed and notice the feeling of complete relaxation in that arm.

Reinforcement

Reinforcement is intended to reward and motivate the child for his or her co-operation during pediatric procedures. Reinforcement may include verbal praise, stickers, or small toys or other incentives. By pairing a positive outcome (e.g., sticker, toy) with an aversive stimulus (e.g., venipuncture), the child develops a positive association with the aversive event. In addition, providing an incentive to engage in cooperative behaviors increases the likelihood that the child will perform the behaviors again in the future (Mednick 2010).

Pediatric Hypnosis

Hypnosis has been used in a number of settings to treat children and adolescent, including children as young as age 3 years. Hypnosis has been found to be helpful in reducing pain and distress in needle procedures (Birnie et al. 2014). Hypnosis has been used to reduce anticipatory nausea related to chemotherapy in oncology patients and to treat procedural anxiety in children undergoing invasive and stressful procedures, including bone marrow aspirations and lumbar punctures. Hypnosis has been shown to result in a decreased need for hypnotic and anxiolytic agents and decreased incidence of anxiety in subsequent procedures (Maldonado and Spiegel 2000). Hypnosis has been associated with lower ratings of postoperative pain and shorter hospital stays (Kuttner and Solomon 2003). Hypnosis can also be used for patients who have phobias about specific medical procedures.

Components of Hypnosis

Hypnosis is a psychophysiological state of attentive, receptive concentration in which there is a relative suspension of peripheral awareness (Spiegel et al. 2000). Hypnotic phenomena occur spontaneously, and the alteration of consciousness that hypnotized individuals may experience has a variety of therapeutic applications (Spiegel and Spiegel 1978). Hypnosis can be used to help alter thoughts, feelings, expectations, attitudes, and perceptions. Although hypnosis is not a treatment in itself, it is often used to complement other types of medical therapy and to facilitate the use of distraction and relaxation to reduce procedural anxiety. Three processes describe the hypnotic experience: absorption, suggestion, and dissociation (Maldonado and Spiegel 2000).

Absorption

Absorption is the tendency to engage in a state of focused attention. It describes a state in which the individual is immersed in a central experience with decreased peripheral awareness. During a state of absorption, peripheral perceptions, thoughts, and memories become less important.

Suggestion

Individuals in a state of hypnosis develop a heightened responsiveness to suggestions provided by the consultant. Individuals will accept instructions in a less critical manner while in a state of hypnosis; they may question the reasons for actions less and respond more automatically. This process may be used by consultants to bypass the defenses of patients in an effort to bring about symptom relief.

Dissociation

During a state of hypnosis, individuals are able to keep many routine experiences out of consciousness. Emotional states and sensory experiences may be dissociated from the individual's conscious experience during a state of hypnosis. The dissociation can prevent access to memories, resulting in states of dissociative amnesia.

Hypnotic Responsiveness in Children

Children are often adept at learning techniques of hypnosis, partly because of their natural ability to enter into states of imagery and imagination (Kuttner and Solomon 2003; Morgan and Hilgard 1978). Children often enter into spontaneous states of self-hypnosis or imaginary play, for example, when they are bored or distracted. Children may spontaneously use fantasy to modify unpleasant situations or to prepare for creative activities and new achievements. In addition, children are often motivated to try out new experiences and are responsive to suggestions during a state of hypnosis.

Responsivity to hypnosis in children is more accurately assessed by looking at the child's ability to engage in active imagination in addition to more formal induction techniques such as eye closure and relaxation, which are the basis of assessment in adults. In particular, eye closure is one of the more difficult items for children because it may trigger negative attitudes and concerns related to sleep as well as limiting opportunities for the child's natural curiosity regarding motor phenomena that may occur during hypnosis. Similarly, elements described as *challenge items* that are used with adult patients, such as arm immobilization, may remove control from the child and provoke oppositional behavior or resistance to hypnosis. Behaviors that suggest susceptibility to hypnosis include quiet wakeful behavior, involvement in vivid imagery, heightened attention to a narrow focus, and the capacity to follow posthypnotic suggestions.

Factors Compromising Hypnotic Responsiveness

Several factors may compromise hypnotic responsiveness in children (Kohen and Olness 2011), including misconceptions about hypnosis, parental attitudes, and situational variables.

Misconceptions

Negative portrayals of hypnosis in the media or misconceptions based on knowledge of hypnosis used for entertainment may interfere with a child's willingness to enter hypnosis. Children may equate hypnosis with loss of autonomy or experience anxiety with certain induction techniques that involve experiences of loss of control. Children may resist hypnosis because of previous negative experiences with the technique, an unwillingness to give up a specific symptom because of secondary gain or defensiveness (Kohen and Olness 2011), or negative feelings directed toward the therapist. Some families may also have objections based on religious beliefs.

Parental Attitudes

Negative attitudes or misinformation on the part of parents and other adult figures may influence the child's responsiveness to hypnosis. Both parents and medical colleagues require education about the use of hypnosis, including education about the need for adequate preparation time for procedures. Last-minute requests for intervention are often associated with failure of the technique in the child for whom the technique might otherwise be helpful. By contrast, positive attitudes on the part of parents may promote the use of hypnosis in children.

Situational Variables

Certain situational variables, such as extreme anxiety or pain or lack of adequate time for training, may interfere with the use of hypnosis in specific clinical situations.

Hypnotic Induction

It is helpful to present hypnosis to children and families as a skill that they may already have but are not aware of using. In pediatric hypnosis, one goal is to help children develop their own abilities and control over the use of the hypnotic techniques. Parents are usually involved to help support the child's efforts, to act as coaches, and to help decrease feelings of anxiety. Children's ability to enter a state of hypnosis results in increased suggestibility to techniques of imagery rather than those of relaxation. Images such as taking part in a sports activity, being in a favorite room of the house, or imagining themselves as a cartoon character are examples of techniques used to help children dissociate themselves psychologically from experiences of pain and anxiety (Maldonado and Spiegel 2000).

Prehypnotic Interview

It is important to introduce the concept of pediatric hypnosis to children and their parents with a full explanation of the applications and techniques. During this didactic discussion, the therapist should elicit and respond to specific concerns of the child and the parents. Any concerns or misconceptions regarding hypnosis should be clarified during this initial interview. It is important to demystify hypnosis and to explore and clarify some of the differences between the use of hypnosis for pediatric versus entertainment purposes. It may be helpful to define hypnosis as a state of mind that combines relaxation and concentration on a specific focus such that undesired thoughts or anxieties fade into the background. The ability to shift attention can be demonstrated by asking the child or parents to focus on sounds in the medical unit that were not previously noticed. The heightened attention that occurs during hypnosis can also be highlighted by describing everyday events that parents may be more attentive to—for example, the cry of an infant in distress.

Further discussion includes emphasizing the specific goals of hypnosis for the child, such as helping the child focus on comfort to reduce the experience of pain. Education about the principles of relaxation training and guided imagery is included.

Inclusion of Parents

Most therapists suggest involving parents in the hypnosis sessions, either from the beginning or after the child has received some training in self-hypnosis.

Younger children generally prefer to have their parents present during the initial sessions because their presence can reduce feelings of anxiety. Older children, by contrast, may find the presence of parents more likely to increase anxiety, and it may be better to conduct initial sessions alone. Parental presence does help to diminish parental anxiety and builds rapport between the family and the consultant. Parents who have observed the sessions are able to act as coaches for their children when they practice the techniques. Many parents will also spontaneously allow themselves to enter into a state of hypnosis during the training or request self-instruction and experience their own benefits from the technique.

Assessment of Hypnotic Responsivity

There is considerable variation in the hypnotizability of individual patients. Patients who are easily hypnotizable can be expected to benefit from techniques of hypnosis, whereas those who are less receptive to this technique should be directed toward other approaches such as biofeedback or relaxation. Objective tests that can be used to determine the patient's level of hypnotic responsivity include a number of clinical scales to assess the patient's ability to enter a state of hypnosis. The Hypnotic Induction Profile (Spiegel and Spiegel 1978) involves a structured hypnotic induction followed by an assessment of the patient's response to suggestions. The Children's Hypnotic Susceptibility Scale (London 1963) has been developed on the basis of the items in the Stanford Hypnotic Susceptibility Scale, Form A (Weitzenhoffer and Hilgard 1959). Morgan and Hilgard (1978) also developed the Stanford Hypnotic Clinical Scale for Children, which has a version for both younger and older children. It is helpful to use a structured script to induce hypnosis that incorporates suggestions for relaxation, imagery, and posthypnotic suggestion prior to efforts to address the child's particular symptom. This exercise may be somewhat less threatening and may help establish a sense of confidence in the technique in both the patient and the parents. After the assessment session, the consultant will debrief with the patient by discussing which components of the induction were most successful with or appealing to the child.

Hypnotic Induction Techniques

A number of different methods that rely on techniques of relaxation and imagery can be used to induce a state of hypnosis (Kohen and Olness 2011).

Children respond to a large variety of hypnotic induction techniques, and the choice depends on the age and personality characteristics of the individual child as well as the experience of the therapist. Techniques need to be adapted on the basis of the age of the child, and success in the induction of hypnosis is enhanced by knowledge of the child's preferences, which should be assessed prior to starting the child's training in hypnosis. Compared with adults, children are more likely to open their eyes, make spontaneous comments, and move around, giving the impression that they are resistant to the procedure. Consultants are likely to be more successful if these behaviors are permitted or reinforced during the induction rather than resisted. It may also be important to deemphasize the use of words such as *sleepy* because younger children may be resistant to falling asleep. It is also important to avoid the use of authoritarian methods and phrases because children generally have a greater need to remain in control than do adults. Use of such phrases as "you may…" rather than "you will…" are likely to be better received.

Visual Imagery Techniques

A number of visual imagery techniques are used to induce hypnosis in children. The child may be asked to imagine a favorite place, either real or imaginary. The consultant may enhance the imagery by adding specific details, including suggestions about sounds, physical sensations, temperature, and color. The child may choose to have friends or family members present in the imaginary place. The child may talk with the therapist about the place he or she is in during hypnosis to help reinforce the cooperative nature of the relationship.

In the cloud-gazing technique, the child is asked to imagine clouds floating in the sky that change in shape and color. The consultant suggests that the child may become part of one of the clouds with feelings of comfort, lightness, and calmness.

In the television fantasy, the child is asked to imagine himself or herself watching a favorite video or television program. The consultant suggests that the child has the remote control for the television and may turn the movie on or off and play out certain scenes, including those of the child involved in pleasurable activities. It is also possible to ask the child to imagine playing different videos, starting with one of the child lying on his or her hospital bed followed by a video of a more pleasurable scene. The child may be asked to notice differences in sensations of pain or anxiety between each video to help the child establish a sense of control over his or her symptoms.

Movement Imagery

In the magic carpet technique, the child is asked to imagine himself or herself sitting on a magic carpet. Suggestions are made that the child will be able to control the movement of the carpet and to take the carpet up into the air and imagine seeing grass, trees, or clouds. The child is able to take the carpet to favorite places or to visit friends. Friends or family members may accompany the child on the magic carpet ride.

In the sports activity technique, the child is asked to imagine himself or herself playing a favorite sport. The child may be prompted to imagine himself or herself at a later age, perhaps playing for a favorite professional team and wearing the team colors. The consultant makes suggestions about the physical sensations experienced by the child as he or she plays the sport. Suggestions may also be made about the response of the crowd and teammates as the child helps the team win the game.

In the bouncing ball technique, the child is asked to imagine himself or herself as a bouncing ball that bounces in any direction the child chooses. The ball may bounce out of the hospital and go on a journey to the child's favorite places.

Ideomotor Techniques

Ideomotor techniques involve suggestions in which the child is asked to imagine particular movements, generally of parts of his or her body, after which the movements generally start to occur. These techniques are particularly effective because they give the child a physical demonstration of his or her own ability to use hypnosis to control a physical movement in his or her body. In the arm levitation technique, a suggestion is made that a balloon is tied around one of the child's wrists. Suggestions about lightness or floating sensations are used to help the child allow his or her arm to float into a vertical position. In the fingers moving together technique, the child is asked to clasp his or her hands together with the two index fingers pointing forward, separated by about 1 inch. The suggestion is made that the fingers become drawn together, either with the image of a rubber band tied around both fingers or of magnets pulling the fingers together. As the fingers slowly move together and touch, suggestions are made for the child to drift off into a state of heightened relaxation.

Application to Pain and Procedural Anxiety

Several techniques and images can be used to help decrease symptoms of pain and anxiety related to invasive procedures. It is important to adapt the technique on the basis of the age and developmental level of the child. It is also helpful for the child to have training in several different techniques of induction and pain relief so that he or she has a choice of techniques to use at the time of the procedure.

Hypnoanesthesia

In this technique, suggestions are made about feelings of numbness that begin in a part of the child's body and then spread to incorporate the area being affected during the procedure. Suggestions may include numbness that can be induced by the image of a cold block of ice, of painting on a local anesthetic, or of pulling a "magic glove" or "magic stocking" over one of the hands or feet of the child. The child may also learn the technique of transferring feelings of numbness from one part of the body to another by touching himself or herself with the "anesthetized" hand. The child may also be asked to imagine nerves that pass from the brain to different areas of the body and are controlled by pain switches in the brain. After the child has identified a specific nerve pathway, which may be designated by a color, the child is asked to imagine a dimmer switch or control that can be used to reduce sensations to and from that particular part of the body.

Distancing Suggestions

The child may be asked to imagine the painful body part floating away and becoming detached from his or her body. As the body part is dissociated, sensations of pain are diminished. Pain may also be transferred from a part of the body, such as the back during a lumbar puncture procedure, to another part, such as a finger, that is then also detached and dissociated. The technique of watching a video can be incorporated, with the child asked to visualize a video of himself or herself undergoing the procedure and then turn off the video and play a video of a favorite place or activity instead. Suggestions are made for decreased experiences of pain while the child is watching the pleasant video.

Conclusion

Although many factors can affect how a child or adolescent reacts to an invasive pediatric intervention, it is apparent that proper preparation can have important short- and long-term benefits (Mednick 2010). Despite numerous studies, it is still unclear which types of intervention are likely to be most effective in preparing a specific child, making it essential to consider the correlates of adjustment in childhood physical illness (see Chapter 2) and the nature of the planned pediatric intervention when determining what type(s) of preparation to implement.

References

Abel CG, Rouleau JL: Behavioral therapy strategies for the medical patients, in Psychiatric Care of the Medical Patient, 2nd Edition. Edited by Stoudemire A, Fogel BS, Greenberg DB. New York, Oxford University Press, 2000, pp 61–71

Bandura A: Social Learning Theory. New York, General Learning Press. 1977

Birnie KA, Noel M, Parker JA, et al: Systematic review and meta-analysis of distraction and hypnosis for needle-related pain and distress in children and adolescents. J Pediatr Psychol 39(8):783–808, 2014 24891439

Blount RL, Davis N, Powers SW, et al: The influence of environment factors and coping styles on children's coping and distress. Clin Psychol Rev 11:93–116, 1991

Butler LD, Symons BK, Henderson SL, et al: Hypnosis reduces distress and duration of an invasive medical procedure for children. Pediatrics 115(1):e77–e85, 2005 15629969

Centers for Disease Control and Prevention: Immunization schedules. October 16, 2018. Available at: www.cdc.gov/vaccines. Accessed March 27, 2019.

Chen E, Zeltzer LK, Craske MG, Katz ER: Alteration of memory in the reduction of children's distress during repeated aversive medical procedures. J Consult Clin Psychol 67(4):481–490, 1999 10450618

Committee on Hospital Care and Child Life Council: Child life services. Pediatrics 133(5):e1471–e1478, 2014, 24777212

Eijlers R, Legerstee JS, Dierckx B, et al: Development of a virtual reality exposure tool as psychological preparation for elective pediatric day surgery: methodological approach to a randomized controlled trial. JMIR Res Protoc 6(9):e174, 2017 28893727

Holland JE, DeMaso DR, Rosoklija I, et al: Self-cathing experience journal: enhancing the patient and family experience in clean intermittent catheterization. J Pediatr Urol 11(4):187.e1–187.e6, 2015 26028181

Jaaniste T, Hayes B, Von Bayer CL: Providing children with information about forthcoming medical procedures: a review and synthesis. Clin Psychol 14:124–143, 2007

Kain ZN, Mayes LC, Caldwell-Andrews AA, et al: Preoperative anxiety, postoperative pain, and behavioral recovery in young children undergoing surgery. Pediatrics 118(2):651–658, 2006 16882820

Kain ZN, Caldwell-Andrews AA, Mayes LC, et al: Family centered preparation for surgery improves perioperative outcomes in children: a randomized controlled trial. Anesthesiology 106(1):65–74, 2007 17197846

Kohen DR, Olness K: Hypnosis and Hypnotherapy With Children, 4th Edition. New York, Routledge/Taylor & Francis Group. 2011, pp 46–53

Koller D, Goldman RD: Distraction techniques for children undergoing procedures: a critical review of pediatric research. J Pediatr Nurs 27(6):652–681, 2012 21925588

Kuttner L, Solomon R: Hypnotherapy and imagery for managing children's pain, in Pain in Infants, Children and Adolescents, 2nd Edition. Edited by Schechter NL, Berde CB, Yaster M. Philadelphia, PA, Lippincott Williams & Wilkins, 2003, pp 317–328

London P: Children's Hypnotic Susceptibility Scale. Palo Alto, CA, Consulting Psychologists Press, 1963

Maldonado JR, Spiegel D: Medical hypnosis, in Psychiatric Care of the Medical Patient, 2nd Edition. Edited by Stoudemire A, Fogel BS, Greenberg DB. New York, Oxford University Press, 2000, pp 73–87

McKenna K, Goodrich L, Forbes PW, et al: Pilot study to examine the clinical utility of biofeedback in solid organ transplant. Clin Pract Pediatr Psychol 2018 [Epub ahead of print]. Available at: https://psycnet.apa.org/record/2018-36379-001. Accessed March 29, 2019.

Mednick L: Preparation for procedures, in Textbook of Pediatric Psychosomatic Medicine. Edited by Shaw RS, DeMaso DR. Washington, DC, American Psychiatric Publishing, 2010, pp 475–485

Melamed BG, Meyer R, Gee C, et al: The influence of time and time of preparation on children's adjustment to hospitalization. J Pediatr Psychol 1:31–37, 1976

Morgan AH, Hilgard JR: The Stanford Hypnotic Clinical Scale for children. Am J Clin Hypn 21(2–3):148–169, 1978 747163

Ruda MA, Ling QD, Hohmann AG, et al: Altered nociceptive neuronal circuits after neonatal peripheral inflammation. Science 289(5479):628–631, 2000 10915627

Rui P, Kang K: National Hospital Ambulatory Medical Care Survey: Emergency Department Summary Tables. 2015. Available at: www.cdc.gov/nchs/data/nhamcs/web_tables/2015_ed_web_tables.pdf. Accessed March 29, 2019.

Spiegel H, Spiegel D: Trance and Treatment: Clinical Use of Hypnosis. New York, Basic Books, 1978

Spiegel H, Greenleaf M, Spiegel D: Hypnosis, in Kaplan and Sadock's Comprehensive Textbook of Psychiatry, Vol 2, 7th Edition. Edited by Sadock BJ, Sadock VA. Philadelphia, PA, Lippincott Williams & Wilkins, 2000, pp 893–904

Weitzenhoffer AM, Hilgard ER: Stanford Hypnotic Susceptibility Scale: Forms A and B for Use in Research Investigation in the Field of Hypnotic Phenomena. Palo Alto, CA, Consulting Psychologists Press, 1959

Index

Page numbers printed in **boldface** type refer to tables or figures.

513